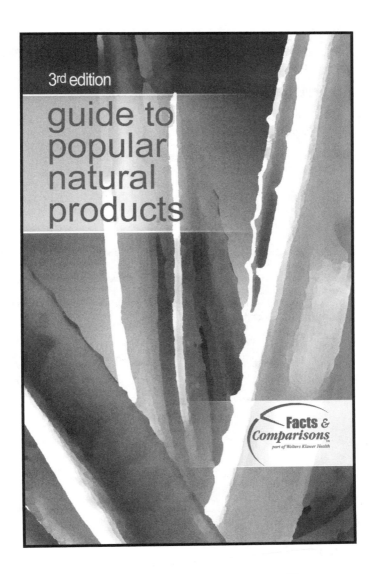

3rd edition

guide to
popular
natural
products

Facts &
Comparisons™
part of Wolters Kluwer Health

D1260688

A Guide to Popular Natural Products, Third Edition

© Wolters Kluwer Health, Inc., 2003

All rights reserved. No part of this publication may be reproduced or transmitted in any form or by any means, electronic or mechanical, including photocopy, recording, stored in a data base or any information storage or retrieval system or put into a computer, without prior permission in writing from Wolters Kluwer Health, Inc., the publisher.

Adapted from *The Review of Natural Products* loose-leaf drug information service through the February 2003 update.

Photography by Martin Wall Botanical Services
Greensboro, North Carolina

ISBN 1-57439-139-9

Printed in the United States of America

The information contained in this publication is intended to supplement the knowledge of health care professionals regarding drug information. This information is advisory only and is not intended to replace sound clinical judgment or individualized patient care in the delivery of health care services. Wolters Kluwer Health, Inc. disclaims all warranties, whether express or implied, including any warranty as to the quality, accuracy or suitability of this information for any particular purpose.

The information contained in *A Guide to Popular Natural Products* is available for licensing as source data. For more information on data licensing, please call 1-800-223-0554.

Facts and Comparisons®
part of Wolters Kluwer Health
111 West Port Plaza Dr., Suite 300
St. Louis, Missouri 63146-3098
www.drugfacts.com
314/216-2100 • 800/223-0554
314/878-3431 Fax

A Guide to Popular Natural Products

Co-Editors

Ara DerMarderosian, PhD
Professor of Pharmacognosy and
  Medicinal Chemistry
Roth Chair of Natural Products
Scientific Director, Complementary
  and Alternative Medicine Institute
University of the Sciences in
  Philadelphia
College of Pharmacy

John A. Beutler, PhD
Natural Products Chemist
National Cancer Institute

Advisory Panel

Michael Cirigliano, MD, FACP
Assistant Professor of Medicine
University of Pennsylvania
School of Medicine

Mary J. Ferrill, PharmD, FASHP
School of Pharmacy
Wingate University
Wingate, North Carolina

Constance Grauds, RPh
President, Association of Natural
  Medicine Pharmacists

Jill E. Stansbury, ND
Chair of the Botanical
  Medical Department
National College of
  Naturopathic Medicine

David S. Tatro, PharmD
Drug Information Analyst

Facts and Comparisons® Publishing Group

Executive Vice President	Kenneth H. Killion
Publisher	Cathy H. Reilly
Senior Managing Editor	Renée M. Wickersham
Managing Editor	Jill A. O'Dell
Associate Editor	Wendy L. Bell
Assistant Editors	Juanito R. Baladad, Jr. Sarah W. Lenzini
Quality Control Editor	Susan H. Sunderman
Senior Composition Specialist	Beverly A. Donnell
Senior SGML Specialist	Linda M. Jones
Manufacturing Services Manager	Susan L. Polcyn
Acquisitions Editor	Teri Hines Burnham
Cover Design	Mark L. Wickersham
Marketing Manager	Cynthia A. Meilink

Facts and Comparisons® Editorial Advisory Panel

LAWRENCE R. BORGSDORF, PharmD, FCSHP
Pharmacist Specialist-Ambulatory Care
Kaiser Permanente
Bakersfield, California

DENNIS J. CADA, PharmD, FASHP, FASCP
Executive Editor, *The Formulary*
Editor in Chief, *Hospital Pharmacy*
Laguna Niguel, California

MICHAEL CIRIGLIANO, MD, FACP
Associate Professor of Medicine
University of Pennsylvania
School of Medicine
Philadelphia, Pennsylvania

TIMOTHY R. COVINGTON, PharmD, MS
Executive Director
Managed Care Institute
Bruno Professor of Pharmacy
McWhorter School of Pharmacy
Samford University
Birmingham, Alabama

JOYCE A. GENERALI, RPh, MS, FASHP
Director, Drug Information Center
Clinical Associate Professor
University of Kansas Medical Center
Department of Pharmacy
Drug Information Service
Kansas City, Kansas

DANIEL A. HUSSAR, PhD
Remington Professor of Pharmacy
Philadelphia College of Pharmacy
University of the Sciences in Philadelphia
Philadelphia, Pennsylvania

LOUIS LASAGNA, MD
Chairman and Adjunct Scholar
Tufts Center for the Study of Drug Development
Boston, Massachusetts

JAMES R. SELEVAN, MD, BSEE
Founder and Member of the Board of Directors
Monarch Healthcare
Vice President of Pharmacy Relations
Syntiro Healthcare Services, Inc.
Laguna Beach, California

RICHARD W. SLOAN, MD, RPh
Chairman
Department of Family Practice
York Hospital
Clinical Associate Professor
Pennsylvania State University
York, Pennsylvania

BURGUNDA V. SWEET, PharmD
Director, Drug Information
Clinical Associate Professor of Pharmacy
University of Michigan
Ann Arbor, Michigan

DAVID S. TATRO, PharmD
Drug Information Analyst
San Carlos, California

THOMAS L. WHITSETT, MD
Professor of Medicine and Pharmacology
Director of Vascular Medicine Program
University of Oklahoma Health Sciences Center
Oklahoma City, Oklahoma

Table of Contents

Publisher's Preface

Natural products are interesting, intriguing, and extremely popular agents. Sometimes controversial, they can be beneficial as well as harmful. Therefore, it is essential that the information provided to health care professionals and consumers be unbiased, accurate, and trusted. The *Guide to Popular Natural Products* is a tool that considers these issues and presents quality information in an easy-to-use format.

Adapted from the widely popular and highly regarded monthly updated publication *The Review of Natural Products*, the *Guide to Popular Natural Products* excerpts the most popular products into an easy-to-use, abridged format, keeping all the features that have made the complete reference source so successful. There are more than 120 monographs on botanicals, herbals, and nutriceuticals (combined under the more general term "natural products") included in this publication. Arranged alphabetically for ease of use, each monograph is comprised of the following sections: scientific name, common name, botany, history, pharmacology, and toxicology.

Each monograph also contains a patient information box, which highlights important factors for the patient such as potential uses, side effects, drug interactions, and dosing. Other unique features of the *Guide to Popular Natural Products* include a comprehensive index, a therapeutic use index, drug interaction appendices, and a full color section of botanical images to aid the reader in identification of the source of the natural product.

Developed under the direction of Ara DerMarderosian, PhD, and John Beutler, PhD, well-known and leading experts in the field of natural products, each monograph is fully referenced to the scientific literature and peer reviewed by a distinctive panel of experts from various areas of the medical community. There is no other publication more thoroughly reviewed and evaluated.

Facts and Comparisons® is proud to include the *Guide to Popular Natural Products* in its distinguished list of reference sources. We hope that the reader finds this a valuable guide in the selection and use of natural products. We encourage comments and suggestions to help us improve the publication for future editions.

Cathy H. Reilly
Publisher

Introduction

This 3rd edition of the *Guide to Popular Natural Products* is a collection of summaries of the scientific research on herbs and other dietary supplements commonly found in stores in the United States. Each monograph includes references to scientific literature that supports the opinions and conclusions made by the authors about the safety and effectiveness of the product. In addition, the monograph describes how the product exerts its effects on the human body and how this translates into its medical uses. Behind these human studies are the pharmacologic insights gained from experiments on animals, cells, and biochemical systems and the elucidation of the chemical compounds present in the product, which are responsible for its effects.

The *Guide to Popular Natural Products* is for the educated layperson who is interested in knowing about the science behind the herb. This is a wider intended audience than its larger relative, the *Review of Natural Products*, which is produced with health professionals, such as doctors, nurses, and pharmacists in mind and which covers three times as many products in greater technical detail. Nonetheless, the *Guide to Popular Natural Products* is based on the same data gleaned from worldwide scientific literature and carries the same authority in its conclusions.

Plants have played a pivotal role in medicine throughout all of recorded history in virtually all human cultures. Indeed, plants are the foundation upon which effective medicine has been built. As science has progressed, so has the knowledge of how plant medicines work. Often, discoveries about plant medicines have catalyzed the progress of basic medical research. For example, opium has been used for centuries to relieve pain; morphine was isolated as the active substance in opium in 1809; morphine and its derivatives have been a mainstay of medicine ever since. Much later, investigation of the human receptors for morphine led to the identification of the endorphins and enkephalins, products of human metabolism that are part of the fundamental process of pain perception.

Different cultures have contributed different medicines to medical science. European herbalists were the first to use the important heart medicine digitalis. The antipsychotic medicine reserpine came from the study of a traditional medicine of India, while ephedrine was isolated from a traditional Chinese herb. The study of how plants are used by different cultures is known as ethnobotany, and many more useful plants undoubtedly are yet to have their medical properties exploited.

Ethnobotany is not the only route to new drugs from natural sources. In some cases, the active ingredient of a plant may be present in amounts too minute for easy detection or be obscured by other, toxic molecules. Sometimes the disease is difficult for folk healers to diagnose. This was the case with taxol, an important cancer drug derived from the Pacific yew. Molecules in yew other than taxol have a profound effect on the heart, thus yew alone is too toxic for use against cancer. However, when the taxol molecule was purified from yew, it was revealed as an important drug for the control of ovarian and breast cancer, substantially reducing mortality.

New methods of analyzing the action of natural substances on biological systems hold the promise of the discovery of many new molecules with the ability to target specific mechanisms of disease. High throughput biology has become common in pharmaceutical companies and is rapidly spreading to academic and government laboratories. When large collections of plants and other natural substances can be examined in short time periods, the chances of important advances improve markedly. Similarly, the speed of chemical separation and analysis has increased, permitting a much more complete chemical examination.

One might question why medicines can be found in plants and other natural sources. The plant has no need to rid itself of human diseases, and the cost of making drug molecules would seem a useless expense. However, plants are quite concerned with their own survival, which means avoiding being eaten by insects or parasitized by fungi. Thus, plants have developed the ability to produce compounds to deter feeding by insects or block the spread of fungi in their tissues. As the genomes of organisms are better understood, it becomes clear that the biochemical "parts" that make up a human, a worm, or a fly are not so different, despite differences in how these parts are put together and how they grow and reproduce. The fact that the parts are effectively recycled means that a compound that helps a plant defend itself against insects may also work to slow the growth of human cancer cells or block release of brain peptides.

So, if plants hold a wealth of medically interesting compounds, why are they not more highly valued by pharmaceutical companies? Why has research into naturally derived medicines been relegated to a marginal activity by the industry? The answers partly lie in the history of drug regulation in the United States.

Herbs and dietary supplements occupy a peculiar legal position in the United States, which can be traced historically to the development and regulation of prescription medicines over the last century. The Pure Food Act of 1906 was enacted in response to widespread perception of unsafe, unsanitary practices in industrial food production, especially meat packing, as recorded by Upton Sinclair in his book "The Jungle" and by other reporters. The Act also resulted in the transformation of the US Pharmacopeia and National Formulary into official, legal standards for drug products.

The law was extended in 1938 by the Food Drug and Cosmetic Act due to concerns over patent medicines and in direct response to the Elixir of Sulfanilamide disaster. Over 100 people died due to reformulation of a sulfa drug in ethylene glycol, a solvent not known to be toxic. The new law called for safety testing of all drugs before they entered the marketplace. A further change was the creation of a class of prescription-only drugs, where safety concerns justified the oversight of a physician.

With medical advances by mid-century including such "wonder drugs" as the sulfas and penicillin, concern shifted from avoiding outright fraud to establishing the safety of the many new drugs beginning to emerge from the scientific reseach catalyzed by the second World War. Drug companies involved in war production of antibiotics developed large research organizations to discover new products for a multitude of diseases, focusing on patentable drugs that could return the large investments being made into research. At the same time, many older drugs derived from plants began to be replaced by newer therapies.

Once again, a catastrophe catalyzed changes in the drug approval process. Thalidomide, a synthetic drug developed in Germany as a tranquilizer, was promoted for use in pregnancy. It rapidly became clear that thalidomide caused fetal malformations when given early in pregnancy, but not before thousands of babies were born with malformed limbs. The skeptical position of FDA official Frances Kelsey delayed approval in the United States, thus, fewer cases were seen in the United States than in Europe. Further additions to the FD&C Act (the Klefauver Amendments) were enacted on the heels of this episode. Requirements for proof of effectiveness became the norm, and it was clear that a balance had to be struck between the risks and benefits of a new medicine.

Older medications were "grandfathered" from these requirements until a review of OTC drugs began in the 1970s. At this point, the economics of drug research and production was radically changed from earlier in the century. Drug companies now invested heavily in research and development, both to discover potential new drugs and to prove their safety and efficacy by costly experimentation. This investment demanded a matching return in sales, and so "blockbusters" became the desired result. Research focused on chronic, widespread diseases in which a large market could be developed. Corresponding investment in biological research by the federal government provided further stimulus to new discoveries.

Because patents were an important factor in protecting blockbuster drugs from competition, medicines that were difficult to patent became undesirable. Drugs derived from natural sources were among those with such difficulties. The OTC reviews required a sponsor to cite research supporting the effectiveness of a product. If each manufacturer of a common product held only a small market share, there was little incentive to invest further in keeping the drug approved. Thus, many economically marginal products, including those with natural origins, were abandoned and forced from the marketplace without proper consideration of their medical value.

Many natural medicines became orphans without a corporate sponsor. The regulatory status of herbs was undefined until passage of the Dietary Supplement Health and Education Act of 1994 (DSHEA). This Act classified herbs and other natural materials as "dietary supplements" along with vitamins and minerals. The definition of a supplement in DSHEA is extremely broad – almost any substance derived from nature, including human hormones, could be considered a supplement. DSHEA allowed for marketing of supplements with no evidence of either safety or efficacy, although liability concerns have prevented widespread marketing of clearly toxic materials. Other provisions of the Act include the establishment of the Office of Dietary Supplements (ODS) within the National Institutes of Health to provide education on supplement use as well as the Office of Alternative Medicine, later renamed the National Center for Complementary and Alternative Medicine (NCCAM), to fund and conduct research on a wide variety of alternative therapies, including herbs. Funding has increased since 1994, with NCCAM currently budgeted for over $113 million yearly. These government organizations have become a focus for funding research on botanicals, with five centers sponsored at different universities, and for opposition from mainstream researchers, who view this as a waste of scientific resources. NCCAM has sponsored several high-profile clinical trials of herbs, including trials of the use of ginkgo for Alzheimers disease and St. John's wort for depression.

These developments reflect the extent of herb use and other alternative medical products in the United States. Many attempts to measure the size of this alternative medical universe have been made. Products such as ephedra, kava, and ginkgo have been heavily promoted and have enjoyed large increases in sales, followed by a decline as safety problems emerged due to wider use. Other products, such as ginseng, saw palmetto, and garlic have steered a steadier course. Overall, growth in the herbal market was very strong from 1994 until 2000, when the market had become saturated with new products and attacks from skeptical medical professionals gained prominence in the media. Herb sales are currently worth several billion dollars per year. Alternative medicine in general generates perhaps five times that much in revenue to practitioners. Surveys have found that up to a third of all respondents have used some form of alternative medicine.

The herb industry faces many challenges. Quality control must be increased. If a product varies in composition from lot to lot, how can its effects possibly be reliable? Labeling must be improved to state clearly what is in each product. Herb-drug interactions must be better understood.

Can this vast alternative medical wilderness be tamed? Can science explain this huge array of products, procedures, and theories? The *Guide to Popular Natural Products* is an effort to compile the scientific information that exists on the most common products, from basic botany, chemistry, and pharmacology to clinical studies in humans. The wilderness is only partly explored, but new methods of analysis and steady funding for research should improve the chances of survival for users and practitioners of herbal therapies. Nonetheless, the old warning, which states "buyer beware," still applies.

Recent developments illustrate the chaotic nature of the herb marketplace. Kava, a sedative used safely by Pacific islanders for centuries, was widely promoted in the herb industry, and sales grew rapidly. In 2002, reports of liver damage linked to kava began to be reported. Regulators began to tighten the screws on kava, and several European countries banned its sale. To date, no convincing evidence has been put forward to explain how or why kava causes liver damage in a very small proportion of people who take it. Is it an interaction with a drug? A peculiarity of metabolism? Or just the wider exposure that a larger market inevitably brings? Recent research points to an alkaloid found in the stems and leaves as the culprit. Natives use only the roots, which do not contain the alkaloid. Theoretically, the overheated market for kava led to sellers salvaging otherwise unsaleable plant parts to meet increased demand.

Ephedra, a useful drug for bronchodilation in asthma, became a huge seller when marketed for weight loss and enhancement of athletic performance. Billions of doses were sold and consumed. But ephedra also has been far and away the most commonly reported herb in the FDA's adverse event reporting system. The death of Baltimore Orioles pitcher Steve Belcher in 2003 spring training from heat stroke, allegedly due to ephedra use, unleashed a firestorm of criticism of the herb. Manufacturers began to remove ephedra from their formulations. Yet what assures the safety of the replacement herbs? We may be on a merry-go-round of toxicology for some time yet.

The allegation that herbs are not drugs is intellectually unsupportable. With any substance there is a balance of risk and benefit that can never be precisely calculated but must always be estimated. As the supplement industry continues to evolve, new products will emerge, have their day in the sun of commerce, and most will fade to a more appropriate role. Others will implode under the force of unexpected adverse effects revealed by wide use. The yearly increases in herb sales seen in the 1990s will not be repeated. The market for herbs is capable of saturation, especially now that it is smaller, because many buyers eschew the unknown risks herbs can represent.

The good news is that products are slowly improving in quality as manufacturers add quality control procedures to the manufacturing process. The FDA has issued regulations for the manufacturing of herb products under Good Manufacturing Procedures (GMPs), as well as guidelines for what must go on labels. Physicians are much more aware of the extent of herb use, and patients are less reluctant to discuss herb use with their physicians. Finally, the progress of clinical trials, though erratic and unpredictable at times, continues.

John A. Beutler, PhD
Co-editor
Braddock Heights, MD
April 2003

Monographs

Alfalfa

SCIENTIFIC NAME(S): *Medicago sativa* L. Common cultivars include Weevelchek, Saranac, Team, Arc, Classic, and Buffalo. Family: Leguminosae

COMMON NAME(S): Alfalfa

❧❧❧❧ PATIENT INFORMATION ❧❧❧❧

Uses: There is a lack of evidence supporting the use of various parts of the alfalfa plant for diuretic, anti-inflammatory, antidiabetic, or antiulcer purposes. Results from 1 small human study showed that the plant might reduce cholesterol levels.

Side Effects: Alfalfa ingestion, especially of the seeds, has been associated with various deleterious effects, and alfalfa seeds and sprouts can be contaminated with bacteria such as *S. enterica* and *E. coli*. The FDA issued an advisory indicating that children, the elderly, and people with compromised immune systems should avoid eating alfalfa sprouts. Ingestion of alfalfa preparations is generally without important side effects in healthy adults.

Dosing: Alfalfa seeds are used commonly as a supplement to lower cholesterol at doses of 0.75 to 3 g/day; however, clinical trials have not been performed to validate this dosage.

BOTANY: This legume grows throughout the world under widely varying conditions. A perennial herb, it has trifoliate dentate leaves with an underground stem that is often woody. Alfalfa grows to approximately 1 m and its blue-violet flowers bloom from July to September.

HISTORY: Alfalfa has played an important role as a livestock forage. Its use probably originated in Southeast Asia. The Arabs fed alfalfa to their horses, claiming it made the animals swift and strong, and named the legume "Al-fal-fa" meaning "father of all foods." The medicinal uses of alfalfa stem from anecdotal reports that the leaves cause diuresis and are useful in the treatment of kidney, bladder, and prostate disorders. Leaf preparations have been touted for their antiarthritic and antidiabetic activity, for treatment of dyspepsia, and as an antiasthmatic. Alfalfa extracts are used in baked goods, beverages, and prepared foods, and the plant serves as a commercial source of chlorophyll and carotene.[1]

PHARMACOLOGY: There is no evidence that alfalfa leaves or sprouts possess effective diuretic, anti-inflammatory, antidiabetic, or antiulcer activity in humans.[2]

In a study of 15 patients, alfalfa seeds added to the diet helped normalize serum cholesterol concentrations in patients with type II hyperlipoproteinemia.[3] *Cholestaid*, a product available in the US containing 900 mg of Esterin patented process alfalfa extract with 100 mg citric acid, is said to neutralize the cholesterol in the stomach before it reaches the liver, thus facilitating the excretion of cholesterol from the body with no side effects or toxicity.[4,5] There is no evidence that canavanine or its metabolites affect cholesterol levels.

INTERACTIONS: The vitamin K found in alfalfa can antagonize the anticoagulant effect of warfarin, resulting in decreased anticoagulant activity and lowered prothrombin time.[6] Based on the potential immunostimulating effect of alfalfa, it has been theorized that alfalfa may interfere with the immunosuppressive action of corticosteroids (eg, prednisone) or cyclosporine.[7]

TOXICOLOGY: The toxicity of L-canavanine is mainly due to its structural similarity to arginine. Canavanine binds to arginine-dependent enzymes interfering with their action. Canavanine may be metabolized to canaline, an analog of ornithine. Canaline may inhibit pyridoxal phosphate and enzymes that require the B_6 cofactor.[3] L-canavanine has also been shown to alter intercellular calcium levels[8] and the ability of certain B- or T-cell populations to regulate antibody synthesis.[9,10] Alfalfa tablets have been associated with the reactivation of SLE in at least 2 patients.[11]

A case of reversible asymptomatic pancytopenia with splenomegaly has been reported in a man who ingested up to 160 g of ground alfalfa seeds daily as part of a cholesterol-reducing diet. His plasma cholesterol decreased from 218 mg/dL to 130 to 160 mg/dL.[12] Pancytopenia was believed to be caused by canavanine.

Alfalfa tablets are part of a popular self-treatment for asthma and hay fever. There is no scientific evidence that this treatment is effective.[13] Fortunately, the occurrence of cross-sensitization between alfalfa (a legume) and grass pollens appears unlikely, assuming the tablets are not contaminated with materials from grasses.[14] One patient died of listeriosis following the ingestion of contaminated alfalfa tablets.[15]

Alfalfa seeds and sprouts can be contaminated with such pathogens as *Salmonella enterica* and *Escherichia coli*.[16-19] Most healthy adults exposed to salmonella or *E. coli* will have symptoms such as diarrhea, nausea, abdominal cramping, and fever that are self-limiting. The *E. coli* infection can lead to hemolytic uremic syndrome with kidney failure or death in children or the elderly. In 1995, 4 outbreaks of *Salmonella* infection occurred in the US because of the consumption of contaminated alfalfa sprouts. In 1995 to 1996, 133 patients in Oregon and British Columbia developed salmonellosis from ingesting alfalfa sprouts contaminated with *S. enterica* (serotype Newport).[16] Also in 1995, 242 patients in the US and Finland developed salmonellosis from ingesting alfalfa sprouts contaminated with *S. enterica* (serotype Stanley).[17] In June and July 1997, simultaneous outbreaks of *E. coli* 0157:H7 infection in Michigan and Virginia were independently associated with eating alfalfa sprouts grown from the same seed lot.[18] The FDA issued an advisory indicating that children, the elderly, and people with compromised immune systems should avoid eating alfalfa sprouts.[19]

[1] Duke J. *Handbook of Medicinal Herbs*. Boca Raton, FL: CRC Press, 1985.

[2] Small E, et al. *Economic Botany*. 1990;44:226.

[3] Molgaard J, et al. *Atherosclerosis*. 1987;65(1-2):173-79.

[4] Levy S. *Drug Topics*. 1999;19:22.

[5] Dewey D. *NuPharma*. 1/1/2001.

[6] Brown CH. *US Pharmacist* online. (http://uspharmacist.com/oldformat.asp?url=newlook/files/feat/mar00druginteractions.html).

[7] Miller LG. *Arch Intern Med*. 1998;158:2200.

[8] Morimoto I. *Kobe J Med Sci*. 1989;35:287-98.

[9] Prete P. *Arthritis Rheum*. 1985;28:1198-1200.

[10] Morimoto I, et al. *Clin Immunol Immunopathol*. 1990;55:97-108.

[11] Roberts J, et al. *N Engl J Med*. 1983;308:1361.

[12] Malinow M, et al. *Lancet*. 1981;I(8220):615.

[13] Polk I. *JAMA*. 1982;247:1493.

[14] Brandenburg D. *JAMA*. 1983;249:3303-304.

[15] Farber J, et al. *N Engl J Med*. 1990;322:338.

[16] VanBeneden C, et al. *JAMA*. 1999;282(2):158-162.

[17] Mahon B, et al. *J Infect Dis*. 1997;175(4):876-82.

[18] CDC. *JAMA*. 1997;278(10):809-10 and *MMWR*. 1997;46:741-44.

[19] Christy C. *Pediatr Infect Dis J*. 1999;18(10):911-12.

Aloe

SCIENTIFIC NAME(S): *Aloe vera* L., *A. perryi* Baker (Zanzibar or Socotrine aloe), *A. barbadensis* Miller (also called *A. vera* Tournefort ex Linne or *A. vulgaris* Lamarck; Curacao or Barbados aloe), or *A. ferox* Miller (Cape aloe). *A. vera* Miller and *A. vera* L. may or may not be the same species. Family: Liliaceae

COMMON NAME(S): Cape, Zanzibar, Socotrine, Curacao, Barbados aloes, aloe vera

---

⋙⋘ PATIENT INFORMATION ⋙⋘

Uses: Aloe appears to inhibit infection and promote healing of minor burns and wounds, and possibly of skin affected by diseases such as psoriasis. Dried aloe latex is used, with caution, as a drastic cathartic.

Side Effects: There has been 1 report that using the gel as standard wound therapy delayed healing. The gel may cause burning sensations in dermabraded skin.

Dosing: As a gel, *A. vera* may be applied externally ad lib. The resin product is cathartic at doses of 250 mg and is not recommended for internal use.[1]

BOTANY: Aloes, of which there are some 500 species, belong to the family Liliaceae.[2] The name, meaning bitter and shiny substance, derives from the Arabic "alloeh." Indigenous to the Cape of Good Hope, these perennial succulents grow throughout most of Africa, southern Arabia, and Madagascar. Although they do not grow in rain forests or arid deserts, they are cultivated in the Caribbean, Mediterranean, Japan, and Americas. Often attractive ornamental plants, their fleshy leaves are stiff and spiny along the edges and grow in a rosette. Each plant has 15 to 30 tapering leaves, each up to 0.5 m long and 8 to 10 cm wide. Beneath the thick cuticle of the epidermis lies the chlorenchyma. Between this layer and the colorless mucilaginous pulp containing the aloe gel are numerous vascular bundles and inner bundle sheath cells from which a bitter yellow sap exudes when the leaves are cut.[3]

HISTORY: In the 4th millennium BC, aloe wall carvings were found in Egyptian temples. Called the "Plant of Immortality," it was a traditional funerary gift for the pharaohs. The *Egyptian Book of Remedies* (ca. 1500 BC) notes aloe use in curing infections, treating the skin, and preparing drugs that were chiefly used as laxatives. The Gospel of John (19:39-40) says that Nicodemus brought a mixture of myrrh and aloes for the preparation of Christ's body. Alexander reportedly conquered the Socotra island to obtain control of its aloe resources. In AD 74, the Greek physician Dioscorides recorded aloe's use in healing wounds, stopping hair loss, treating genital ulcers, and eliminating hemorrhoids. In the 6th century AD, Arab traders carried aloe to Asia, and in the 16th century, it was carried to the New World by the Spaniards. Its clinical use began in the 1930s as a treatment for roentgen dermatitis.[3]

PHARMACOLOGY: Aloe latex has been used for centuries as a drastic cathartic. The aloinosides exert strong purgative effects by irritating the large intestine. These should be used with caution in children.

The most common use of the gel remains the treatment of minor burns and skin irritations. The activity of aloe in treating burns may stem from its moisturizing effect, which prevents air from drying the wound.[4] Current theory sug-

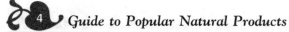

gests healing is stimulated by the mucopolysaccharides contained in aloe in combination with sulfur derivatives and nitrogen compounds. Topical aloe treatment for burns has not been adequately documented. Two FDA advisory panels found insufficient evidence to show that *A. vera* is useful in the treatment of minor burns and cuts or vaginal irritations.

More recent studies have found preparations containing aloe to accelerate wound healing, even in frostbitten patients.[5] In patients undergoing dermabrasion, aloe accelerated skin healing by approximately 72 hours compared to polyethylene oxide gel dressing.[6] However, at least 1 study found that aloe delayed wound healing (83 days vs 53 days).[7]

One study using *A. vera* gel[8] found no activity against *S. aureus* and *E. coli*. Other tests[9] found that *A. chinensis* inhibited growth of *S. aureus*, *E. coli*, and *M. tuberculosis*, but that *A. vera* was inactive. Further, these extracts lost their in vitro activity when mixed with blood. The latex has shown some activity against pathogenic strains.[10] Two commercial preparations (*Aloe gel* and *Dermaide Aloe*) exerted antimicrobial activity against gram-negative and -positive bacteria as well as *Candida albicans* when used in concentrations greater than 90%.[11] Aloe has been found to be more effective than sulfadiazine and salicylic acid creams in promoting wound healing and as effective as sulfadiazine in reducing wound bacterial counts.[12]

Aloe-emodin is antileukemic in vitro;[13] other studies showed *A. vera* gel to be less cytotoxic[14] than indomethacin or prednisolone in tissue cultures.

An emulsion of the gel was reported to cure 17 of 18 patients with peptic ulcers, but no control agent was used in the study.[15]

A Chinese study found that parenteral administration of aloe extract protects the liver from chemical injury and ameliorates ALT levels dramatically in patients with chronic hepatitis.[16]

Only the dried latex is approved for internal use as a cathartic. In some cases, *A. vera* is sold as a food supplement. The FDA has only approved *A. perryi*, *A. vera*, *A. ferox*, and certain hybrids for use as natural food flavorings.[17]

TOXICOLOGY: Since aloe is used extensively as a folk medicine, its adverse effects have been well documented. Except for the dried latex, aloe is not approved as an internal medication. Aloe-emodin and other anthraquinones may cause severe gastric cramping and are contraindicated in children and pregnant women.[18] The external use of aloe usually has not been associated with severe adverse reactions. Reports of burning skin following topical application of aloe gel to dermabraded skin have been described.[19] Contact dermatitis from the related *A. arborescens* has been reported.[2]

[1] Claus E, ed. *Pharmacognosy.* 3rd ed. Philadelphia, PA: Lea & Febiger; 1956.

[2] Nakamura T, et al. *Contact Dermatitis.* 1984;11(1):50.

[3] Grindlay D, et al. *J Ethnopharmacol.* 1986;16:117.

[4] Ship AG. *JAMA.* 1977;238(16):1770.

[5] McCauley RL, et al. *Postgrad Med.* 1990;88(8):67.

[6] Fulton JE, Jr. *J Dermatol Surg Oncol.* 1990;16(5):460.

[7] Schmidt JM, et al. *Obstet Gynecol.* 1991;78(1):115.

[8] Fly, K. *Economic Bot.* 1963;14:46.

[9] Gottshall, et al. *J Clin Invest.* 1949;28:920.

[10] Lorenzetti LJ, et al. *J Pharm Sci.* 1964;53:1287.

[11] Haggers JP, et al. *J Am Med Technol.* 1979;41:293.

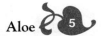

[12] Rodriguez-Bigasm, et al. *Plast Reconstr Surg.* 1988;81(3):386.

[13] Kupchan, K. *J Nat Prod.* 1976;39:223.

[14] Fischer JM. *US Pharmacist.* 1982;7(8):37.

[15] Blitz JJ, et al. *J Am Osteopath Assoc.* 1963;62:731.

[16] Fan YJ, et al. *Chung Kuo Chung Yao Tsa Chih.* 1989;14(12):746.

[17] Hecht A. *FDA Consum.* 1981(July-Aug):27.

[18] Spoerke DG, et al. *Vet Hum Toxicol.* 1980;222:418.

[19] Hunter D, et al. *Cutis.* 1991;47(3):193.

Angelica

SCIENTIFIC NAME(S): *Angelica archangelica* L., synonymous with *Archangelica officinalis* Hoffm. Family: Apiaceae (carrots)

COMMON NAME(S): European angelica, Echt engelwurz (German)

✥✥✥ PATIENT INFORMATION ✥✥✥

Uses: Often used as a flavoring or scent, angelica has been used medicinally to stimulate gastric secretion, treat flatulence, and topically treat rheumatic and skin disorders; however, there is little documentation to support these uses.

Interactions: Avoid using angelica root concurrently with warfarin.

Side Effects: Furanocoumarins in the plant may cause photodermatitis. Poisoning has been reported with high doses of angelica oils.

Dosing: Angelica root typically is given at doses of 3 to 6 g/day of the crude root.[1]

BOTANY: Angelica is a widely cultivated, aromatic biennial, northern European herb with fleshy, spindle-shaped roots, an erect stalk, and many greenish-yellow flowers arranged in an umbel. The seeds are oblong and off-white. It is similar to and sometimes confused with the extremely toxic water hemlock, *Cicuta maculata*.

There are several recognized varieties of *A. archangelica*, wild and cultivated. In the US, *A. atropurpurea* L. is often cultivated in place of the European species.

HISTORY: Angelica has been cultivated as a medicinal and flavoring plant in Scandinavian countries since the 12th century and in England since the 16th century. The roots and seeds are used to distill about 1% of a volatile oil used in perfumery and as a flavoring for gin and other alcoholic beverages. The candied leaves and stems are used to decorate cakes. The oil has been used medicinally to stimulate gastric secretion, treat flatulence, and topically treat rheumatic and skin disorders.

PHARMACOLOGY: Angelic acid was formerly used as a sedative. The angular furanocoumarin angelicin has also been reported to have sedative proper-

ties, although recent experimental evidence of this is limited. The carminative action of the volatile oil is caused by an unremarkable monoterpene content. Angelica root oil was preferentially relaxant on tracheal smooth muscle preparations compared with ileal muscle.[2] The oil had no effect on skeletal muscle in a second study.[3] The calcium-blocking activity of angelica root has been examined relative to solvent used in extraction, and furanocoumarins were identified as the likely active species.[4] The root oil has been found to have antifungal and antibacterial activity.[5]

INTERACTIONS: Theoretically, there is a possible increased risk of bleeding when using angelica root concurrently with warfarin. The additive or synergistic effects of coumarin or coumarin derivatives may be possibly present in angelica root.[6,7] Because warfarin has a narrow therapeutic index, it would be prudent to avoid concurrent use.

TOXICOLOGY: The linear furanocoumarins are well-known dermal photosensitizers, while the angular furanocoumarins are less toxic.[8] The presence of linear furanocoumarins in the root indicates that the plant parts should be used with caution if exposure to sunlight is expected. The coumarins are not important constituents of the oil, which therefore gives the oil a greater margin of safety in that respect. However, poisoning has been recorded with high doses of angelica oils.

[1] Blumenthal M, Brinckmann J, Goldberg A, eds. *Herbal Medicine: Expanded Commission E Monographs.* Newton, MA: Integrative Medicine Communications; 2000.

[2] Reiter M, et al. *Arzneimittelforschung.* 1985;35(1A):408-14.

[3] Lis-Balchin M, et al. *J Ethnopharmacol.* 1997;58:183-87.

[4] Härmälä P, et al. *Planta Med.* 1992;58:176-82.

[5] Opdyke D. *Food Cosmet Toxicol.* 1975;13:713.

[6] Miller L. *Arch Intern Med.* 1998;158:2200-11.

[7] Heck A. *Am J Health Syst Pharm.* 2000;57:1221-27.

[8] Ceska O, et al. *Experientia.* 1986;42:1302-04.

L-arginine

COMMON NAME(S): L-arginine

❧❧❧ PATIENT INFORMATION ❧❧❧

Uses: L-arginine has been beneficial in several cardiovascular diseases (eg, congestive heart failure [CHF], peripheral artery disease, angina, hypertension, hyperlipidemia) and type 2 diabetes. It plays an important role in healing and increases nitric oxide concentrations.

Side Effects: L-arginine has few reported side effects. Nausea and diarrhea have been reported infrequently. Parenteral administration at high doses has caused metabolic acidosis or electrolyte alterations.

Dosing: L-arginine has been studied at oral doses of 6 to 17 g/day for a variety of conditions.[1-5]

SOURCE: Amino acids are the major components of protein. Animal and plant products contain several amino acids, including arginine. Some of these sources are meats, milk, and eggs.[6] The physiologically active form, L-arginine, is the natural product obtained by hydrolysis of proteins. Because L-arginine can be synthesized endogenously from L-citrulline, it is classified as a nonessential amino acid in adults. However, in children and in certain conditions (eg, trauma, infection), L-arginine synthesis may become compromised and then may be considered "semi-essential."[7]

HISTORY: L-arginine is commonly sold as a health supplement claimed to be capable of improving vascular health and enhancing sexual function in men.

PHARMACOLOGY: Nitric oxide is produced by a variety of animal and human cells and is involved in many physiological and pathophysiological processes.[8] Nitric oxide is a free radical, generated from L-arginine by the enzyme nitric oxide synthase.[9] L-arginine supplementation to raise nitric oxide levels has been suggested to be beneficial in many areas.

Nutritional/Metabolic/Immunostimulatory: Arginine is classified as a nonessential amino acid but may become essential in stressful situations, including periods of growth (during childhood or pregnancy) or trauma to the body (eg, severe sepsis, wound healing, liver disease).[10-12] L-arginine is a human growth stimulant and has been used in bodybuilding.[13] Anabolic actions also can be confirmed in many studies concerning L-arginine supplementation and improved wound healing,[8,14-16] including healing of burns,[17] tendons,[9] GI tract,[18] and bone.[19] One mechanism suggested may be because of the enzyme arginase, which produces a favorable environment for fibroblast and collagen production.[20] In another report, exogenous L-arginine produced nitric oxide, resulting in a decrease of hepatic ischemia/reperfusion injury.[21]

Cardiovascular health: Many cardiovascular diseases originate in the vascular endothelial cells, which, if unhealthy, can cause vasoconstriction, inflammation, thrombolytic activity, and cell proliferation. These abnormalities are due in part to enhanced degradation of nitric oxide. By having increased concentrations of L-arginine available to maintain nitric oxide, it may improve certain vascular disease states. Some diseases include the following: CHF, peripheral artery disease, angina, hypertension, and hyperlipidemia.[22-24] Several articles are available on this topic and include the following findings: 1) Increased flow-induced vasodilation in isolated guinea pig hearts was dependent on L-arginine to maintain nitric oxide concentrations;[25] 2) L-arginine produced nonstereo-specific peripheral vasodilation and improves endothelium-dependent vasodilation in coronary heart disease (CHD) patients;[26] 3) Patients with peripheral artery disease experienced a 150% improvement in walking distance with L-arginine supplementation of 8 g twice daily for 14 days;[27] 4) An intermediate compound of L-arginine was found to be reduced in plasma concentrations of patients with cardiovascular risk factors, including impairment of endothelial function;[28] 5) L-arginine has improved cardiac performance in severe CHF patients;[29] 6) CHD patients with angina demonstrated improvement after L-arginine supplementation,[30] as have angina patients who experienced improved exercise tolerance with L-arginine.[31] In 1 clinical trial, oral L-arginine therapy was ineffective in improving nitric oxide bioavailability in coronary artery disease (CAD) patients.[1]

L-arginine also has been beneficial in similar disease states including hypertension and hypercholesterolemia. According to 1 report, L-arginine supplementation in humans significantly lowered blood pressure in 6 patients.[32] Certain mechanisms in this area have been investigated, suggesting that nitric oxide-mediated vasodilator tone is deficient in hypertension[33] and salt-sensitive patients with mild essential hypertension reduce the ability of L-arginine to produce nitric oxide in vascular endothelium.[34] Nitric oxide possesses antithrombotic and antiatherosclerotic actions in the vasculature. In human microvascular endothelial cells, nitric oxide (with L-arginine substrate) regulates tissue factor as well, reducing endotoxin and cytokine-induced expression of tissue factor.[35]

L-arginine supplementation in other vascular disease states has been beneficial. L-arginine's ability to increase nitric oxide availability has improved transplantation diabetes, renal disease, and other perfusion-type injuries.

The substrate for nitric oxide synthesis by the endothelium is limited in diabetes but can be overcome with L-arginine supplementation.[36] L-arginine counteracts lipid peroxidation, reducing damage to the blood vessels.[37] Hyperglycemia in patients with type 2 diabetes causes hemodynamic changes (eg, reduction of blood pressure), which can be reversed by L-arginine.[38] L-arginine also may play a role in insulin resistance.[39]

L-arginine is a precursor for polyamines required for proliferative responses characteristic of many renal diseases. It is also the nitric oxide precursor that is a vasodilator in the endothelium, which is beneficial in reducing intraglomerular pressure and disease.[40] L-arginine has been proven effective in nephrosclerosis and progressive renal failure.[41] L-arginine's ability to raise nitric oxide levels relaxes bladder muscle spasms, as well, and controls the pain in interstitial cystitis.[42]

Relaxation of cavernous smooth muscle in the penis requires nitric oxide synthesized by L-arginine. This suggests that L-arginine may be beneficial in erectile dysfunction. It has been advertised that L-arginine in the form of dietary supplements improves sexual performance in men. However, in a clinical, controlled, crossover study no statistical difference in impotence scores was found in 32 patients administered 500 mg L-arginine 3 times a day vs placebo.[43]

Other effects of L-arginine include increasing quantity and cytotoxic capability of lymphokine activated and natural-killer T-cells in breast cancer.[44] Another source suggests that individuals with genital herpes should decrease their intake of arginine (while increasing lysine). Arginine assists herpes simplex in multiplying, while lysine breaks down arginine.[45]

TOXICOLOGY: Parenteral administration of L-arginine in high doses has caused metabolic acidosis including elevated potassium levels due to effects on intra- and extracellular potassium balance.[7] Oral administration of L-arginine in humans has not caused any major adverse effects. L-arginine may exacerbate sickle cell crisis. Doses up to 30 g/day are well tolerated, with infrequent reports of nausea and diarrhea.[46] No adverse effects were reported with 9 g/day L-arginine over 6 months.[30] Arginine may trigger onset of herpes infection, although there is no solid evidence to confirm this.[46]

[1] Blum A, et al. *Circulation.* 2000;101(18):2160-64.

[2] Piatti PM, et al. *Diabetes Care.* 2001;24:875-880.

[3] Mullen MJ, et al. *J Am Coll Cardiol.* 2000;36:410-416.

[4] Langkamp-Henken B, et al. *JPEN J Parenteral Enteral Nutr.* 2000;24:280-287.

[5] Clark RH, et al. *JPEN J Parenteral Enteral Nutr.* 2000;24:133-139.

[6] Wild R, ed. *The Complete Book of Natural and Medicinal Cures.* Emmaus, PA:Rodale Press, Inc., 1994:124-27.

[7] http://www.uspharmacist.com/NewLook/CE/larginine/default.htm

[8] Wang R, et al. *J Invest Dermatol.* 1996;106(3):419-27.

[9] Murrell G, et al. *Inflamm Res.* (Switzerland) 1997;46(1):19-27.

[10] Visek W. *J Nutr.* 1986;116(1):36-46.

[11] Cynober L, et al. *Nutrition Clinique et Metabolisme.* (France) 1996;10(2):89-95.

[12] Evoy D, et al. *Nutrition.* 1998;14(7-8):611-17.

[13] http://ghr15-canada.com/amino_acids.html

[14] Noiri E, et al. *Am J Physiol Cell Physiol.* 1996;270(3):39-43.

[15] Schaffer M, et al. *J Am Coll Surg.* 1997;184(1):37-43.

[16] Cooper M, et al. *J Burn Care Rehabil.* 1996;17(2):108-16.

[17] Mertz P, et al. *J Burn Care Rehabil.* 1996;17(3):199-206.

[18] Thornton F, et al. *J Surg Res.* 1997;69(1):81-86.

[19] Fini M, et al. *Ann Ital Chir.* 1996;67(1):77-83.

[20] Shearer J, et al. *Am J Physiol.* 1997;272(2 Pt 1):E181-90.

[21] Higa T, et al. *Surg Today.* 2000;30(4):352-59.

[22] Drexler H. *Prog Cardiovasc Dis.* 1997;39(4):287-324.

[23] Giugliano D. *Nutr Metab Cardiovasc Dis.* 2000;10(1):38-44.

[24] Sanders D, et al. *Perfusion.* 2000;15(2):97-104.

[25] Wascher T, et al. *Eur J Clin Invest.* 1996;26(8):707-12.

[26] Quyyumi A. *J Am Coll Cardiol.* 1998;32(4):904–911.

[27] Boger R, et al. *J Am Coll Cardiol.* 1998;32:1336-44.

[28] Garlichs C, et al. *J Lab Clin Med.* 2000;135(5):419-25.

[29] Bocci E, et al. *Clin Cardiol.* 2000;23(3):205-10.

[30] Lerman A, et al. *Circulation.* 1998;97:2123-28.

[31] Ceremuzynski L, et al. *Am J Cardiol.* 1997;80:331-33.

[32] Siani A, et al. *Am J Hypertens.* 2000;13(5 Pt 1):547-51.

[33] Calver A, et al. *J Hypertens.* 1992;10:1025-31.

[34] Higashi Y, et al. *Hypertension.* 1996;27(3 Pt 2):643-48.

[35] Yang Y, et al. *Circulation.* 2000;101(18):2144-48.

[36] Pieper G, et al. *Eur J Pharmacol.* 1996;317(2-3):317-20.

[37] Lubec B, et al. *Free Radic Biol Med.* 1997;22(1-2):355-57.

[38] Marfella R, et al. *Diabetes Care.* 2000;23(5):658-63.

[39] Kelly G. *Altern Med Rev.* 2000;5(2):109-32.

[40] Peters H, et al. *Semin Nephrol.* 1996;16(6):567-75.

[41] Sanders P. *Blood Purif.* 1995;13:219-27.

[42] Smith S, et al. *J Urol.* 1997;158(3 Pt 1):703-708.

[43] Klotz T, et al. *Urol Int.* 1999;63(4):220-23.

[44] Brittenden J, et al. *Br J Cancer.* 1994;69:918-21.

[45] Althoff S, et al. *A Guide to Alternative Medicine.* Lincolnwood, IL: Publications International, 1997:100-01.

[46] Anderson S, et al, eds. Federation of the American Society for Experimental Biology/Life Sciences Research Office. Safety of amino acids used as dietary supplements. Center for Food Safety and Applied Nutrition. 1992;FDA Contract #223–88–2124, Task No. 8.

SCIENTIFIC NAME(S): *Cynara scolymus* L., *C. cardunculus*, Family: Compositae or Asteraceae

COMMON NAME(S): Globe artichoke, garden artichoke, alcachofra (Brazil)

❧❧❧ PATIENT INFORMATION ❧❧❧

Uses: Artichoke has been used for its antioxidant and GI soothing effects. It also may have cytoprotective actions in the liver and hypocholesterolemic effects.

Side Effects: Artichoke can cause allergic reactions, most commonly dermatitis.

Dosing: Artichoke leaf extract at 1.5 g/day was found to lower serum cholesterol and triglycerides in a post-marketing survey study.[1]

BOTANY: The artichoke is a member of the daisy family. It is a perennial herb, widely cultivated in the Mediterranean regions and adjoining parts of central Europe. This well-known plant grows to a height of approximately 2 meters. It has a strong, erect stem and its large leaves are lobed and gray-green. The edible flower bud is purple-green in color, and has scales or bracts that enclose it. The plant blooms from July to August.[2-4]

HISTORY: The artichoke has been cultivated for thousands of years.[2] In the first century AD, Dioscorides recommended applying mashed roots on the body to sweeten offensive odors.[3]

The artichoke was used as food and medicine by ancient Egyptians, Greeks, and Romans. The artichoke appeared in Europe in the 15th century.[4] The botanical name is derived in part from the tradition of fertilizing the plant with ashes, and partly from the Greek *skolymos*, meaning "thistle" from the spines found on the bracts (they are not leaves) that enclose the flower heads forming the edible portion of the plant.[5] The French have used artichoke juice as a liver tonic. The herb's abilities to break down fat and improve bile flow have been recognized.[6] Artichoke has been used traditionally to treat a variety of conditions including hepatic diseases,

jaundice, dyspepsia, and chronic albuminuria. It has also been used as a diuretic and to manage postoperative anemia.[3] The flower head is cooked and eaten as a delicacy. The flower contains a sweetener that enhances flavor perception, while the leaves contain bitter principles that are used in the preparation of aperitif liqueurs.[7]

PHARMACOLOGY: Artichoke possesses many properties, including antioxidant effects, hepatoprotective ability, GI soothing qualities, and cholesterol-lowering effects.

Antioxidant activity: The flavonoid constituents in artichoke (eg, luteolin) demonstrate antioxidant activity.[8]

GI effects: GI effects of artichoke include beneficial actions in digestive and dyspeptic ailments, loss of appetite, and gallbladder problems.[3,9] Artichoke flavonoids and caffeoylquinic acids are responsible for these actions, including hepatobiliary dysfunction and digestive complaints.[10] Naturally occurring fructose-containing oligosaccharides in artichoke act as prebiotics in the gut.[11]

Cholesterol-lowering effects: Artichoke has been found to possess cholesterol-lowering effects. Leaf extracts were found to inhibit cholesterol biosynthesis. Constituents cynaroside and its aglycone luteolin were mainly responsible for this effect, while chlorogenic, caffeic dicaffeoylquinic acids, and cynarin demonstrated little or no inhibitory effects.[12,13] Another report also concluded the ineffectiveness of cynarin, demonstrating no hypolipidemic actions in 17 patients with familial type II hyperlipoproteinemia.[14] A prospective study investigating 143 patients with total cholesterol more than 280 mg/dL reported that patients given 1800 mg dry extract/day vs placebo over a 6-week period experienced statistically significant changes in total and LDL cholesterol. Total cholesterol was decreased 18.5% vs 8.6% and LDL cholesterol was reduced 22.9% vs 6.3% in patients using the dry artichoke extract vs placebo, respectively. Thus, dry artichoke extract was recommended to treat hyperlipoproteinemia, preventing atherosclerosis and coronary heart disease.[15]

Other uses: A review on artichoke leaf extract is available, discussing digestive, antioxidative, hepatoprotective, lipid-lowering, and other effects.[1]

Other reported effects of artichoke include analgesic/anti-inflammatory[16] and hypoglycemic.[17] The artichoke is a good source of nutrition, including protein and fiber.[2,8,9,11] Artichoke extracts also may exert mild diuretic activity. Cynarase has been used commercially to curdle milk during cheese-making processes, clotting milk at a dilution of 1 part in 150,000.[7]

Artichoke seed oil was suggested to be of use as a component in making soaps, shampoos, resins, and polishes.[18]

TOXICOLOGY: In a 143-patient study, no adverse events were reported from artichoke administration, indicating excellent tolerability of dry extract.[16] Frequent contact with artichoke and other compositae family plants; however, has caused allergic reactions in sensitive individuals. Reports of contact dermatitis[20] and urticaria syndrome from occupational contact with artichoke have been documented, identifying the responsible components as cynaropicrin and other sesquiterpene lactones.[19-21]

According to the German Commission E Monographs, contraindications to the use of artichoke include allergy to compositae family plants and any bile duct obstruction. Presence of gallstones warrants a physician's consultation.[15] Lack of toxicity data suggests limiting use of artichoke during pregnancy and lactation.[14]

[1] Kraft K. *Phytomedicine.* 1997;4(4):369-78.

[2] Ensminger A, et al. *Foods and Nutrition Encyclopedia.* 2nd ed. Boca Raton, FL: CRC Press; 1994:116-118, 964-965.

[3] Chevallier A. *The Encyclopedia of Medicinal Plants.* New York, NY: DK Publishing; 1996:96-97.

[4] Online. (http://www.rain-tree.com/artichoke.htm)

[5] Bianchini F. *Health Plants of the World.* Milan, Italy: Arnoldo Mondadori Editore; 1975.

[6] Online. (http://www.prweb.com/releases/1998/prweb3080.htm)

[7] Schauenberg P, et al. *Guide to Medicinal Plants.* New Canaan, CT: Keats Publishing; 1977.

[8] Brown J, et al. *Free Radic Res.* 1998;29(3):247-55.

[9] Blumenthal M, ed. *The Complete German Commission E Monographs.* Boston, MA: American Botanical Council. 1998;169.

[10] Wegener T, et al. *Wien Med Wochenschr.* 1999;149(8-10):241-47. [German.]

[11] Gibson G. *Br J Nutr.* 1998;80(4):S209-12.

[12] Gebhardt R. *J Pharmacol Exp Ther.* 1998;286(3):1122-28.

[13] Anonymous. *Forsch Komplementarmed.* 1999;6(3):168-69. [German.]

[14] Heckers H, et al. *Atherosclerosis.* 1977;26(2):249-53.

[15] Englisch W, et al. *Arzneimittelforschung.* 2000;50(3):260-65. [German.]

[16] Ruppelt B, et al. *Mem Inst Oswaldo Cruz.* 1991;86 Suppl 2:203-205.

[17] Barbetti P, et al. *Ars Pharm.* 1992;33(1-4 vol 1):433-439.

[18] Miceli A, et al. *Bioresour Technol.* 1996;57(3):301-302.

[19] von Schneider G, et al. *Planta Med.* 1974;25:149.

[20] Meding B. *Contact Dermatitis.* 1983;9(4):314.

[21] Quirce S, et al. *J Allergy Clin Immunol.* 1996;97(2):710-11.

Barberry

SCIENTIFIC NAME(S): *Mahonia aquifolium* (Pursh.) Nutt., *Berberis vulgaris* L., and *B. aquifolium* Pursh. Family: Berberidaceae

COMMON NAME(S): Barberry, Oregon grape, Oregon barberry, Oregon grapeholly, trailing mahonia, berberis, jaundice berry, woodsour, sowberry, pepperidge bush, sour-spine[1,2]

⊷⊷⊷ PATIENT INFORMATION ⊷⊷⊷

Uses: The fruits have been used in jams, jellies, and juices. Plant alkaloids have been found to be antibacterial, antifungal, anti-inflammatory, antioxidant, and antidiarrheal. Berberine is a uterine stimulant. It also has current use for psoriasis.[3,4]

Side Effects: Barberry can produce stupor, daze, diarrhea, and nephritis and is contraindicated during lactation and pregnancy. Hypersensitivity reactions (eg, burning, itching, redness) have occurred in some patients using topical dosage forms.

Dosing: Barberry berries and root bark have been used as an alternative source of berberine. Daily doses of 2 g of the berries have been used, but there are no clinical studies to substantiate barberry's varied uses.[5]

BOTANY: The barberry grows wild throughout Europe but has been naturalized to many regions of the eastern US. *M. aquifolium* is an evergreen shrub native to the northwestern US and Canada. Barberry grows to more than approximately 3 meters with branched, spiny, holly-like leaves and is widely grown as an ornamental. Its yellow flowers bloom from May to June and develop into red to blue-black oblong berries.[6]

HISTORY: The plant has a long history of use, dating back to the Middle Ages. Salishan native elders have used *M. aquifolium* to treat acne[7] and native American Indians utilized Mahonia berries to treat scurvy.[8] A decoction of the root plant has been used to treat GI ailments and coughs.[6] The alkaloid berberine was included as an astringent in eye drops, but its use has become rare from lack of availability.

The edible fruits have been used to prepare jams, jellies, and juices. The use of the plant in traditional medicine has been limited by the bitter taste of the bark and root. However, more than 3 dozen medicinal uses for barberry, including cancer, cholera, and hyperten-

sion have been listed.[9,10] Other reported uses of *M. aquifolium* include the treatment of the following conditions: Fever, gout, renal and biliary diseases, rheumatic symptoms, diarrhea, gastric indigestion, and dermatosis.[11,12]

PHARMACOLOGY: *M. aquifolium* is valued for its antipsoriatic effects and its antibacterial, antifungal, anti-inflammatory, and antioxidant activity. It also has been used for treating acne, eczema, and candida infection.

Products of lipoxygenase metabolism enhance the pathophysiology of psoriasis. Each of the 6 bisbenzylisoquinoline alkaloids (oxyacanthine, armoline, baluchistine, berbamine, obamegine, aquifoline) isolated from *M. aquifolium* exhibited various lipoxygenase inhibitory activity resulting in an anti-inflammatory and antioxidant effect.[13]

Additional studies suggest that the antiproliferative effect is caused by the berberine content of *M. aquifolium*. Berbamine may reduce the synthesis of 5-lipoxygenase and cyclooxygenase,

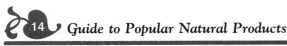

thereby reducing the activity of these enzymes in the arachidonic acid cascade.[14]

Berberine and several related alkaloids are bactericidal, in 1 study exceeding chloramphenicol (eg, *Chloromycetin*) against *Staphylococcus epidermidis*, *Neisseria meningitidis*, *Escherichia coli*, and other bacteria.[2] Another study reported that a methanolic extract (containing 80 mg of dried plant material) from the root of *M. aquifolium* exhibited antifungal activity against *Trichoderma viridae* and was considered more effective than nystatin.[15]

Several alkaloids (eg, berbamine, oxyacanthine) in Mahonia reportedly block the influx of calcium. The mechanism of the vasodilation is postulated to also involve alpha-adrenoreceptors.[16,17]

Berberine (100 mg 4 times/day), given alone or together with tetracycline, has been found to improve acute watery diarrhea and excretion of vibrios after 24 hours, compared with placebo in patients with noncholera diarrhea.[18] Berberine does not appear to exert its antidiarrheal effect by astringency, and the mechanism of action has not been defined.[19]

Berberine has anticonvulsant, sedative, and uterine stimulant properties. Local anesthesia can occur following SC injection of berberine.[9] Berbamine also produces a hypotensive effect.[8]

TOXICOLOGY: Symptoms of poisoning are characterized by lethargy, stupor and daze, vomiting and diarrhea, and nephritis.[20] *M. aquifolium* is contraindicated during lactation and pregnancy because some of the alkaloids (eg, berberine, palmatine) may stimulant uterine contractions.[20] It is also contraindicated in patients with hypersensitivity to *M. aquifolium*. Burning, redness, and itching have been reported in some patients using the topical dosage forms.[11,12]

[1] Windholz M, ed. *The Merck Index.* 10th ed. Rahway, NJ: Merck and Co; 1983.

[2] Leung AY. *Encyclopedia of Common Ingredients Used in Food, Drugs, and Cosmetics.* New York, NY: J Wiley and Sons; 1980.

[3] Wiesenauer, Ludtke. *Phytomedicine.* 1996;3:231-235.

[4] Muller Z, Ziereis K, Gawlik I. *Planta Med.* 1995;61:74-75.

[5] Gruenwald J, ed. *PDR for Herbal Medicines.* 2nd ed. Montvale, NJ: Thomson Medical Economics; 2000: 61-62.

[6] Schauenberg P, Paris F. *Guide to Medicinal Plants.* New Canaan, CT: Keats Publishing, Inc; 1977.

[7] Turner NJ, Hebda RJ. *J Ethnopharmacol.* 1990;29:59-72.

[8] Foster S, Tyler VE. *Tyler's Honest Herbal.* 4th ed. Binghamton, NY: Haworth Press; 1999.

[9] Duke JA. *Handbook of Medicinal Herbs.* Boca Raton, FL: CRC Press; 1985.

[10] Hartwell JL. *Lloydia.* 1968;31:71.

[11] Gieler U, von der Weth A, Heger M. *Ars Med.* 1995;14:1018-1019.

[12] Gieler U, von der Weth A, Heger M. *J Dermatol Treat.* 1995;6:31-34.

[13] Bezakova L, Misik V, Malekova L, et al. *Pharmazie.* 1996;51:758-761.

[14] Augustin M, Andrees U, Grimme H, et al. *Forsch Komplementarmed.* 1999;6(suppl 2):19-21.

[15] McCutcheon AR, Ellis SM, Hancock RE, et al. *J Ethnopharmacol.* 1994;44:157-169.

[16] Sotnikova R, Kettmann V, Kostalova D, et al. *Methods Find Exp Clin Pharmacol.* 1997;19:589-597.

[17] Sotnikova R, Kostalova D, Vaverkova S. *Gen Pharmacol.* 1994;25:1405-1410.

[18] Khin-Maung-U, Myo-Khin, Nyent-Nyent-Wai, et al. *BMJ.* 1985;291:1601-1605.

[19] Akhter MH, Sabir M, Bhide NK. *Indian J Med Res.* 1979;70:233-241.

[20] Blumenthal M, ed. *The Complete German Commission E Monographs: Therapeutic Guide to Herbal Medicines.* Austin, TX: American Botanical Council; 1998.

SCIENTIFIC NAME(S): Beta-1,3-glucan, beta-1,3/1,6-glycan

COMMON NAME(S): Beta glycans, beta glucans

❧❧❧ PATIENT INFORMATION ❧❧❧

Uses: Although few studies in humans are available (and are primarily in HIV patients), beta glycans are sold as supplements to boost the immune system and have also been studied in animals for their antitumor actions.

Side Effects: The FDA classifies baker's yeast beta-1,3/1,6-glycan as GRAS (generally recognized as safe), but reports show beta glycans may potentiate airway allergic responses and worsen symptoms in patients with existing disease.

Dosing: In an HIV trial, patients were given 2 to 10 mg of the beta-glucan lentinan IV once a week for 8 weeks. In a second trial, 1 to 5 mg of lentinan was given IV twice a week for 12 weeks.[1]

HISTORY: Beta-1,3/1,6-glycan has been studied for more than 30 years. It has immune system stimulant properties. In the 1980s, beta glycans were used to make salmon more disease resistant.[2]

PHARMACOLOGY: Norwegian beta glycan is sold as an all-natural dietary supplement to boost the immune system and protect against colds and flu. It is claimed to strengthen the body's ability to fight disease-causing organisms. Because of its molecular shape, it binds specifically to macrophage surfaces, activating the immune system and increasing resistance.[2] In another product claim, beta glycans are said to be acid-resistant and pass through the stomach unchanged. Once in the intestine, macrophages attach to activate them.[3] Other product claims include beta glycans' ability to heal bed sores, nail fungus, and ear infections.[4]

Beta glycan's role in HIV appears promising in phase I and II human trials but needs confirmation.[1]

TOXICOLOGY: Baker's yeast beta-1,3/1,6-glycan has a "GRAS" rating by the FDA.[3] A report on Norwegian beta glycans noted that if a patient with an existing disease takes beta glycans, symptoms may actually worsen for a couple of days.[2] In a clinical trial testing beta glycans use in AIDS patients, side effects severe enough to be reported to the FDA were anaphylactoid reaction, back pain, leg pain, depression, rigor, fever, chills, granulocytopenia, and elevated liver enzymes (1 case each); 4 of 98 patients discontinued therapy because of side effects.[1] Beta glycans may potentiate airway allergic responses.[5,6]

A preclinical safety evaluation of soluble glycan in mice, rats, guinea pigs, and rabbits is available. Data from this report indicate that "administration of soluble glycan over a wide dose range does not induce mortality or significant toxicity."[7]

---

[1] Gordon M, et al. *J Med.* 1998;29(5-6):305-330.
[2] Levy S. *Drug Topics.* 2000 Apr 17:73.
[3] http://www.immunehealthsystems.com/questions.htm.
[4] http://www.immunehealthsystems.com/beta.htm.

[5] Wan G, et al. *Eur J Immunol.* 1999;29(8):2491-2497.
[6] Tarlo S. *Occup Med.* 2000;15(2):471-484.
[7] Williams D, et al. *Int J Immunopharmacol.* 1988;10(4):405-414.

Bitter Melon

SCIENTIFIC NAME(S): *Momordica charantia* L. Family: Cucurbitaceae

COMMON NAME(S): Bitter melon, balsam pear, bitter cucumber, balsam apple, "art pumpkin," cerasee, carilla cundeamor

---

⋙⋙ PATIENT INFORMATION ⋙⋙

Uses: Bitter melon's effects include hypoglycemic, antimicrobial, antifertility, and others.

Side Effects: Use with caution in hypoglycemic patients. The red arils around bitter melon seeds are toxic to children. The plant is not recommended in pregnant women because it may cause uterine bleeding and contractions or may induce abortion.

Drug Interactions: Increased hypoglycemic effect when *M. charantia* and chlorpropamide are coadministered.

Dosing: Bitter melon juice has been recommended for diabetes at daily doses of 50 to 100 mL; 900 mg of fruit given 3 times/day also has been given for the same indication. There are no clinical trials available to substantiate these doses.

BOTANY: Bitter melon is an annual plant growing to approximately 1.8 m tall. It is cultivated in Asia, Africa, South America, and India and is considered a tropical fruit. The plant has lobed leaves, yellow flowers, and edible (but bitter-tasting), orange-yellow fruit. The unripe fruit is green and is cucumber-shaped with bumps on its surface. The parts used include the fruit, leaves, seeds, and seed oil.[1-3]

HISTORY: Bitter melon has been used as a folk remedy for tumors, asthma, skin infections, GI problems, and hypertension.[4] The plant has been used as a traditional medicine in China, India, Africa, and southeastern US.[3] The plant has been used in the treatment of diabetes symptoms. In the 1980s, the seeds were investigated in China as a potential contraceptive.[1]

PHARMACOLOGY: Beneficial effects of bitter melon have been studied and reviewed.[3,6-8] These effects include hypoglycemic, antimicrobial, antifertility, and others.

The hypoglycemic effects of bitter melon have been clearly established in animal and human studies.[9,10] Constituents of the plant that contribute to its hypoglycemic properties include charantin, polypeptide P, and vicine.[2,5,11,12] Reduction of blood glucose and improvement of glucose tolerance are the mechanisms by which the plant exerts its actions.

Animal studies document the hypoglycemic effects and include reports in diabetic mice;[13-15] studies in rats,[16-19] including improvement in glucose tolerance,[20] sustained decrease in blood glucose levels even after 15 days of discontinuation of bitter melon treatment (as well as a decrease in serum cholesterol levels),[21] and a suggested oral hypoglycemic mechanism involving the presence of viable beta cells;[22] and a study in diabetic rabbits, which also confirmed the plant's consistent hypoglycemic effects.[23]

Other mechanisms for hypoglycemic effects include extrapancreatic actions such as increased glucose uptake by tissues, glycogen synthesis in liver and muscles, triglyceride production in adipose tissue, and gluconeogenesis.[24] Another report suggests the activity to be partly caused by increased glucose use in the liver, rather than an insulin secretory effect.[25] Hepatic enzyme studies demonstrate bitter melon's hypoglycemic activity without glucose tolerance improvement in mice;[26] hypoglycemic activity by depression of blood glucose synthesis through depression of enzymes glucose-6-phosphatase and fructose-1,6-bisphosphatase, along with enhancement of glucose oxidation by enzyme G6PDH pathway;[27] and hypoglycemic actions involving hepatic cytochrome P450 and glutathione S-transferases in diabetic rats.[28] One report finds retardation of retinopathy (a diabetic complication) in diabetic rats administered a fruit extract of bitter melon.[29] At least 1 animal study finds no hypoglycemic effects in diabetic rats given a freeze-dried preparation of the plant for 6 weeks.[30]

Bitter melon improved glucose tolerance in humans.[20] Another study reported improved glucose tolerance in 18 type 2 diabetic patients with 73% success from a juice preparation of bitter melon.[31] Another report observed a 54% decrease in postprandial blood sugar, as well as a 17% reduction in glycosylated hemoglobin in 6 patients taking 15 g of aqueous bitter melon extract.[2] A report is available on patients taking a powder preparation of the plant.[32] Clinical trials using fresh fruit juice in 160 diabetic patients controlled diabetes. Bitter melon did not promote insulin secretion but did increase carbohydrate use.[4] A review describing the antidiabetic activity of bitter melon discusses in vitro, animal, and human studies, mechanisms of action, and the phytochemicals involved.[5]

Antimicrobial effects of bitter melon have been documented. Roots and leaf extracts have shown antibiotic activity.[3,4] One study reports cytostatic activity from bitter melon aqueous extract,[33] as constituents momorcharins

have antitumor properties and can inhibit protein synthesis.[34] Similarly, the plant also inhibits replication of viruses, including polio, herpes simplex 1, and HIV.[3,5] A study on antipseudomonal activity reports bitter melon to be effective, but not promising, in overall results.[35] Antiviral and other effects of bitter melon have been reviewed.[3]

Bitter melon exhibits genotoxic effects in *Aspergillus nidulans*.[36] It is cytotoxic in leukemia cells as a guanylate cyclase inhibitor.

Bitter melon's role in fertility has been reported. A protein found in the plant was found to show antifertility activity in male rats.[37] Oral administration of the fruit (1.7 g/day extract) to male dogs caused testicular lesions and atrophy of spermatogenic aspects. In female mice, the plant exhibited similar, but reversible, antifertility effects.[5] Momorcharins are capable of producing abortions.[34] Uterine bleeding has been induced in pregnant rats given the juice, as well as in rabbits, but not in nonpregnant females.[5] The ripe fruit has been said to induce menstruation.[1]

Other effects of bitter melon include the following: Dose-related analgesic activity in rats and mice,[38] anti-inflammatory actions,[5] and treatment for GI ailments, such as gas, ulcer, digestion, constipation, dysentery,[1,4] or hemorrhoids.[39] The plant has also been used for skin diseases (eg, boils, burns, infections, scabies, psoriasis),[4] and for its lipid effects[5] and hypotensive actions.[4,5] The plant has also been used as an insecticide.[3,4]

TOXICOLOGY: Bitter melon as an unripe fruit is commonly eaten as a vegetable[2,3] Bitter melon extract is said to be nontoxic.[3] The plant is relatively safe at low doses and for a duration of up to 4 weeks.[1] There are no published reports of serious effects in adults given the "normal" oral dose of 50 mL. In general, bitter melon has low clinical toxicity, with some possible adverse GI effects.[5]

Because of the plant's ability to reduce blood sugar, some caution is warranted in susceptible patients who may experience hypoglycemia.[1] Two small children experienced hypoglycemic coma resulting from intake of a tea made from the plant. Both recovered upon medical treatment.[5] Another report concerning increased hypoglycemic effect noted an interaction between *M. charantia* (a curry ingredient) and chlorpropamide in a 40-year-old diabetic woman taking concurrently for her condition.[40]

The red arils around bitter melon seeds are toxic to children. The juice given to a child in 1 report caused vomiting, diarrhea, and death.[4]

Bitter melon's hepatotoxic effects have been demonstrated in animals, in which enzymes became elevated following plant administration. The momorcharin constituents may induce morphological changes in hepatocytes as well.[5]

The seed constituent, vicine, is a toxin said to induce "favism," an acute condition characterized by headache, fever, abdominal pain, and coma[3,5]

Bitter melon is not recommended in pregnant women because of its reproductive system toxicities (see Pharmacology, antifertility section), including induction of uterine bleeding and contractions or abortion induction.[3,5,37]

[1] Chevallier A. *Encyclopedia of Medicinal Plants.* New York, NY: DK Publishing, 1996:234.

[2] Murray M. *The Healing Power of Herbs, 2 ed.* Rocklin, CA: Prima Publishing, 1995;357-358.

[3] Cunnick J, et al. *J Nat Med.* 1993;4(1):16-21.

[4] Duke J. *CRC Handbook of Medicinal Herbs.* Boca Raton, FL: CRC Press Inc., 1989;315-316.

[5] Raman A, et al. *Phytomedicine.* 1996;2(4):349-362.

[6] Sankaranaravanan J, et al. *Indian J Pharm Sci.* 1993;55(1):6-13.

[7] Platel K, et al. *Nahrung.* 1997;41(2):68-74.

[8] Avedikian J. *California Pharmacist.* 1994 Aug;42:15.

[9] Lei Q, et al. *J Tradit Chin Med.* 1985 Jun;5(2)99-106.

[10] Aslam M, et al. *Internat Pharm J.* 1989 Nov-Dec;3:226-229.

[11] Wong C, et al. *J Ethnopharmacology.* 1985 Jul;13:313-321.

[12] Handa G, et al. *Indian J Nat Prod.* 1990;6(1):16-19.

[13] Bailey C, et al. *Diabetes Res.* 1985;2(2):81-84.

[14] Day C, et al. *Planta Med.* 1990 Oct;56(5):426-429.

[15] Cakici I, et al. *J Ethnopharmacology.* 1994;44(2):117-121.

[16] Karunanayake E, et al. *J Ethnopharmacology.* 1984 Jul;11:223-231.

[17] Chandrasekar B, et al. *Indian J Med Res.* 1989;90:300-305.

[18] Higashino H, et al. *Nippon Yakurigaku Zasshi.* 1992 Nov;100(5):415-421.

[19] Ali L, et al. *Planta Med.* 1993 Oct;59(5):408-412.

[20] Leatherdale B, et al. *Br Med J (Clin Res Ed).* 1981 Jun 6;282(6279):1823-1824.

[21] Singh N, et al. *Indian J Physiol Pharmacol.* 1989 Apr-Jun;33(2):97-100.

[22] Karunanayake E, et al. *J Ethnopharmacology.* 1990;30(2):199-204.

[23] Akhtar M, et al. *Planta Med.* 1981;42(3):205-212.

[24] Welihinda J, et al. *J Ethnopharmacology.* 1986 Sep;17:247-255.

[25] Sarkar S, et al. *Pharmacol Res.* 1996 Jan;33(1):1-4.

[26] Tennekoon K, et al. *J Ethnopharmacology.* 1994;44(2):93-97.

[27] Shibib B, et al. *Biochem J.* 1993 May 15;292(Pt. 1):267-270.

[28] Raza H, et al. *Biochem Pharmacol.* 1996 Nov 22;52(10):1639-1642.

[29] Srivastava Y, et al. *Indian J Exp Biol.* 1987 Aug;25(8):571-572.

[30] Platel K, et al. *Nahrung.* 1995;39(4):262-268.

[31] Welihinda J, et al. *J Ethnopharmacology.* 1986 Sep;17:277-281.

[32] Akhtar M. *JPMA J Pak Med Assoc.* 1982 Apr;32(4):106-107.

[33] Rojas N, et al. *Revista Cubana de Farmacia.* 1980 May-Aug;14:219-225.

[34] Bruneton J. Pharmacognosy, PhytoChemistry, Medicinal Plants. Paris, France: Lavoisier, 1995;192.

[35] Saraya A, et al. *Mahidol Univ J Pharm Sci.* 1985 Jul-Sep;12:69-73.

[36] Ramos R, et al. *J Ethnopharm.* 1996;52(3):123-127.

[37] Chang F, et al. *Chin Traditional and Herbal Drugs.* 1995 Jun;26:281-284.

[38] Biswas A, et al. *J Ethnopharmacology.* 1991;31(1):115-118.

[39] Hocking G. A Dictionary of Natural Products. Medford, NJ: Plexus Publishing Inc., 1997;504-505.

[40] Aslam M, et al. *Lancet.* 1979 Mar 17;1:607.

Black Cohosh

SCIENTIFIC NAME(S): *Cimicifuga racemosa* (L.) Nutt. Family: Ranunculaceae. Plants associated with cohosh (although white cohosh and blue cohosh are quite distinct) include other *Cimicifuga* species, *Macrotys actaeoides*, and *Actaea racemosa* L.

COMMON NAME(S): Black cohosh, baneberry, black snakeroot, bugbane, squawroot, rattle root[1]

❧❧❧ PATIENT INFORMATION ❧❧❧

Uses: Black cohosh has been used to help manage some symptoms of menopause and as an alternative to hormone replacement therapy (HRT). It may be useful for hypercholesterolemia treatment or peripheral arterial disease.

Side Effects: Overdose causes nausea, dizziness, nervous system and visual disturbances, reduced pulse rate, and increased perspiration.

Dosing: The crude root has been administered at daily doses of 40 to 200 mg/day in clinical studies, although historically, higher doses of 1 g of root have been used. Standardized extracts such as *Remifemin* (Schaper & Brummer) standardized to 1 mg triterpene glycosides in 20 mg of extract, have been administered at doses from 2 to 8 mg/day of glycosides for menopause and related conditions.[2-5]

BOTANY: Black cohosh grows in open woods at the edges of dense forests from Ontario to Tennessee and west to Missouri. This perennial grows to 240 cm and is topped by a long plume of white flowers that bloom from June to September. Its leaflets are shaped irregularly with toothed edges. The term "black" refers to the dark color of the rhizome. The name "cohosh" comes from an Algonquian word meaning "rough," referring to the feel of the rhizome.[6]

HISTORY: The roots and rhizomes of this herb are used medicinally. Traditional uses include the treatment of dysmenorrhea, dyspepsia, and rheumatisms. A tea from the root has been recommended for sore throat. The Latin name *cimicifuga* means "bug-repellent" for which the plant has been used. American Indians used the plant to treat snakebites.

The old-time remedy "Lydia Pinkham's Vegetable Compound" from the early 1900s contained many natural ingredients, one of which was black cohosh.[7]

PHARMACOLOGY: *Remifemin*, the brand name of the standardized extract of the plant, has been used in Germany for menopausal management since the mid-1950s.[8]

In women treated for 8 weeks with *Remifemin* and luteinizing hormone, but not follicle-stimulating hormone, levels were reduced significantly. This product is used for the management of menopausal hot flashes. Analysis of the commercial product identified at least 3 fractions that contribute synergistically to the suppression of LH and bind to estrogen receptors. These data suggest that black cohosh has a measurable effect on certain reproductive hormones.[2] The product may offer an alternative to conventional HRT. In patient populations with a history of estrogen-dependent cancer (although it possesses some estrogenic activity), *Remifemin* shows no stimulatory effects on established breast tumor cell lines dependent on estrogen's presence. Instead, inhibitory actions were seen. In addition, the product exerts no effect on endometrium, so there is no need to oppose therapy with progesterone as with conventional HRT. The plant extract's action proves to be more like estriol than estradiol. Estradiol is associated with a higher risk for breast, ovarian, and endometrial cancers. Estriol mainly exerts its effects on the vaginal lining rather than the uterine lining as estradiol does. However, more studies are needed to address osteoporosis and bone health with use of the product.[8]

One report finds no signs of uterine growth and vaginal cornification in ovariectomized rats given black cohosh extract. This helps to confirm that the plant's beneficial effects on menopausal discomfort cannot be explained as estrogenic's typical effects.[9]

A clinical and endocrinologic study has been performed in 60 patients less than 40 years of age who had undergone hysterectomies. Four randomized treatment groups included estriol, conjugated estrogens, estrogen-gestagen sequential therapy, or black cohosh extract. Results of this report showed no significant differences between groups in success of therapy.[3]

Other actions of black cohosh include the following: Constituent actein that has been shown to have a hypotensive effect in rabbits and cats and causes peripheral vasodilation in dogs;[10,11] antimicrobial activity both by black cohosh[12] and related species *Cimicifuga dahurica*;[13] in vivo hypocholesterolemic activity; and therapy for patients with peripheral arterial disease by causing peripheral vasodilation and increase in blood flow from constituent actein.[13]

TOXICOLOGY: Overdose of black cohosh may cause nausea, vomiting, dizziness, nervous system and visual disturbances, reduced pulse rate, and increased perspiration. The constituent actein does not possess toxicity in animal studies.[13]

Large doses of the plant may induce miscarriage.[6] Black cohosh is contraindicated in pregnancy and may cause premature birth in large doses.[13]

A case report describes a 45-year-old woman who experienced seizures, possibly related to consumption of an herbal preparation containing black cohosh.[14]

[1] Meyer JE. *The Herbalist*. Hammond, IN: Hammond Book Co., 1934.

[2] Duker E, et al. *Planta Med*. 1991;57(5):420-424.

[3] Lehmann-Willenbrock E, et al. *Zentralbl Gynakol*. 1988;110(10):611-618.

[4] McKenna DJ, et al. *Natural Dietary Supplements Desktop Reference*. Marine on St. Croix, MN: Institute for Natural Products Research; 1998.

[5] Warnecke G. *Med Welt*. 1985;36:871-874.

[6] Dobelis IN, ed. *Magic and Medicine of Plants*. Pleasantville, NY: Reader's Digest Association, 1986.

[7] Tyler V. *Pharmacy in History*. 1995;37(1):24-28.

[8] Murray M. *Am J Nat Med*. 1997;4(3):3-5.

[9] Einer-Jensen N, et al. *Maturitas*. 1996;25(2):149-153.

[10] Genazzani E, et al. *Nature*. 1962;194:544.

[11] Corsano S, et al. *Gazz Chim Ital*. 1969;99:915.

[12] Bukowiecki H, et al. *Acta Pol Pharm*. 1972;29:432.

[13] Newall C, et al. *Black Cohosh Herbal Medicines*. London, England: Pharmaceutical Press, 1996;80-81.

[14] Shuster J. *Hosp Pharm*. 1996;31:1553-1554.

SCIENTIFIC NAME(S): *Juglans nigra* Family: Juglandaceae

COMMON NAME(S): Black walnut

◄◄◄◄ PATIENT INFORMATION ►►►►

Uses: Black walnut has been used as a wood source. It can also be beneficial in certain skin disorders, for constipation, and as an anti-infectant or vermifuge. It has nutritional value and its essential fatty acids (EFAs) help protect against heart disease and reduce cholesterol. There are no human trials to support these effects.

Side Effects: Do not use during pregnancy or chronic gastrointestinal tract disease. Juglone, the naphthaquinone found in black walnut and many others in the family Juglandaceae, is regarded as a toxin. Allergic reactions have occurred.

BOTANY: There are about 15 species of Juglans. "Walnut" refers to several varieties, most commonly the English or Persian walnut and the black walnut (*J. nigra*). Walnut trees have short trunks with round-topped crowns, and can grow to 45 m in height. The black walnut is native to the deciduous forests of the eastern US (central Mississippi, Appalachian regions) and Canada. Its wood is valued for its rich beauty and yields valuable lumber, prized for furniture, cabinets, and gun stocks. The fruit is an elongated drupe, containing a 4-ribbed edible nut within a thick, hard, black shell (smaller in size than the English walnut).[1-4]

HISTORY: Walnuts have been found in prehistoric deposits dating from the Iron Age in Europe. They are mentioned in the Bible; King Solomon's nut garden dates back to 940 BC.[4] Black walnuts were an important food for American Indians and early settlers.[2] The genus name, *Juglans*, comes from the Latin *Jovis glans*, meaning "nut of Jupiter" or nut of the gods. Many legends have been associated with the walnut. Greeks and Romans regarded it as a symbol of fertility. In the Middle Ages, walnuts were thought to ward off witchcraft, the evil eye, and epileptic fits from evil spirits lurking in the walnut branches. Medicinal uses of walnuts included treatments for swollen glands, shingles, and sores. The oil was used for intestinal discomfort.[4]

PHARMACOLOGY: Aside from the use of its wood as a valuable lumber, black walnut has been employed in other ways; extract of black walnut was used to dye the hair,[1,3] skin, and clothing.[4] Black walnut as a food is common, including its presence in baked goods, candies, and frozen foods.[2,4] Even its shells, after hulling, have been used as fillers in glues, roofing materials, and tiles. They are also employed as stuffing for toys and as abrasives. Walnut shells are even burned for energy.[4]

The black walnut is important for its nutritional value. The nuts are high in calories, a good protein source, and rich in dietary fiber and EFAs, which protect against heart disease and reduce cholesterol. EFAs reduce platelet adhesion and may also play a role in reducing arrhythmias and cardiac arrest.[5-8] Dietary fiber content not only helps reduce cholesterol but aids in relieving constipation.[8,9]

Black walnut is beneficial in certain skin problems, including eczema, pruritus, psoriasis, and blistering.[3,9] It has been used as an astringent to shrink tissues and as a tonic restorative.[3] Black walnut has been shown to kill skin parasites due to its disinfectant qualities. Constituent juglone is antimicrobial and antiparasitic.[3,10] Black walnut has been used for warts. Eye irritations and styes have been relieved by black walnut as well.[3] Internally, black walnut is beneficial for these same conditions. It is mentioned by many sources as a vermifuge. The anthelmintic properties are said to be due to high tannin content. The bark (including kernel and green hull) has been used by Asians and certain American Indian tribes to expel worms. Other fungal and parasitic infections including ringworm and tapeworm have been eliminated by black walnut.[1,9] Other uses for black walnut include reduction of fluid secretion in glandular disturbances, treatment of gout and rheumatism, and for purported anticancer effects.[3,11] The toxic nature of juglone makes it a possible candidate for chemotherapy.[12]

No major human clinical trials regarding black walnut and its claimed uses have been found through a search of medical literature.

TOXICOLOGY: Juglone, the naphthaquinone found in black walnut and many others in the family Juglandaceae, is regarded as a toxin. Induced toxicosis in horses has been studied.

Juglone 1 g orally administered in horses caused inconsistent mild signs of laminitis, in which inflammation of the feet around the hooves occurs, resulting in lameness from the pain.[13] Other studies have confirmed this type of toxicosis from black walnut,[14,15] including a detailed description in a case report.[16] In contrast, 1 report confirms the laminitis to be from black walnut but not from the constituent juglone, because the heartwood of black walnut, which is devoid of this component, was used.[17] Black walnut's effects on equine vasculature have been evaluated.[18-20] One mechanism suggested in another report is that black walnut increases capillary pressure, causing transvascular fluid movement, resulting in edema and possible eventual ischemia.[21]

Allergic reactions to black walnut in animals and humans have occurred.[22] Allergy studies involving skin testing with black walnut pollen (and other pollens) finds moderate allergic reactions in certain individuals.[23] Reports on dermatitis from black walnut[24,25] and on *Escherichia coli* in black walnut[26] are available.

Black walnut is contraindicated in pregnancy because of possible cathartic effects at higher doses and in patients with chronic disease of the GI tract.[27,28]

[1] Hocking G. *A Dictionary of Natural Products.* Medford, NJ: Plexus Publishing, Inc., 1997:409.

[2] Ensminger A, et al. *Foods and Nutrition Encyclopedia.* 2nd ed. Boca Raton, FL: CRC Press, 1994:2277-2278.

[3] D'Amelio F. *Botanicals: A Phytocosmetic Desk Reference.* Boca Raton, FL: CRC Press, 1999:209.

[4] Rosengarten F. *The Book of Edible Nuts.* New York, NY: Walker and Company, 1984:239-262.

[5] Abbey M, et al. *Am J Clin Nutr.* 1994;59:995-999.

[6] Berry E, et al. *Am J Clin Nutr.* 1991;53:899-907.

[7] Simon J, et al. *Stroke.* 1995;26:778-782.

[8] Sabate J, et al. *N Engl J Med.* 1993;328:603-607.

[9] http://www.metromkt.net/viable/1bwalnut.shtml

[10] Chevallier A. *The Encyclopedia of Medicinal Plants.* London, England: DK Publishing, 1996:222-223.

[11] http://thriveonline.oxygen.com/health/Library/vitamins/vitamin102.html

[12] Segura-Aguilar J, et al. *Leuk Res.* 1992;16(6-7):631-637.

[13] True R, et al. *Am J Vet Res.* 1980;41(6):944-945.

[14] Ralston S, et al. *J Am Vet Med Assoc.* 1983;183(10):1095.

[15] Uhlinger C. *J Am Vet Med Assoc.* 1989;195(3):343-344.

16 Thomsen M, et al. *Vet Hum Toxicol.* 2000;42(1):8-11.

17 Minnick P, et al. *Vet Hum Toxicol.* 1987;29(3):230-233.

18 Galey F, et al. *Am J Vet Res.* 1990;51(1):83-88.

19 Galey F, et al. *Am J Vet Res.* 1990;51(4):688-695.

20 Galey F, et al. *J Comp Pathol.* 1991;104(3):313-326.

21 Eaton S, et al. *Am J Vet Res.* 1995;56(10):1338-1344.

22 MacDaniels L. *Cornell Vet.* 1983;73(2):204-207.

23 Lewis W, et al. *Ann Allergy.* 1975;35(2):113-119.

24 Schwartz L. *Publ Health Rep.* 1931;46:1938.

25 Siegel J. *Arch Derm Syph.* 1954;70-511.

26 Meyer M, et al. *Appl Microbiol.* 1969;18(5):925-931.

27 http://www.healthgate.com/choice/uic/cons/mdx-books/vit/herb22.shtml

28 McGuffin M, et al, ed. *American Herbal Products Association's Botanical Safety Handbook.* Boca Raton, FL: CRC Press, 1997.

SCIENTIFIC NAME(S): *Sanguinaria canadensis* L. Family: Papaveraceae (poppies)

COMMON NAME(S): Bloodroot, red pucoon, red root, coon root, paucon, sweet slumber, tetterwort, snakebite, Indian paint

---

ᕕᕗᕗᕗ PATIENT INFORMATION ᕗᕗᕗᕗ

Uses: Bloodroot was used historically as a treatment for skin cancers, polyps, and warts, although there are no clinical trials to support these uses. It was marketed in the early 1980s in toothpastes and mouthwashes for the prevention of gum disease and plaque; however, more recent studies have found it inferior to drugs such as doxycycline and chlorhexidine.

Side Effects: Recent studies have found a strong correlation between the use of sanguinarine dental products and oral leukoplakia, a possible precursor to oral cancer. Bloodroot is contraindicated during pregnancy.

Dosing: Bloodroot is emetic at doses of 30 to 125 mg in humans. It was formerly an ingredient in toothpastes and mouthwashes, but its use has been discontinued because of toxicity concerns.[1]

BOTANY: Bloodroot is an early spring wildflower that grows in the woodlands of the eastern US and Canada. Its single white flower emerges from the ground folded within a grey-green leaf and the delicate petals rapidly detach as the seed pod matures. The stout rhizome yields a bright red latex when cut, giving the plant its common name. The root and rhizome are collected in the fall for medicinal use.

HISTORY: Bloodroot was used by eastern American Indian tribes as a red dye and in the treatment of ulcers, skin conditions, and as a blood purifier. All of these medicinal uses apparently derive from the appearance of the blood-red latex exuded from the fresh root. The juice was also used for coughs and sore throats, with the bitter taste masked by placing the juice on a lump of maple sugar that was then sucked. Higher oral doses were observed to have expectorant and emetic properties. The root entered 19th century medicine as a caustic topical treatment for skin cancers, polyps, and warts. In 1983 an extract of bloodroot was marketed in toothpaste and mouthwashes for preven-

tion of gum disease and plaque (see Pharmacology).

PHARMACOLOGY:

Biochemistry: Sanguinarine has been found to intercalate with DNA[2-4] favoring GC-rich sequences.[3,5] It has also been found to inhibit NaK-ATPase[6-8] in several systems, including human erythrocytes.[9] A431 cancer cells were found to undergo apoptosis at lower doses of sanguinarine than normal cells.[10] Other documented effects are inhibition of tubulin function by sanguinarine and chelerythrine,[11] and protein kinase C inhibition.[12] This latter effect has been shown to depend on reaction of the alkaloids with critical thiol groups.[13] Such a mechanism may also underlie some of these alkaloids' other diverse effects, including inhibition of liver aminotransferase,[13] inhibition of phosphorylation of a mitochondrial protein from rat heart,[14] inhibition of NFκB activation,[15] and induction of calcium release from sarcoplasmic reticulum.[16]

Antimicrobial activity: Sanguinarine has long been known to have antibiotic activity in vitro.[17] An ecological role in chemical defense of the plant against microorganisms and herbivores has been postulated;[18] given the broad variety of bioactivity noted above and the high concentration of alkaloids, this hypothesis is quite reasonable. The cholera bacterium, for example, is sensitive to sanguinarine.[19] More relevant are studies of oral cavity microbes. Virtually all isolates from human dental plaque were growth-inhibited by sanguinarine at 16 mcg/mL;[20] consequently, shifts in the spectrum of species in the oral flora were not observed.[21] Clinical studies using bacterial counts of saliva did not show reductions in *S. mutans* or *S. salivarius* with sanguinarine, while chlorhexidine was effective using the same measures.[22] Another similar clinical study of sanguinarine with zinc chloride found reductions in plaque bacteria over a 6-month trial compared to placebo.[23] A transient overgrowth of sanguinarine-resistant bacteria, but not fungi, in the mouth was observed in a further clinical study.[24] Consistent with this result, 6 yeast species were not efficiently killed by sanguinarine, while other mouthwash ingredients were effective.[25]

Antiplaque and gingivitis clinical studies:
Early reports of small clinical studies indicated that sanguinarine might have use in plaque reduction.[26-29] Other studies using different methods questioned this efficacy,[30] while the addition of zinc was claimed to increase the efficacy of sanguinarine.[31] These studies were conducted over relatively short time periods. A 6-month, double-blind trial of sanguinarine toothpaste against plaque and gingivitis found no advantage over placebo.[32] When compared with a chlorhexidine mouthwash in a crossover trial, a sanguinarine-zinc mouthwash was less effective.[33] A direct comparison of sanguinarine with sodium fluoride toothpaste demonstrated equal activity against plaque and gingivitis.[34] A further 6-month trial showed moderate antiplaque and gingivitis activity for a sanguinarine mouthwash, but it was less effective than chlorhexidine.[35] A 6-month study of combined toothpaste and mouthwash in an orthodontic population showed benefit from sanguinarine by a variety of endpoints.[36] A review of studies from 1983 to 1990 suggested that the design of the clinical studies may have skewed results and proposed guidelines for improving further trials, including larger study populations, avoidance of crossover designs, and selection of appropriate controls.[37] Other studies have remained mixed. A small effect on plaque was seen for sanguinarine mouthwash compared with chlorhexidine[38] while safety and efficacy were reported in another study with combined sanguinarine toothpaste and mouthwash.[39] A further review concluded that sanguinarine was ineffective.[40] A comparison of sanguinarine-containing regimens with and without fluoride found a modest additional benefit for sanguinarine.[41] Attempts to market sanguinarine-containing products in the United Kingdom and Australia have met with skepticism.[42,43]

The most recent extensive trials of sanguinarine-containing dental products have used new delivery systems. A biodegradable matrix was used to achieve modest plaque and gingivitis control with sanguinarine; however, it was not more effective than supragingival mechanical plaque control.[44] A 9-month study of subgingivally delivered sanguinarine versus doxycycline in periodontitis found doxycycline superior to sanguinarine,[45,46] as did another study.[47] A French clinical study suggested combined use of chlorhexidine and sanguinarine.[48] In summary, the current clinical status of sanguinarine in dental plaque and gingivitis prevention and treatment is that while modestly effective, it is inferior to chlorhexidine, doxycycline, and other newer agents under development.

TOXICOLOGY: Short-term toxicity studies of sanguinarine and *Sanguinaria* extracts in rats found minimal oral toxicity (LD50 1200 to 1700 mg/kg), probably because of its very limited gastric absorption, while sanguinarine was considerably more toxic via acute intravenous administration (LD50 29 mg/kg).[49] A dermal LD50 of greater than 200 mg/kg in rabbits was estimated.[50] No reproductive or developmental effects in rats and rabbits were reported.[50] An expert panel reviewed the toxicological literature on bloodroot in 1990 and found no cause for concern.[51] Despite its DNA intercalating ability, sanguinarine was not mutagenic in the Ames test.[52] Phototoxic effects against mosquito larvae have been reported.[53]

Other cause for concern stems partly from reports of "epidemic dropsy" in India, where contamination of edible cooking oils with sanguinarine-containing *Argemone mexicana* seeds has been responsible for toxicity.[54-57] Further concerns were stimulated by reports of cytotoxicity of sanguinarine to cultured cells from oral tissue[58] and inhibition of neutrophil function.[59] Recent epidemiological work found a strong correlation of use of sanguinarine dental products with oral leukoplakia, a condition considered to be a possible precursor of oral cancer.[60,1]

Bloodroot is contraindicated during pregnancy and has uterine-stimulating action.

[1] Eversole L, et al. *Oral Surg Oral Med Oral Pathol Oral Radiol Endod.* 2000;89:455-464.
[2] Maiti M, et al. *FEBS Lett.* 1982;142:280-284.
[3] Nandi R, et al. *Biochem Pharmacol.* 1985;34:321-324.
[4] Sen A, et al. *Biochem Pharmacol.* 1994;48:2097-2102.
[5] Bajaj N, et al. *J Mol Recognit.* 1990;3:48-54.
[6] Straub K, et al. *Biochem Biophys Res Commun.* 1975;62:913-922.
[7] Cohen H, et al. *Biochem Pharmacol.* 1978;27:2555-2558.
[8] Seifen E, et al. *Eur J Pharmacol.* 1979;60:373-377.
[9] Cala P, et al. *J Membr Biol.* 1982;64:23-31.
[10] Ahmad N, et al. *Clin Cancer Res.* 2000;6:1524.
[11] Wolff J, et al. *Biochemistry.* 1993;32:13334-13339.
[12] Gopalakrishna R, et al. *Methods Enzymol.* 1995;252:132-146.
[13] Walterová D, et al. *J Med Chem.* 1981;24:1100-1103.
[14] Lombardini J, et al. *Biochem Pharmacol.* 1996;51:151-157.
[15] Chaturvedi M, et al. *J Biol Chem.* 1997;272:30129-30134.
[16] Hu C, et al. *Br J Pharmacol.* 2000;130:299-306.
[17] Mitscher L, et al. *Lloydia.* 1978;41:145-150.
[18] Schmeller T, et al. *Phytochemistry.* 1997;44:257-266.
[19] Nandi R, et al. *Experientia.* 1983;39:524-525.
[20] Dzink J, et al. *Antimicrob Agents Chemother.* 1985;27:663-665.
[21] Godowski K. *J Clin Dent.* 1989;1:96-101.

[22] Hoover J, et al. *J Can Dent Assoc.* 1990;56:325-327.
[23] Harper D, et al. *J Periodontol.* 1990;61:359-363.
[24] Godowski K, et al. *J Periodontol.* 1995;66:870-877.
[25] Giuliana G, et al. *J Periodontol.* 1997;68:729-733.
[26] Southard G, et al. *J Am Dent Assoc.* 1984;108:338-341.
[27] Wennstrom J, et al. *J Clin Periodontol.* 1985;12:867-872.
[28] Wennstrom J, et al. *J Clin Periodontol.* 1986;13:86-93.
[29] Parsons L, et al. *J Clin Periodontol.* 1987;14:381-385.
[30] Etemadzadeh H, et al. *J Clin Periodontol.* 1987;14:176-180.
[31] Southard G, et al. *J Clin Periodontol.* 1987;14:315-319.
[32] Mauriello S, et al. *J Periodontol.* 1988;59:238-243.
[33] Moran J, et al. *J Clin Periodontol.* 1988;15:612-616.
[34] Mallatt M, et al. *J Periodontol.* 1989;60:91-95.
[35] Grossman E, et al. *J Periodontol.* 1989;60:435-440.
[36] Hannah J, et al. *Am J Orthod Dentofacial Orthop.* 1989;96:199-207.
[37] Laster L, et al. *J Can Dent Assoc.* 1990;56:19-30.
[38] Quirynen M, et al. *J Clin Periodontol.* 1990;17:223-227.
[39] Harper D, et al. *J Periodontol.* 1990;61:352-358.

40 Balanyk T. *Clin Prev Dent.* 1990;12:18-25.

41 Kopczyk R, et al. *J Periodontol.* 1991;62:617-622.

42 Grenby T. *Br Dent J.* 1995;178:254-258.

43 Cullinan M, et al. *Aust Dent J.* 1997;42:47-51.

44 Polson A, et al. *J Clin Periodontol.* 1996;23:782-788.

45 Polson A, et al. *J Periodontol.* 1997;68:110-118.

46 Polson A, et al. *J Periodontol.* 1997;68:119-126.

47 Drisko C, *J Clin Periodontol.* 1998;25:947-952, 978-979.

48 Tenenbaum H, et al. *J Periodontol.* 1999;70:307-311.

49 Becci P, et al. *J Toxicol Environ Health.* 1987;20:199-208.

50 Keller K, et al. *J Clin Dent.* 1989;1:59-66.

51 Frankos V, et al. *J Can Dent Assoc.* 1990;56:41-47.

52 Kevekordes S, et al. *Mutat Res.* 1999;445:81-91.

53 Arnason J, et al. *Photochem Photobiol.* 1992;55:35-38.

54 Shenolikar I, et al. *Food Cosmet Toxicol.* 1974;12:699-702.

55 Dalvi R. *Experientia.* 1985;41:77-78.

56 Sachdev M, et al. *Arch Ophthalmol.* 1988;106:1221-1223.

57 Das M, et al. *Crit Rev Toxicol.* 1997;27:273-297.

58 Babich H, et al. *Pharmacol Toxicol.* 1996;78:397-398.

59 Agarwal S, et al. *J Periodontal Res.* 1997;32:335-344.

60 Damm D, et al. *Oral Surg Oral Med Oral Pathol Oral Radiol Endod.* 1999;87:61-66.

SCIENTIFIC NAME(S): *Caulophyllum thalictroides* (L.) Michx. Family Berberidaceae (barberries)

COMMON NAME(S): Blue cohosh, squaw root, papoose root, blue ginseng, yellow ginseng

---

ᴥᴥᴥ PATIENT INFORMATION ᴥᴥᴥ

Uses: Blue cohosh has been used to induce uterine contractions. It is widely advertised on the Internet, but is dangerous (see Toxicology).

Side Effects: Blue cohosh root is a dangerous product. Its toxicity appears to outweigh any medical benefit.

Dosing: Blue cohosh has traditionally been used at doses of 0.5 to 3 g/day; however, its potential for teratogenicity makes it unsuitable for women who are or may become pregnant. Because its principal indications are for gynecological disorders, avoid its use.[1]

BOTANY: Blue cohosh is an early spring perennial herb whose yellowish-green flowers mature into bitter, bright blue seeds. It is found throughout woodlands of the eastern and midwestern US, especially in the Allegheny Mountains. The matted, knotty rootstock, collected in the autumn, is used for medicinal purposes. The root of an Asian species, *C. robustum* Maxim., has also been used medicinally.

HISTORY: Blue cohosh was used by American Indians; the name "cohosh" comes from the Algonquin name of the plant. It was used by Menomini, Meskawi, Ojibwe, and Potawatomi tribes for menstrual cramps, to suppress profuse menstruation, and to induce contractions in labor.[2] It was widely used in 19th century Eclectic medicine as an emmenagogue, parturient, and antispasmodic. It continues to be used for regulating the menstrual cycle and for inducing uterine contractions.

PHARMACOLOGY: N-methyl-cytisine (caulophylline) was found to be a nicotinic agonist in animals[3] and to displace [3H]nicotine from nicotinic acetylcholine receptors with 50 nm potency.[4] It was essentially inactive at muscarinic receptors. Other quinolizidine alkaloids were considerably less potent nicotinic ligands, with anagyrine having IC50 values greater than 100 mcm in these test systems.[4]

Magnoflorine has its own pharmacological properties, decreasing arterial blood pressure in rabbits and inducing hypothermia in mice, as well as inducing contractions in the isolated pregnant rat uterus and stimulating isolated guinea pig ileal preparations in cell membranes.[5] The blue cohosh saponins have uterine stimulant effects, as well as cardiotoxicity presumably due to vasoconstriction of coronary blood vessels.[6] Extracts of *Caulophyllum* given to rats were found to inhibit ovulation and affect the uterus.[7] The saponins of the Siberian species *C. robustum* (caulosides) have antimicrobial activity.[8] A mechanism for cytotoxicity has been suggested for cauloside C involving formation of pH-dependent channels.[9]

TOXICOLOGY: Blue cohosh berries are poisonous to children when consumed raw although the roasted seeds have been used as a coffee substitute.[10] The root can cause contact dermatitis.[10] The alkaloid anagyrine is a teratogen in ruminants,[11] causing "crooked calf syndrome." Another quinolizidine alkaloid in the plant, N-methylcytisine, was teratogenic in a rat embryo culture.[12] The skeletal malformations seen in calves have been postulated to be caused by the action of the quinolizidine alkaloids on muscarinic and nicotinic receptors of the fetus, preventing normal fetal movements required for proper skeletal development.

A case was reported in which a newborn human infant, whose mother was administered blue cohosh to promote uterine contractions, was diagnosed with acute myocardial infarction associated with CHF and shock. The infant eventually recovered after being critically ill for several weeks.[13] The FDA Special Nutritionals Adverse Event Monitoring System notes fetal toxicity cases of stroke and aplastic anemia following ingestion by the mother.

[1] Claus E, ed. *Pharmacognosy*. 3rd ed. Philadelphia, PA: Lea & Febiger; 1956.

[2] Kennelly E, et al. *J Nat Prod*. 1999;62:1385-1389.

[3] Scott C, et al. *J Pharmacol Exp Ther*. 1943;79:334.

[4] Schmeller T, et al. *J Nat Prod*. 1994;57:1316-1319.

[5] El-Tahir K. *Int J Pharmacognosy*. 1991;29:101.

[6] Ferguson H, et al. *J Am Pharm Assoc (Sci Ed)*. 1954;43:16.

[7] Chandrasekhar K, et al. *J Reprod Fertil*. 1974;38:236-237.

[8] Anisimov M. *Antibiotiki*. 1972;17:834-837. Russian.

[9] Likhatskaya G, et al. *Adv Exp Med Biol*. 1996;404:239-249.

[10] Hardin J, et al. *Human poisoning from native and cultivated plants*. Durham, NC: Duke University Press,1974;60.

[11] Keeler R. *J Toxicol Environ Health*. 1976;1:887-898.

[12] Erichsen-Brown C. *Medicinal and other uses of North American plants. A historical survey with special reference to the Eastern Indian tribes*. NY: Dover Press, 1980;355.

[13] Jones T, et al. *J Pediatr*. 1998;132:550-552.

SCIENTIFIC NAME(S): *Borago officinalis* L. Family: Boraginaceae (borage family)

COMMON NAME(S): Borage, burrage, common bugloss, bee-bread, bee fodder, star flower, ox's tongue, cool tankard

---

‌PATIENT INFORMATION‌

Uses: Borage has been used in European herbal medicine since the Middle Ages and may be useful either alone or in combination with fish oil in the treatment of rheumatoid arthritis, atopic eczema, diabetic neuropathy, and osteoporosis, although limited information is available.

Side Effects: No adverse effects have been found in topical use or with seed oil. Do not ingest the leaves and flowers because they may contain hepatotoxic compounds.

Dosing: Borage seed oil has been given in doses of 1.4 to 2.8 g/day in several clinical trials for arthritis and other inflammatory conditions.[1] The content of gamma-linolenic acid is between 20% and 26% of the oil.[2,3]

BOTANY: Borage is an annual that grows to about 0.6 meters in height. The stem and leaves are covered with coarse, prickly hairs, and the flowers are large, star-shaped, and bright blue, with contrasting black anthers. It is a native of Europe but has been widely naturalized in other areas. The fresh plant has a salty flavor and a cucumber-like odor.

HISTORY: Borage leaves have been used as a potherb and in European herbal medicine since the Middle Ages, and are mentioned by Pliny, Dioscorides, and Galen. The name "borage" derives from the medieval Latin "burra," meaning rough-coated, which refers to the hairs. An alternative explanation suggests a corruption of the Latin "corago" (courage), as in Gerard's rhyme *"ego borago gaudia semper ago"* (I, borage, bring alwaies courage), in line with its reputation as an herb to dispel melancholy. Borage leaves and flowers were added to wine and lemon juice to make the popular beverages "claret cup" and "cool tankard." Borage leaves also have been used for rheumatism, colds, and bronchitis, as well as to increase lacta-tion in women. Infusions of the leaves were used to induce sweating and diuresis.[4]

PHARMACOLOGY: The 18-carbon fatty acid linoleic acid is considered an essential fatty acid in human nutrition because it must be obtained from the diet. It is converted by the enzyme delta-6-desaturase to gamma linolenic acid (GLA), and this enzyme is considered rate-limiting in the pathway. GLA is further elaborated to the 20-carbon fatty acid dihomogamma-linolenic acid (DGLA), a key metabolite for the synthesis of the anti-inflammatory prostaglandins of the 1-series (eg, PGE1) and 15-(S)-hydroxy-8,11,13-eicosatrienoic acid (15HETrE) by different types of cells.[5] Therefore, supplementation with GLA might bypass the rate-limiting step in biosynthesis, providing more of these anti-inflammatory modulators. In addition, pathophysiological conditions have been found to alter the ability to convert linoleic acid to GLA.[5] The current commercial sources of GLA include borage seed oil, evening primrose oil, and black currant seed oil, with the oil from the fungus *Mucor javanicus* in development as well.[6] Cloning of delta-6-

desaturase enzymes into plants not normally possessing them has been proposed as a means to increase dietary GLA; although, has been opposed by concerned parties.[7]

Investigations in humans have followed a similar pattern. Borage seed oil increased plasma phospholipid GLA and DGLA levels, while augmenting the arterial baroreflex control of vascular resistance in healthy humans, actions that may be useful in the treatment of hypertension.[8] Proportions of different phospholipid types were unchanged but DGLA was increased in platelets when borage seed oil was administered for 42 days.[9] Neutrophils from subjects whose diets were supplemented with GLA mobilized 3-fold more DGLA after ionophore stimulation than controls.[10] In older subjects, GLA had no effect on natural killer cell activity, while fish oil reduced it by half.[11] T-lymphocyte proliferation, in contrast, was decreased by both GLA and fish oil in the same type of population.[12] This effect on lymphocytes was reproduced by a second group for GLA in borage seed oil, where increases in plasma GLA and DGLA were observed.[1] The release of pro-inflammatory leukotriene B_4 from neutrophils with ionophore stimulation was reduced, while DGLA was elevated in healthy adults. The effects were greater at the higher of 2 doses.[13]

Clinical trials have been performed with borage seed oil or purified GLA in several diseases. A 24-week randomized, double-blind, placebo-controlled trial of borage seed oil (1.4 g/day of GLA) in rheumatoid arthritis found clinically important reduction in symptoms compared with a cotton seed oil placebo.[2] A larger (n = 56) trial using a higher dose (2.8 g/day GLA) included a 6-month double-blind phase and a second 6-month single-blind trial. Improvement was found in arthritis symptoms

for both groups, with the cohort receiving 12 months of GLA supplementation improving throughout both phases.[3] All of these regimens detected no adverse effects. Reviews of trials in rheumatoid arthritis have evaluated efficacy of GLA as beneficial,[14,15] an opinion shared by a Cochrane Review.[16]

A multicenter trial of borage seed oil in atopic eczema found modest improvement in the supplement group; however, the effect did not reach statistical significance.[17] The dose was 0.5 g/day GLA, given over 24 weeks, which may be too small to detect a significant effect. The trial also may have been confounded by varying use of steroids by some centers.[18,19]

A multicenter trial of fish oil and borage seed oil added to enteral feeding mixtures in patients with acute respiratory distress syndrome found improvement in outcomes, with further major organ failures reduced, shorter intensive care unit stay, and less ventilator support required compared with controls.[20]

A pilot study of fish oil plus borage seed oil in elderly osteoporotic women found improved bone density in the treatment arm compared with placebo, and improvement after crossover to all treatment in both groups.[21] A review of trials of GLA for impaired nerve function in diabetics concluded that GLA may hold promise for treatment of diabetic neuropathy.[22]

TOXICOLOGY: Clinical studies of borage seed oil have not found adverse effects when doses up to 2.4 g/day of GLA equivalents were administered. The presence of unsaturated pyrrolizidine alkaloids in leaves, flowers, and seeds of borage[23,24] requires that seed oils be tested for content, and that other parts not be ingested to avoid the potential for hepatotoxicity.[25,26]

1 Rossetti RG, Seiler CM, DeLuca P, Laposata M, Zurier RB. *J Leukoc Biol.* 1997;62:438-443.

2 Leventhal LJ, Boyce EG, Zurier RB. *Ann Intern Med.* 1993;119:867-873.

3 Zurier RB, Rossetti RG, Jacobson EW, et al. *Arthritis Rheum.* 1996;39:1808-1817.

4 Awang DVC. *Can Pharm J.* 1990;123:121-126.

5 Fan Y-Y, Chapkin RS. *J Nutr.* 1998;128:1411-1414.

6 Lawson LD, Hughes BG. *Lipids.* 1988;23:313-317.

7 Palombo JD, DeMichele SJ, Liu J-W, Bistrian BR, Huang Y-S. *Lipids.* 2000;35:975-981.

8 Mills DE, Mah M, Ward RP, Morris BL, Floras JS. *Am J Physiol.* 1990;259(6 Pt 2):R1164-R1171.

9 Barre DE, Holub BJ. *Lipids.* 1992;27:315-320.

10 Chilton-Lopez T, Surette ME, Swan DD, Fonteh AN, Johnson MM, Chilton FH. *J Immunol.* 1996;156:2941-2947.

11 Thies F, Nebe-von-Caron G, Powell JR, Yaqoob P, Newsholme EA, Calder PC. *Am J Clin Nutr.* 2001;73:539-548.

12 Thies F, Nebe-von-Caron G, Powell JR, Yaqoob P, Newsholme EA, Calder PC. *J Nutr.* 2001;131:1918-1927.

13 Ziboh VA, Fletcher MP. *Am J Clin Nutr.* 1992;55:39-45.

14 Belch JJF, Hill A. *Am J Clin Nutr.* 2000;71(suppl):352S-356S.

15 Rothman D, DeLuda P, Zurier RB. *Semin Arthritis Rheum.* 1995;25:87-96.

16 Little C, Parsons T. *Cochrane Database Syst Rev.* 2001;(1):CD002948.

17 Henz BM, Jablonska S, Van de Kerkhof PCM, et al. *Br J Dermatol.* 1999;140:685-688.

18 Kapoor R, Klimaszewski A. *Br J Dermatol.* 2000;143:200-201.

19 Henz BM. *Br J Dermatol.* 2000;143:201.

20 Gadek JE, DeMichele SJ, Karlstad MD, et al. *Crit Care Med.* 1999;27:1409-1420.

21 Kruger MC, Coetzer H, de Winter R, Gericke G, van Papendorp DH. *Aging (Milano).* 1998;10:385-394.

22 Horrobin DF. *Diabetes.* 1997;46:S90-S93.

23 Larson KM, Roby MR, Stermitz FR. *J Nat Prod.* 1984;47:747-748.

24 Dodson CD, Stermitz FR. *J Nat Prod.* 1986;49:727-728.

25 Langer T, Franz C. *Sci Pharm.* 1997;65:321-328.

26 Mierendorff HJ. *Fett Wiss Technol.* 1995;97:33-37.

SCIENTIFIC NAME(S): Bovine colostrum

COMMON NAME(S): Cow milk colostrum

❧❧❧ PATIENT INFORMATION ❧❧❧

Uses: Bovine colostrum has been used to treat diarrhea, to improve GI health, and to boost the immune system.

Side effects: Bovine colostrum appears to be safe and effective.

Dosing: Bovine colostrum is a difficult preparation to standardize because its antibody content may vary widely. Some clinical studies have been performed with hyperimmune colostrum, which may have a specific antibody titer; however, most products do not meet this criterion. Studies administering 25 to 125 mL of liquid formulations or 10 to 20 g of dry powder have been reported.[1-4]

SOURCE: Colostrum is the premilk fluid produced from mammary glands during the first 2 to 4 days after birth. It is a rich natural source of nutrients, antibodies, and growth factors for the newborn.[5]

PHARMACOLOGY: Bovine colostrum, with its rich pool of nutrients, has successfully supported and maintained a variety of cell cultures.[6-10] Various concentrations of bovine colostral constituents, including certain immunoglobulins, have been studied in calves fed colostrum or colostral supplement products.[11-15] Certain immune factors and antibodies also fight a variety of organisms, allergens, or toxins including pneumonia, candida, and flu. Constituent lactoferrin prevents pathogens from getting the iron they need to flourish. Lactalbumins and cytokines (interleukin 1 and 6, interferon γ) are also important as antivirals and anticancer agents.[16]

Several studies show how bovine colostrum concentrates, including G immunoglobulin isolates, are highly successful alternative agents used to improve GI health and to treat diarrhea caused by a variety of pathogens. In more than 50% of AIDS patients, diarrhea and subsequent weight loss pose a problem. The severity of symptoms in some cases and sometimes unidentifiable pathogens unaffected by antibiotics welcome alternative therapy with bovine colostrum.

In 1 study, 29 AIDS patients received a bovine colostrum preparation. The average stool per day decreased from 7.4 before therapy to 2.2 after treatment.[17] Another report finds similar results in animals, including high capacity for neutralization of bacterial toxins and high effectiveness in treating severe diarrhea, using a specialized colostrum preparation.[18] A 25-patient study of HIV subjects with chronic diarrhea administered bovine colostrum preparation also confirms therapeutic effectiveness, resulting in 64% of patients experiencing complete (40%) or partial (24%) remission of diarrhea.[19] *Cryptosporidium*, a human GI parasite, can also cause life-threatening diarrhea in immunodeficient patients when antibiotics or other antidiarrheals may be ineffective. Bovine colostrum therapy has reduced significantly oocyst excretion of pathogen in stools vs placebo and relieved a previously untreatable AIDS patient of severe *cryptosporidium*-associated diarrhea.[20,21] *Lactobin*, a registered bovine colostral product, shows antibody reactivity and neutralization against certain *E. coli* strains and shiga-like toxins.[22]

Immunoglobulin preparation supplementation was found to protect against *Shigellosis* (*S. flexneri*), and suggests its usefulness in high-risk groups including travelers and military personnel during *Shigella* outbreaks.[23] Bovine colostrum use against organisms *Yersinia enterocolitica* and *Campylobacter jejuni* has also been reported.[24] Bovine colostrum also inhibits *Helicobacter pylori* and *Helicobacter mustelae* by binding to certain lipid receptors, which may modulate the interaction of these pathogens to their target sites.[25] One report investigates the bovine colostral immunoglobulin proteins and how they are subject to degradation by gastric acid and intestinal enzymes under certain conditions.[26] Bovine colostrum supplementation, in another report, has been shown to prevent NSAID-induced gut injury in various in vivo and in vitro models, suggesting its possible usefulness for certain ulcerative bowel conditions.[5]

The immune-boosting properties of bovine colostrum have been greatly proclaimed as performance enhancers and anti-aging/healing supplements. Certain Web pages, for instance, promote significant fitness gains for athletes, noting its "anabolic effects" and claiming it can "promote muscle growth." [27] One clinical trial finds bovine colostrum supplement to increase serum IGF-1 concentration in athletes.[28] IGF-1 is a growth factor that speeds up protein synthesis and slows catabolism.[22]

TOXICOLOGY: A few symptoms, including mild nausea and flatulence, were seen in certain trials, but most have reported bovine colostrum to be well tolerated.[17-19] At least 2 allerginicity studies have been performed in humans.[29,30]

[1] Playford RJ, et al. *Clin Sci (Lond).* 2001;100:627-633.
[2] Antonio J, Sanders MS, Van Gammeren D. *Nutrition.* 2001;17:243-247.
[3] Sarker SA, Casswall TH, Mahalanabis D, et al. *Pediatr Infect Dis J.* 1998;17:1149-1154.
[4] Mero A, Miikkulainentti, Riski J, Pakkanen R, Aalto J, Tahala T. *J Appl Physiol.* 1997;83:1144-1151.
[5] Playford R, et al. *Gut.* 1999;44:653-658.
[6] Steimer KS, et al. *J Cell Biol.* 1981;88(2):294-300.
[7] Steimer KS, et al. *J Cell Physiol.* 1981;109(2):223-234.
[8] Tseng MT, et al. *Cell Tissue Kinet.* 1983;16(1):85–92.
[9] Pakkanen R, et al. *J Immunol Methods.* 1994;169(1):63-71.
[10] Viander B, et al. *Biotechniques.* 1996;20(4):702-707.
[11] Garry FP, et al. *J Am Vet Med Assoc.* 1996;208(1):107-110.
[12] Mee JF, et al. *J Dairy Sci.* 1996;79(5):886-894.
[13] Morin DE, et al. *J Dairy Sci.* 1997;80(4):747-753.
[14] Hopkins BA, et al. *J Dairy Sci.* 1997;80(5):979-983.
[15] Quigley J, III, et al. *J Dairy Sci.* 1998;81(7):1936-1939.
[16] Fauci A, et al. *Harrison's Principles of Internal Medicine.* 14th ed. New York, NY: McGraw Hill. 1998;1753,1760.
[17] Rump JA, et al. *Clin Investig.* 1992;70(7):588-594.
[18] Stephan W, et al. *J Clin Chem Clin Biochem.* 1990;28(1):19-23.
[19] Plettenberg A, et al. *Clin Investig.* 1993;71:42-45.
[20] Okhuysen P, et al. *Clin Infect Dis.* 1998;26:1324-1329.
[21] Ungar B, et al. *Gastrenterology.* 1990;98:486-489.
[22] Lissner R, et al. *Infection.* 1996;24(5):378-383.
[23] Tacket CO, et al. *Am J Trop Med Hyg.* 1992;47:3,276-283.
[24] Lissner R, et al. *Int J Clin Pharmacol Ther.* 1998;36(5):239-245.
[25] Bitzan M, et al. *J Infect Dis.* 1998;177:955-961.
[26] Petschow BW, et al. *J Pediatr Gastroenterol Nutr.* 1994;19:228-35.58.
[27] http://www.metafoods.com/athletic.htm.
[28] Mero A, et al. *J Appl Physiol.* 1997;83(4):1144-1151.
[29] Savilahti E, et al. *Acta Paediatr Scand.* 1991;80(12):1207-1213.
[30] Lefranc- Millot C, et al. *Int Arch Allergy Immunol.* 1996;110(21):56-62.

Brahmi

SCIENTIFIC NAME(S): *Bacopa monnieri* (L.) Wettst. family: Scrophulariaceae (figworts); also known as *Bacopa monniera, Herpestis monniera,* or *Moniera cuneifolia*

COMMON NAME(S): Brahmi, Jalnaveri, Jalanimba, Sambrani chettu, thyme-leaved gratiola

---

✿✿✿ PATIENT INFORMATION ✿✿✿

Uses: Brahmi is used as a nerve tonic and an aid to learning.

Side Effects: Brahmi has no reported side effects.

Drug Interactions: Use caution when coadministering with phenothiazine.

Dosing: A single clinical trial of brahmi's effects on cognition reported a daily dose of 300 mg of extract.[1]

BOTANY: *Bacopa monnieri* is a creeping herb that grows in marshy places and is frequently planted in freshwater aquaria. It is native to India but has spread throughout the tropics. The name brahmi has also been applied to *Centella asiatica* (better known as *gotu kola*), as well as *Merremia gangetica*; however, most authorities consider it most appropriate for *B. monnieri*.[2] A tissue culture method has been developed for the plant.[3]

HISTORY: Brahmi is a well-known drug in the Ayurvedic medical tradition in India, and is used in many Ayurvedic herbal preparations. It has been traditionally used to treat asthma, hoarseness, insanity, epilepsy, and as a nerve tonic, cardiotonic, and diuretic.[2] It was prominently mentioned in Indian texts as early as the 6th century AD.[4]

PHARMACOLOGY: In mice, the ethanolic extract of *B. monnieri* was found to increase cerebral levels of GABA 15 minutes after administration.[5] Oral treatment of rats with the extract of *B. monnieri* for 24 days facilitated their ability to learn mazes.[6] A saponin fraction of *B. monnieri* reduced spontaneous motor activity in rats, and lowered rectal temperatures in mice.[7] The same extract showed tranquilizing effects in rats but did not block the conditioned avoidance response. It also protected against audiogenic seizures.[8] More recently, the extract was found to improve the performance of rats in various behavioral models of learning.[4] Furthermore, the purified bacosides A and B showed dose-dependent effects in the same rat models, as well as in a taste aversion response test.[9] Bacosine, a free triterpene isolated from the aerial parts of *B. monnieri*, was found to have analgesic effects operating through opioidergic pathways.[10] The ethanolic extract of *B. monnieri* relaxed smooth muscle preparations of guinea pig and rabbit pulmonary arteries, rabbit aorta, and guinea pig trachea by a mechanism that was postulated to involve prostacyclins.[11] The same investigators found spasmolytic effects of the ethanol extract in guinea pig ileum and rabbit jejuenum to be nonspecifically mediated through calcium channels.[12] The saponins were found to have anthelmintic activity using *C. elegans* as a test organism.[13] They are also reported to be hemolytic.[14]

TOXICOLOGY: Brahmi appears to be free of reported side effects. Its CNS actions do not include serious sedation, although the potentiation of chlorpromazine's effect on conditioned avoidance responses may indicate caution with phenothiazine coadministration.[8]

[1] Stough C, Lloyd J, Clarke J, et al. *Psychopharmacology (Berl)*. 2001;156:481-484.

[2] *The Wealth of India: A Dictionary of Indian Raw Materials and Industrial Products*. Vol 2:B. Delhi: Council of Scientific and Industrial Research; 1948;2-3.

[3] Tiwari V, et al. *Plant Cell Rep*. 1998;17:538.

[4] Singh H, et al. *J Ethnopharmacol*. 1982;5:205.

[5] Dey P, et al. *Indian J Exp Biol*. 1966;4:216.

[6] Dey C, et al. *Indian J Physiol Allied Sci*. 1976;30:88

[7] Ganguly D, et al. *Indian J Physiol Pharmacol*. 1967;11:33.

[8] Ganguly D, et al. *Indian J Med Res*. 1967;55:473.

[9] Singh H, et al. *Phytother Res*. 1988;2:70.

[10] Vohora S, et al. *Fitoterapia*. 1997;68:361.

[11] Dar A, et al. *Phytother Res*. 1997;11:323.

[12] Dar A, et al. *J Ethnopharmacol*. 1999;66:167.

[13] Renukappa T, et al. *J Chromatogr A*. 1999;847:109.

[14] Basu N, et al. *Indian J Chem*. 1967;5:84.

Bupleurum

SCIENTIFIC NAME(S): *Bupleurum chinense* DC., related species include *B. falcatum* L., *B. scorzoneraefolium*, *B. fruticosum* L., *B. ginghausenii*, *B. rotundifolium* L., *B. stewartianum*. Family: Umbelliferae[1]

COMMON NAME(S): Thoroughwax, hare's ear root, chai hu (Chinese)

ঌ৵৶ PATIENT INFORMATION ঌ৵৶

Uses: Bupleurum has been found beneficial as a liver protectant and possesses positive effects on the immune system, including treatment for cold and flu, inflammatory disorders, and certain cancers. It is also useful in gastrointestinal ailments, certain brain disorders, and for gynecological problems.

Side Effects: Bupleurum has caused sedative effects in some patients, along with increased flatulence and bowel movements in large doses. Some combinations with bupleurum may have certain undesirable effects such as induction of pneumonitis, or nausea and reflux in sensitive patients.

Dosing: Dosage of bupleurum root is 1.5 to 6 g/day; however, no clinical trials have been performed to validate this range as safe and effective.

BOTANY: Bupleurum is a perennial herb that grows mainly in China, but also is cultivated in other areas. The plant grows to approximately 1 m in height and requires plenty of sun to flourish. The leaves are long and sickle-shaped with parallel veining. Terminal clusters of small, yellow flowers appear in autumn.[2,3]

HISTORY: Bupleurum is a traditional Chinese herb dating back to the first century BC. It is one of China's "harmony" herbs purported to effect organs and energy in the body. Bupleurum has been used as a liver tonic, with spleen and stomach toning properties as well. The plant has also been said to clear fevers and flu, promote perspiration, and alleviate female problems.[1-3]

PHARMACOLOGY: Bupleurum's traditional role as a liver tonic has been substantiated by research. The saikosides are known liver protectants, and bupleurum has been found to be beneficial in both acute and chronic liver disease.[2,4] Doses of saikosaponins demonstrate marked hepatoprotective activity in several animal models.[5-8] IV injection of bupleurum provided beneficial therapeutic outcomes in 100 cases of infectious hepatitis in adults and children.[9]

Bupleurum's effects on the immune system have been widely reported. Traditional use of the plant for acute infection, cold with chills and fever, headache, vomiting, and malaria treatment have been discussed.[3,4] Bupleurum was also found to possess antitussive effects.[10] The saikosides stimulate corticosteroid production, thus increasing the anti-inflammatory effects.[2] Bupleurum inactivated enveloped viruses including measles and herpes, but had no effect on naked viruses such as polio.[11] Bupleurum demonstrated cytotoxic effects in certain human cell lines in vitro.[4] Mitogenic activity has been shown from certain extracts of the plant.[12] Other immune problems may benefit from bupleurum including SLE, inflammatory disorders, and autoimmune disease.[4]

Improvement in certain GI conditions has also been seen with bupleurum. Constituents bupleurans and saikosaponins have been shown to decrease gastric ulcer development.[4]

A Chinese medicinal treatment including *B. chinense* was found to be comparable to methylphenidate (eg, *Ritalin*) in a 100-patient study of children 7 to 14 years of age with minimal brain dysfunction (MBD). The group that was administered the Chinese combination had far fewer side effects, as well as more improvement in parameters such as intelligence or enuresis than the methylphenidate group.[13]

Bupleurum is often used as part of the popular Japanese herbal remedy Sho-saiko-to (Tj-9, Xino-chai-hu-tang), which is used extensively for the treatment of various liver diseases. In one study, this product was found to reduce the incidence of hepatocellular carcinoma in patients.[14]

Other ailments for which bupleurum is used include irregular menstruation, PMS, hot flashes, prolapsed uterus,[1,3] kidney problems (protectant), high cholesterol (saponins decrease cholesterol by increasing excretion in bile),[4] and hemorrhoids.[2]

TOXICOLOGY: Bupleurum has produced sedative effects in some patients, along with increased flatulence and bowel movements in large doses. Some combinations with bupleurum may have certain undesirable effects such as induction of pneumonitis, or nausea and reflux in sensitive patients. Some reports are unclear as to whether or not the ill effects are due specifically to bupleurum.[4]

[1] Hocking, G. *A Dictionary of Natural Products.* Plexus Publ. Inc.: Medford NJ, 1997;132-133.

[2] Chevallier, A. *Encyclopedia of Medicinal Plants.* DK Publishing: New York, NY, 1996;68.

[3] *A Barefoot Doctor's Manual.* (American translation of official Chinese paramedical manual). Running Press: Philadelphia, PA, 1977;848.

[4] Bone, K. *Can J Herbalism.* 1996;22-25,41.

[5] Chiu H, et al. *Am J Chin Med.* 1988;16(3-4):127-137.

[6] Lin C, et al. *Am J Chin Med.* 1990;18(3-4):105-112.

[7] Lin C, et al. *Am J Chin Med.* 1990;18(3-4):113-120.

[8] Yen M, et al. *J Ethnopharmacol.* 1991;34(2-3):155-165.

[9] Chang H, et al. *Pharmacology and Applications of Chinese Materia Medica.* World Scientific: Singapore, 1987.

[10] Takagi K, et al. *Yakugaku Zasshi.* 1969;89(5):712-720.

[11] Ushio Y, et al. *Planta Med.* 1992;58(2):171-173.

[12] Ohtsu S, et al. *Biol Pharm Bull.* 1997;20(1):97-100.

[13] Zhang H, et al. *Chung Hsi I Chieh Ho Tsa Chih.* 1990;10(5):278-279, 260.

[14] Oka H, et al. *Cancer.* 1995;76(5):743-749.

Butterbur

SCIENTIFIC NAME(S): *Petasites hybridus* (L.) Gaertner, Meyer & Scherb. Family: *Asteraceae* (daisies)

COMMON NAME(S): Butterbur, pestwurz (German), pestilence-wort, blatterdock, bog rhubarb, butter-dock, bogshorns, butterfly dock, exwort

❧❧❧❧ PATIENT INFORMATION ❧❧❧❧

Uses: Butterbur extract has shown activity against hayfever, migraines, and other types of pain in 2 small studies.

Side Effects: Pyrrolizidine alkaloids are known liver toxins. Dosage forms must be certified as free of hepatotoxic pyrrolizidine alkaloids.

Dosing: Butterbur cannot be recommended for human use because of the presence of hepatotoxic pyrrolizidine alkaloids. An extract was used in a clinical trial for migraine at 100 mg/day; however, unless a product is demonstrated to be free of alkaloids, its use would be contraindicated.[1]

BOTANY: Butterbur is a perennial shrub native to Europe that has very large, downy leaves. It commonly grows in wet, marshy ground or on sandbars of streams. The distinctive pink-lilac flowers grow on large spikes, and appear before the leaves in spring. The related species *P. albus* is also native to Europe and has been used medicinally. The Japanese species *P. japonicus* is used as a rhubarb-like vegetable and in medicine.

HISTORY: The generic name *Petasites* is derived from the Greek word *petasus*, a type of broad-brimmed hat worn by shepherds, referring to the broad, downy leaves. The name butterbur relates to the use of the leaves to wrap butter. During the Middle Ages, butterbur leaves and roots were used to treat plague (hence *pestwurz*) and fevers. Other traditional uses include the treatment of cough, asthma, and gastric ulcer.[2]

PHARMACOLOGY: Petasin was initially isolated as the antispasmodic constituent of butterbur.[3] The iso- series of compounds was less potent than the parent compounds. Since the iso- series is thermodynamically more stable, rearrangement during storage would lead to lower potency.[4] The mechanism of action was described as nonspecific;[5] however, later studies by the same group found that S-petasin blocked calcium channels in vascular smooth muscle cells.[6]

Further investigation of mechanism found inhibition of peptido-leukotriene synthesis in macrophages (a calcium-dependent process) without an effect on prostaglandins.[7] Isopetasin and 3 oxopetasan esters were found to be responsible for this effect, while petasin was inactive as a peptido-leukotriene synthesis inhibitor.[8] On the contrary, anti-inflammatory assays in primed human eosinophils and neutrophils found that petasin was able to block early events leading to leukotriene generation.[9]

Two randomized double-blind clinical trials have demonstrated efficacy for butterbur extracts. In the first, a super-critical fluid (SCF) carbon dioxide extract of butterbur was found to have equal efficacy against seasonal allergic rhinitis (hayfever) compared with the antihistamine cetirizine, with butterbur displaying no sedative side effects.[10] The extract was standardized to 8 mg of petasin per tablet. A second trial, also with an SCF extract, found butterbur to be superior to placebo in migraine prophylaxis over a 12-week period.[11]

TOXICOLOGY: Pyrrolizidine alkaloids are known liver toxins, and the *German Commission E* set upper limits of pyrrolizidine dosage to a maximum of 1 mcg/day. Because butterbur roots normally contain as much as 100 mcg/ g, while leaves contain considerably less,[12,13] using the leaves is one method for reducing toxicity. The use of SCF extraction to produce extracts with little or no pyrrolizidine content is another promising possibility.

[1] Grossman W, Schmidramsl H. *Altern Med Rev.* 2001;6:303-310.

[2] Monograph. *Petasites hybridus. Altern Med Rev.* 2001;6:207-209.

[3] Aebi A, Waaler T, Büchi J. *Pharm Weekbl.* 1958;93:397-406.

[4] Debrunner B, Neuenschwander M. *Pharm Acta Helv.* 1995;70:315-323.

[5] Ko WC, Lei CB, Lin YL, Chen CF. *Planta Med.* 2001;67:224-229.

[6] Wang GJ, Shum AY, Lin YL, et al. *J Pharmacol Exp Ther.* 2001;297:240-246.

[7] Brune K, Bickel D, Peskar BA. *Planta Med.* 1993;59:494-496.

[8] Bickel D, Röder T, Bestmann HJ, Brune K. *Planta Med.* 1994;60:318-322.

[9] Thomet OA, Wiesmann UN, Schapowal A, Bizer C, Simon H. *Biochem Pharmacol.* 2001;61:1041-1047.

[10] Schapowal A. *BMJ.* 2002;324:144-146.

[11] Grossmann M, Schmidramsl H. *Int J Clin Pharmacol Ther.* 2000;38:430-435.

[12] Langer T, Möstl E, Chizzola R, Gutleb R. *Planta Med.* 1996;62:267-271.

[13] Wildi E, Langer T, Schaffner W, Büter KB. *Planta Med.* 1998;64:264-267.

Calendula

SCIENTIFIC NAME(S): *Calendula officinalis* L. Family: Compositae

COMMON NAME(S): Calendula, garden marigold, gold bloom, holligold, marygold, pot marigold, marybud[1]

ᴥᴥᴥ PATIENT INFORMATION ᴥᴥᴥ

Uses: Calendula has been used topically in folk medicine to treat wounds and internally to reduce fever, treat cancer, and control dysmenorrhea. Extracts have proved antibacterial, antiviral, and immunostimulating in vitro. Petals are consumed as a seasoning. The plant has been used to repel insects.

Side Effects: Allergic reactions to the botanical family and one case of anaphylaxis have been reported.

Dosing: One to 4 g of herb has been used to make a tea for sore throat and peptic ulcer; however, clinical trials have not validated this dose. An ointment containing 2% to 5% flower extract is used for topical wound healing.[2]

BOTANY: Believed to have originated in Egypt, this plant has almost world-wide distribution. There are numerous varieties of this species, each one varying primarily in flower shape and color. Calendula grows to about 60 cm in height, and the wild form has small, bright yellow-orange flowers that bloom from May to October. It is the ligulate florets, mistakenly called the flower petals, that have been used medicinally. This plant should not be confused with several other members of the family that also carry the "marigold" name.

HISTORY: The plant has been grown in European gardens since the 12th century and its folkloric uses are almost as old. Tinctures and extracts of the florets had been used topically to promote wound healing and reduce inflammation. Systemically, they have been used to reduce fever, control dysmenorrhea, and treat cancer. The dried petals have been used like saffron as a seasoning and to adulterate saffron.[3]

The pungent odor of the marigold has been used as an effective pesticide. Marigolds are often interspersed among vegetable plants to repel insects.[4]

PHARMACOLOGY: Despite the historical use of calendula and the detailed studies of its chemistry, there are almost no studies regarding its efficacy in the treatment of human disorders.

Calendula extracts have been used topically to promote wound healing, and experiments in rats have shown this effect is measurable. An ointment containing 5% flower extract in combination with allantoin was found to "markedly stimulate" epithelialization in surgically induced wounds. On the basis of histological examination of the wound tissue, it was concluded that the ointment increased glycoprotein, nucleoprotein, and collagen metabolism at the site.[5]

Russian investigators found that sterile preparations of calendula extracts alleviated signs of chronic conjunctivitis and ocular inflammatory conditions in rats.[6] The extracts also had a systemic anti-inflammatory effect. Other Russian investigators have used plant extract mixtures containing calendula for the treatment of chronic hyposecretory gastritis.

Calendula extracts have in vitro antibacterial, antiviral,[7,8] and immunostimulating properties.[9] Published reports of small clinical trials conducted in Poland

and Bulgaria suggest that extracts of the plant may be useful in the management of duodenal ulcers, gastroduodenitis, and gum disease.

TOXICOLOGY: Despite its widespread use, there have been no reports in the Western literature describing serious reactions to the use of calendula preparations. A report of anaphylactic shock in a patient who gargled with a calendula infusion has been reported in Russia.

Allergies to members of the family Compositae (chamomile, feverfew, dandelion) have been attributed to the pollens of these plants. There is a potential for allergic reactions with calendula use.

In animals, doses of up to 50 mg/kg of extract had essentially no pharmacologic effect and induced no histopathologic changes following either acute or chronic administration.[10] Saponin extracts of calendula showed antimutagenic activity.[11]

[1] Meyer JE. *The Herbalist*. Hammond, IN: Hammond Book Co, 1934.

[2] Gruenwald J, ed. *PDR for Herbal Medicines*. 2nd ed. Montvale, NJ: Thomson Medical Economics; 2000: 497-498.

[3] Duke JA. *Handbook of Medicinal Herbs*. Boca Raton, FL: CRC Press, 1985.

[4] Lewis WH, et al. *Medical Botany: Plants Affecting Man's Health*. New York: John Wiley & Sons, 1977.

[5] Klouchek-Popava E, et al. *Acta Physiol Pharmacol Bulg*. 1982;8:63.

[6] Marinchev VN, et al. *Oftalmol Zh*. 1971;26:196.

[7] Dumenil G, et al. *Ann Pharm Fr*. 1980;38:493.

[8] De Tommasi N, et al. *J Nat Prod*. 1990;53(4):830.

[9] Wagner H, et al. *Arzneimittelforschung*. 1985;35:1069.

[10] Iatsyno AI, et al. *Farmakol Toksikol*. 1978;41:556.

[11] Elias R, et al. *Mutagenesis*. 1990;5(4):327.

SCIENTIFIC NAME(S): *Capsicum frutescens* L., *Capsicum annuum* L., and a large number of hybrids and varieties of the species. Family: Solanaceae

COMMON NAME(S): *C. frutescens*: capsicum, cayenne pepper, red pepper, African chilies, green pepper; *C. annuum*, var. *conoides*: tabasco pepper, paprika, pimiento, Mexican chilies; *C. annuum*, var. *longum*: Louisiana long pepper or hybridized to the Louisiana sport pepper.

ᶺᵎᵃᵃᵃ PATIENT INFORMATION ᶺᵎᵃᵃᵃ

Uses: Many varieties are eaten as vegetables and spices. The component capsaicin is an irritant and analgesic, used in self-defense sprays, and in pain treatments for postsurgical neuralgia, shingles, osteoarthritis, rheumatoid arthritis, and others.

Interactions: When given to rats, capsaicin caused impaired elimination of antipyrene but had no effects on the pharmacokinetics of theophylline or quinine. Human studies are necessary to investigate whether capsaicin interferes with the cytochrome P450 hepatic drug metabolizing enzymes.

Side Effects: Topical, mucosal, and GI irritations are common. Allergies to latex, bananas, kiwi, chestnut, avocado, or having "mugwort-celery-spice-syndrome" may predispose people to capsicum (pepper) allergy.

Dosing: For internal use, a typical dose of cayenne powder is 30 to 120 mg as a digestive aid. The pungency of hot peppers can vary widely, influencing the dose required, and much higher doses (1 to 20 g) occasionally have been recommended;[1,2] however, high doses of pungent peppers may induce gastritis. For external uses, capsaicin and capsicum creams are available in several strengths, from 0.025% to 0.075% capsaicin.[3]

BOTANY: *C. frutescens* is a small spreading annual shrub that is indigenous to tropical America. It yields an oblong, pungent fruit, while *C. annuum* (the common green pepper) yields paprika. At one time, it was believed that all peppers derived from *C. frutescens*, *C. annuum*, or their hybrids. However, it is now recognized that approximately 5 species and their hybrids contribute as sources of "peppers."[4] Capsicum peppers should not be confused with the black and white pepper spices derived from the unripened fruit of *Piper nigrum*.

HISTORY: Capsicum was first described in the mid-1400s by a physician who accompanied Columbus to the West Indies. The plants derive their names from the Latin *capsa*, meaning box, referring to the partially hollow, box-like fruit. Capsicum has been highly desired as a spice and has been cultivated in some form in almost every society. Peppers are among the most widely consumed spices in the world, with an average daily per capita consumption in some Southeast Asian countries approaching 5 g of red pepper (approximately 50 mg of capsaicin).[5] Preparations of capsicum have been used as topical rubefacients, and extracts have been ingested as a stomachic, carminative, and GI stimulant.

PHARMACOLOGY:

Irritant: Capsicum is a powerful irritant because of the effect of the oleoresin and capsaicin. Solutions of capsaicin applied topically can produce sensations varying from warmth to burning, depending on the concentration; with repeated applications, an apparent desensitization to the burning occurs. This effect has been studied in detail and has resulted in the elucidation of capsaicin's mechanism of action.

In 1 study, 4 applications of a 0.1% solution of capsaicin were applied topically to the skin of healthy subjects and compared with untreated skin. Histamine was injected intradermally at the application site to test for chemical responsiveness. As expected, injection at the untreated area evoked a wheal, flare, and itching. The capsaicin-treated areas developed a wheal but no flare. The flare response, also called axon reflex vasodilation, is believed to be mediated by the release of the vasoactive compound, substance P. This compound is involved in the transmission of painful stimuli from the periphery to the spinal cord. Following an initial application, substance P is released, causing the sensation of pain. However, upon repeated administration, the compound is depleted and a lack of pain sensation ensues. This effect usually occurs within 3 days of regular application. Pretreatment with capsaicin also abolishes airway edema and bronchoconstriction induced by cigarette smoke and other irritants.[6]

Pain treatment: Capsaicin has become a valuable "pharmacologic probe" for studying the reception and transmission of painful or injurious stimuli. Because capsaicin-evoked mechanical allodynia and hyperalgesia cross nerve territories, organic and psychogenic mechanisms must be considered in the differential diagnosis of chronic pain.[7] The use of capsaicin ointments for the treatment of pain caused by herpes zoster (shingles) has been of more practical importance. In patients affected with shingles, often excruciating pain may persist around the infected nerve tracts for months to years after the initial flare. Zostrix cream (Bioglan Pharma, Inc.), containing ei-

ther 0.025% or 0.075% capsaicin, has been found to be effective when applied topically in the management of postherpetic neuralgia.[8,9] It also has been found to be effective in the management of trigeminal and diabetic neuralgia, causalgia, postmastectomy, postsurgical neuralgias, rheumatoid arthritis, and osteoarthritis. A preliminary study using high-dose (5% to 10%) topical capsaicin brought relief to patients with intractable pain, thus warranting further investigation.[10]

Pruritus: Topical capsaicin has been shown to effectively treat pruritus associated with psoriasis,[11,12] pityriasis rubra pilaris,[13] PUVA (photochemotherapy with psoralen),[14] and prurigo nodularis.[15]

Densitization of nasal nerves: The inhalation of a capsaicin solution can desensitize nasal nerves that cause runny nose, sneezing, and congestion. In a small study at Johns Hopkins Asthma & Allergy Center, such symptoms were alleviated in 8 volunteers who received repeated nasal sprays of capsaicin.[16] In a placebo-controlled study, intranasal capsaicin was shown to be effective in reducing nasal symptomatology in nonallergic, noninfectious perennial rhinitis without affecting cellular homeostasis up to 9 months after treatment.[17,18]

Tonsillitis/Cough: In Germany, *C. annuum* in a fixed combination with *Guajacum officinale* and *Phytolacca americana* has been successfully used to treat tonsillitis;[19,20] and used along with other homeopathic remedies to treat otitis media in children.[21]

Cough response to capsaicin (concentration that caused 5 coughs) has been used to assess the cough susceptibility in a wide range of diseases.[22]

Decreased bladder pain/Hyperreflexia: Intravesical capsaicin has decreased frequency and nocturia of patients with severe bladder pain.[23] Repeated instillations of intravesical capsaicin were shown to be effective for 3 to 5 years in treating detrusor hyperreflexia because of spinal cord disease.[24] Intraureteric capsaicin instillation was shown to provide dramatic symptomatic relief in some patients with loin pain hematuria syndrome.[25]

Birdseed use: Capsaicin has been used in birdseed to discourage squirrels, as birds do not have capsaicin receptors, while squirrels do.

INTERACTIONS: Studies in humans are necessary to investigate whether capsaicin interferes with the cytochrome P450 hepatic drug metabolizing enzymes.

TOXICOLOGY: The most well-known adverse effect of peppers is the often intolerable burning sensation that occurs following contact with moist mucous membranes. For this reason, it is a common component of many self-defense sprays. When sprayed into an attacker's eyes, it causes immediate blindness and irritation for up to 30 minutes, with no permanent damage. If mucous membranes come in contact with capsicum, they should be flushed with water. Anecdotal reports suggest that flushing the area with milk may be beneficial.

Topical irritation is common, particularly with the use of commercial creams. One clinical study in patients with postherpetic lesions was terminated early because approximately one-third of the patients experienced "unbearable" burning.[26]

The intense GI burning that often accompanies the ingestion of peppers may be reduced by removing the seeds from the pepper pods before ingestion[27] or by ingesting bananas along with the peppers.[28] One study found no difference in the healing rate of duodenal ulcers among patients who ingested 3 g of capsicum daily compared with untreated controls,[29] and another study found that chili protects against aspirin-induced gastroduodenal mucosal injury,[1] disproving a commonly held idea that peppers always exacerbate GI problems. Low-dose capsaicin may stimulate the swallowing reflex and prevent aspiration pneumonia in elderly patients with swallowing disorders.[30] Capsaicin has been referred to as a "double-edged sword" because it enhances postprandial heartburn; however, capsaicin decreases gastric liquid emptying, which could provide mucosal protection.[31]

Allergic reaction to paprika has been seen in patients with "mugwort-celery-spice-syndrome."[32] These patients exhibit allergy to mugwort, birch-pollen, celery, anise, coriander, cumin, fennel, and green and black peppercorns, along with fresh bell peppers and dried bell-pepper fruits (paprika).[32]

Patients sensitive to latex, banana, kiwi, chestnut, and avocado can also exhibit sensitization to peppers.[33]

"Hunan hand" is a contact dermatitis resulting from the direct handling of capsaicin found in chili peppers.[34] Controversy exists regarding capsaicin's mutagenicity and tumorigenicity.[35,36]

A review of the literature, including a study that showed lack of tumor promoting activity in mouse skin, concluded that capsaicin is a carcinogen, cocarcinogen, and anticarcinogen.[35,36]

[1] Yeoh KG, Kang JY, Yap I, et al. *Dig Dis Sci.* 1995;40:580-583.

[2] Lim K, Yoshioka M, Kikuzato S, et al. *Med Sci Sports Exerc.* 1997;29:355-361.

3 Altman RD, et al. *Sem Arthritis Rheumatism.* 1994;23(6 suppl 3):25-33.

4 Leung AY. *Encyclopedia of Common Natural Ingredients Used in Food, Drugs and Cosmetics.* New York, NY: John Wiley and Sons, 1980.

5 Buck SH, et al. *Tips.* 1983;4:84.

6 Hot peppers and substance P [editorial]. *Lancet.* 1983;B335:1198.

7 Sang CN, et al. *Anesthesiology.* 1996;85:491-496.

8 Bernstein JE, et al. *J Am Acad Dermatol.* 1987;17:93-96.

9 Hebel S, Burnham T, eds. *Drug Facts and Comparisons.* St. Louis, MO: Facts and Comparisons, Jul 1992:632.

10 Robbins WR, et al. *Anesth Analg.* 1998;86(3):579-583.

11 Ellis CN, et al. *J Am Acad Dermatol.* 1993;29:438-442.

12 Krogstad AL, et al. *Br J Dermatol.* 1999;141:87-93.

13 Neess CM, et al. *Clin Exp Dermatol.* 2000;25:209-11.

14 Kirby B, et al. *Br J Dermatol.* 1997;137:152.

15 Stander S, et al. *J Am Acad Dermatol.* 2001;44:471-478.

16 Snider M. *USA Today.* March 18, 1992:A1.

17 Blom HM, et al. *Clin Exp Allergy.* 1997;27:796-801.

18 Blom HM, et al. *Clin Exp Allergy.* 1998;28:1351-1358.

19 Wiesenauer M. *Adv Ther.* 1998;15:362-371.

20 Rau E. *Adv Ther.*2000;17:197-203.

21 Friese KH, et al. *Int J Clin Pharmacol Ther.* 1997;35:296-301.

22 Doherty MJ, et al. *Thorax.* 2000;55:643-649.

23 Lazzeri M, et al. *J Urol.* 1996;156:947-952.

24 De Ridder D, et al. *J Urol.* 1997;158:2087-2092.

25 Armstrong T, et al. *BJU Int.* 2000;85:233-237.

26 GenDerm capsaicin for shingles pain relief. *F-D-C Reports.* Feb 27, 1989.

27 Prevost, RJ. *Lancet.* 1982;8277(1):917.

28 Roberts RM. *Lancet.* 1982;8270:519.

29 Kumar N, et al. *BMJ.* 1984;288:1803-1804.

30 Ebihara T, et al. *Lancet.* 1993;341:432.

31 Rodriguez-Stanley S, et al. *Aliment Pharmacol Ther.* 2000;14:129-134.

32 Ebner C, et al. *Allergy.* 1998;53(46 Suppl):52-54.

33 Gallo R, et al. *Contact Dermatitis.* 1997;37:36-37.

34 Williams SR, et al. *Ann Emerg Med.* 1995;25:713-715.

35 Park KK, et al. *Anticancer Res.* 1998;18:4201-4205.

36 Surh YJ, et al. *Food Chem Toxicol.* 1996;34:313-316.

SCIENTIFIC NAME(S): *Uncaria tomentosa* (Willd.) DC and *Uncaria guianensis* (Aubl.) Gmel. Family: Rubiaceae

COMMON NAME(S): Cat's claw, life-giving vine of Peru, samento, uña de gato

---

⠆⠆⠆⠆ PATIENT INFORMATION ⠆⠆⠆⠆

Uses: Various species have been used as an astringent, anti-inflammatory, contraceptive, for gastric ulcers, rheumatism, cancer treatment, and as a general tonic. Studies have verified some anticancer and immunostimulant properties. The major alkaloid is hypotensive.

Side Effects: Data suggest little hazard in ingestion.

Dosing: One gram of root bark given 2 to 3 times is a typical dose, while 20 to 30 mg of a root bark extract has been recommended. A standardized extract based on a particular chemotype of this species (C-Med-100, *Krallendorn*, Immodal Pharmaka GmbH) containing 8% to 10% carboxy alkyl esters, and less than 0.5% oxindole alkaloids has been used for clinical trials as an immunostimulant at doses from 250 to 300 mg.[1,2]

BOTANY: Cat's claw, or uña de gato (Spanish), is a tropical vine of the madder family (Rubiaceae). The name describes the small curved-back spines on the stem at the leaf juncture. The genus *Uncaria* is found throughout the tropics, mainly in Southeast Asia, the Asian continent, and South America. The two species of current interest, *Uncaria tomentosa* (Willd.) DC and *Uncaria guianensis* (Aubl.) (Gmel.), are found in South America. These species are lianas or high-climbing, twining, woody vines.[3,4] Both species are known in Peru as uña de gato.

There are 34 reported species of *Uncaria*. One Asian species, known as gambir or pole catechu (*Uncaria gambir* [Hunter] Roxb.), is a widely used tanning agent which has long medicinal use as an astringent and antidiarrheal.[5]

HISTORY: *U. guianensis* has long folkloric use in South America as a wound healer and for treating intestinal ailments.[4] Large amounts of *U. guianensis* are collected in South America for the European market, while American sources prefer *U. tomentosa*.[3]

The bark decoction of *U. guianensis* is used in Peru as an anti-inflammatory, antirheumatic, and contraceptive, as well as in treating gastric ulcers and tumors, gonorrhea (by the Bora tribe), dysentery (by the Indian groups of Colombia and Guiana), and cancers of the urinary tract in women.[4]

The Ashanica Indians believe that samento (also *U. tomentosa*) has "life-giving" properties, and use a cup of the decoction each week or two to ward off disease, treat bone pains, and cleanse the kidneys.[6] Recent interest in uña de gato stems from a reference to the plant in a popular book, *Witch Doctor's Apprentice, Hunting for Medicinal Plants in the Amazonian.*[7]

Reviews and scientific studies by the National Cancer Institute in the last decade have led to verification of some of the anticancer and immunostimulant properties.[4] Some of the demand for the bark has been attributed to European reports on its clinical use with AZT in AIDS treatment. The demand for the bark in the US is based on the purported usefulness of its tea in treating diverticulitis, hemorrhoids, peptic ulcers, colitis, gastritis, parasites, and leaky bowel syndrome.[6]

PHARMACOLOGY: Both species, *U. tomentosa* and *U. guianensis*, have been used folklorically in the form of a bark decoction for a wide range of disorders, including gastric ulcers, inflammation, rheumatism, tumors, and as a contraceptive. Specifically, *U. guianensis* has been employed to treat dysentery, gonorrhea, and cancer of the urinary tract in women.[3]

Recent reports have demonstrated *Uncaria*'s role in improving immunity in cancer patients,[6] as well as its antimutagenic properties.[8] All the individual alkaloids of *U. tomentosa*, with the exception of hynchophylline and mitraphyllin, have immunostimulant properties[9] and the ability to enhance phagocytosis in vitro. Other researchers have shown pteropodine and isopteropodine to have immune-stimulating effects.[6]

The major alkaloid rhynchophylline has been shown to be antihypertensive, to relax the blood vessels of endothelial cells, dilate peripheral blood vessels, inhibit sympathetic nervous system activities, lower the heart rate, and lower blood cholesterol.[6,10] The alkaloid mytraphylline has diuretic properties,[6] while the alkaloid hirsutine inhibits urinary bladder contractions and possesses local anesthetic properties.[6,11] At higher dosages, hirsutine showed a "curarelike" ability on neuromuscular transmission.[6,12] The Oriental crude drug "chotoko" (the dried climbing hooks of *Uncaria* species) has hypotensive properties.[13] Six quinovic acid glycosides in *U. tomentosa* have antiviral activity *in vitro*.[14,15] The alkaloid gambirine isolated from *U. callophylla* has cardiovascular properties.[16]

TOXICOLOGY: Plant extracts and fractions of *U. tomentosa* exhibit no mutagenic effects, but show a protective antimutagenic property in vitro and decreased the mutagenicity in a smoker who had ingested a decoction of the plant for 15 days.[8] While there is little published data on the toxicology of uña de gato, there is an international patent (1982) and a German dissertation (1984) which indicate low toxicity for this material.[6] The scattered pharmacological studies also seem to indicate little hazard in ingesting the plant decoction.

[1] Lehmann-Willenbrock E, Riedel HH. *Zentralbl Gynakol.* 1988;110:611-618.

[2] Sheng Y, Li L, Holmgren K, Pero RW. *Phytomedicine.* 2001;8:275-282.

[3] Duke J, et al. *Amazonian Ethobotanical Dictionary.* Boca Raton, FL: CRC Press, 1994.

[4] Foster S. *Health Food Bus.* 1995(Jun);24.

[5] Duke JA. *Handbook of Medicinal Herbs.* Boca Raton, FL: CRC Press, 1985.

[6] Jones K. *Am Herb Assoc.* 1994;10(3):4.

[7] Maxwell, N. *Witch Doctor's Apprentice, Hunting for Medicinal Plants in the Amazonian.* 3rd ed. New York: Citadel Press, 1990.

[8] Wagner H, et al. *Planta Med.* 1985:419.

[9] Hemingway SR, et al. *J Pharm Pharmacol.* 1974;26(Suppl):113P.

[10] Harada M, et al. *Chem Pharm Bull.* 1979;27(5):1069.

[11] *Peruvian Cat's Claw: A Gift from Nature.* Gilroy, CA: Bour-Man Medical.

[12] Harada M, Ozaki Y. *Chem Pharm Bull.* 1976;24(2):211.

[13] Endo K, et al. *Planta Med.* 1983;49:188.

[14] Aquino R, et al. *J Nat Prod.* 1989;52(4):679.

[15] Aquino R, et al. *J Nat Prod.* 1990;53(3);559.

[16] Rizzi R, et al. *J Ethnopharmacol.* 1993;38(1):63.

SCIENTIFIC NAME(S): *Matricaria chamomilla* L. and *Anthemis nobilis*. Sometimes referred to as *Chamaemelum nobile* (L.) All. Family: Compositae (Asteraceae)

COMMON NAME(S): *M. chamomilla* is known as German, Hungarian, or genuine chamomile, and *A. nobilis* is called English or Roman chamomile (common chamomile).

♣♣♣♣ PATIENT INFORMATION ♣♣♣♣

Uses: Teas and extracts of the flower heads have been used as anti-inflammatories, gastrointestinal antispasmodics, and sedatives. Research has found chamomile components with these effects and antiallergic activity.

Side Effects: Although toxicity appears to be low, sensitive individuals have experienced contact dermatitis, anaphylaxis, and other reactions. Inhibition of GI activity may slow drug absorption.

Dosing: Chamomile has been used to make a tea for diarrhea and as a sleep aid. Typical doses have been 9 to 15 g/day. An extract of chamomile with apple pectin, *Diarrhoesan* (Dr. Loges) standardized to 3.5 mg chamazulene/100 g extract and 50 mg bisabolol/100 g extract has been studied for treatment for diarrhea.

BOTANY: *M. chamomilla* grows as an erect annual and *A. nobilis* is a slow-growing perennial. The fragrant flowering heads of both plants are collected and dried for use as teas and extracts.

HISTORY: Known since Roman times for their medicinal properties, the plants have been used as antispasmodics and sedatives in the folk treatment of digestive and rheumatic disorders. Teas have been used to treat parasitic worm infections and as a hair tint and conditioner. The volatile oil has been used to flavor cigarette tobacco.

PHARMACOLOGY: Bisabolol, a chamomile compound, exerts numerous pharmacologic effects that may account for the many traditional uses of chamomile. The compound effectively reduces inflammation, and is antipyretic in yeast-induced fever in rats.[1] It shortens the healing time of cutaneous burns in guinea pigs.[2] The compound also inhibits the development of gastric ulcers in rats, induced by indomethacin, stress, and ethanol, and shortens the healing time of acetic acid-induced ulcers.[3]

Chamomile infusions have been used traditionally as GI antispasmodics. Alcohol extracts of *M. chamomilla* showed antispasmodic effects in vitro.[4] Bisabolol and the lipophilic compounds bisabolol oxides A and B, as well as the essential oil, have a papaverine-like antispasmodic effect. Bisabolol is about as potent as papaverine and twice as potent as the oxides.[5] The chamomile flavones apigenin, luteolin, patuletin, and quercitin also have marked antispasmodic effects as do the coumarins umbelliferone and herniarine.

The hydrophilic components of chamomile, principally the flavonoids, also contribute to the anti-inflammatory process. The most active flavonoids are apigenin and luteolin, with potencies similar to that of indomethacin.[6]

Because of the low water solubility of the essential oil, teas prepared from chamomile flowers contain only approximately 10% to 15% of the oil present in the plant. Despite the relatively low concentration of lipophilic components in water infusions, chamomile teas are generally used over long periods of time, during which a cumulative therapeutic effect may result.[7]

TOXICOLOGY: The toxicity of bisabolol is low following oral administration in animals. The acute LD-50 is approximately 15 mL/kg in rats and mice. In a 4-week subacute toxicity study, the administration of bisabolol (1 to 2 mL/kg body weight) to rats caused no significant toxicity. No teratogenicity or developmental abnormalities were noted in rats and rabbits after chronic administration of 1 mL/kg bisabolol.[8]

The tea, prepared from the pollen-laden flower heads, has resulted in contact dermatitis,[9] anaphylaxis,[10] and other severe hypersensitivity reactions in people allergic to ragweed, asters, chrysanthemums, and other members of the family Compositae.[11] Although some experts suggest that people with allergies to ragweed pollens should refrain from ingesting chamomile, good evidence for this cross-sensitivity remains to be established.

The dried flowering heads are emetic when ingested in large quantities.[12]

[1] Jakovlev V, et al. *Planta Medica*. 1979;35:125.
[2] Isaac O. *Planta Medica*. 1979;35:118.
[3] Szelenyi I, et al. *Planta Medica*. 1979;35:218.
[4] Forster HB, et al. Antispasmodic effects of some medicinal plants. *Planta Medica*. 1980;40:309.
[5] Achterrath-Tuckerman U, et al. *Planta Medica*. 1980;39:38.
[6] Hamon NW. *Can Pharm J*. 1989(Nov):612.
[7] Farnsworth NR. *JAMA*. 1972;221:410.
[8] Habersang S, et al. *Planta Medica*. 1979;37:115.
[9] Rowe AH. *J Allergy*. 1934;5:383.
[10] Benner MH, et al. *J Allergy Clin Immunol*. 1973;52:307.
[11] *Med Lett Drugs Ther*. 1979;21:29.
[12] Lewis WH, et al. *Medical Botany*. New York, NY: John Wiley and Sons, 1977.

SCIENTIFIC NAME(S): *Larrea divaricata* Cav. [synon. with L. *tridentata* (DC) Coville], also referred to as *L. glutinosa* Engelm. Family: Zygophyllacea

COMMON NAME(S): Chaparral, creosote bush, greasewood, hediondilla[1]

⊱⊰⊱⊰ PATIENT INFORMATION ⊱⊰⊱⊰

Uses: Chaparral tea has been widely used in folk medicine to treat conditions ranging from the common cold to snakebite pain. A derivative was formerly used as a food preservative. Anecdotal and in vitro evidence suggests antineoplastic effects.

Side Effects: No longer classified as safe. Chaparral may cause liver damage, contact dermatitis, and stimulate most malignancies.

Dosing: Chaparral has been documented to be hepatotoxic at doses of crude herb from 1.5 to 3.5 g/day. Therefore, its use is discouraged.[2-4]

BOTANY: The chaparrals are a group of closely-related wild shrubs found in the arid regions of the southwestern US and Mexico. Chaparral found in health food stores usually consists of leaflets and twigs. This branched bush grows to 270 cm. Its leaves are bilobed and have a resinous feel and strong smell.

HISTORY: Chaparral tea was used as a remedy by American Indians and has been suggested for the treatment of bronchitis and the common cold, to alleviate rheumatic pain, stomach pain, chicken pox, and snakebite pain. A strong tea from the leaves has been mixed with oil as a burn salve.[5] It is an ingredient in some OTC weight loss teas.

In 1959, the National Cancer Institute (NCI) was informed through lay correspondence that several cancer patients claimed beneficial effects on their cancers from drinking chaparral tea. Years later, a similar treatment was brought to the attention of physicians at the University of Utah, when an 85-year-old man with a proven malignant melanoma of the right cheek with a large cervical metastasis refused surgery and treated himself with chaparral tea. Eight months later he returned with marked regression of the tumor.[6] Additional cases observed by the physicians at the University of Utah included four patients who responded to some degree to treatment with the tea, including two with melanoma, one with metastatic choriocarcinoma, and one with widespread lymphosarcoma. After 2 days of treatment, the patient with lymphosarcoma discontinued chaparral treatment, despite the disappearance of 75% of his disease. The choriocarcinoma patient, who had not responded well to other therapies, responded well to chaparral tea for 2 months after which the disease became progressive. Of the melanoma patients, one experienced a 95% regression and the remaining disease was excised; the other, after remaining in remission for 4 months, subsequently developed a new lesion.[7]

Reports subsequently appeared in the lay literature describing the virtues of chaparral tea as an antineoplastic treatment.

PHARMACOLOGY: Nordihydroguaiaretic acid (NDGA) is believed to be responsible for the biological activity of chaparral. Up until 1967, when more effective antioxidants were introduced, NDGA was used in the food industry as a food additive to prevent fermentation and decomposition. It is theorized that any anticancer effect of chaparral tea is caused by the ability of NDGA to block cellular respiration. NDGA and its related compounds inhibit the beef heart mitochondrial nicotinuamide adenine dinucleotide (NADH) oxidase system and succinoxidase system, and therefore, exert some antioxidant activity at the cellular level.[8] NDGA also inhibits collagen- and ADP-induced platelet aggregation and platelet adhesiveness in aspirin-treated patients.[9]

Studies conducted by the NCI found that in vitro, NDGA was an effective anticancer agent, being described as "the penicillin of the hydroquinones and the most potent antimetabolite in vitro."[10] However, this activity is almost completely abolished in vivo. Chaparral failed to show any significant anticancer activity in two separate NCI chemotherapy screening tests in mice.[7] There is some evidence that when combined with ascorbic acid, NDGA shows some inhibitory effect against small Ehrlich ascites tumors in mice.

Other disconcerting data from 34 cancer patients treated for varying periods of time with chaparral suggest that a majority of malignancies are stimulated by NDGA, while some go on to regress.[7]

TOXICOLOGY: The creosote bush can induce contact dermatitis.[11] NDGA has been found to induce mesenteric lymph node and renal lesions in rats;[12] and because of these problems, it was removed from the Generally Recognized as Safe (GRAS) list in 1970.[13]

Several reports have linked the ingestion of chaparral tea with the development of liver damage.[12,14] In all 3 cases, the patients took chaparral tablets or capsules for 6 weeks to 3 months. They developed signs of hepatic damage as evidenced by liver enzyme abnormalities; these resolved following discontinuation of the plant material. These reports indicate that chronic ingestion of chaparral may be associated with liver damage.

[1] Dobelis IN, ed. *Magic and Medicine of Plants*. Pleasantville, NY: Reader's Digest Association, Inc., 1986.

[2] *MMWR*. 1992;43:812.

[3] Sheikh N, Philen RM, Love LA. Chaparral-associated hepatotoxicity. *Arch Intern Med*. 1997;157:913-919.

[4] Grant KL, et al. *Integrative Med*. 1998;1;83-87.

[5] Sweet M. *Common Edible and Useful Plants of the West*. Healdsburg, CA: Naturegraph Publications, 1976.

[6] Smart CR, et al. *Cancer Chemother Rep*. 1969;53:147.

[7] *Unproven Methods of Cancer Management*. American Cancer Society, 1970.

[8] Gisvold O, Thaker E. *J Pharm Sci*. 1974;63:1905.

[9] Gimeno MF, et al. *Prostaglandin Leukotrein Med*. 1983;111:109.

[10] Burk D, Woods M. *Radiat Res Suppl*. 1963;3:212.

[11] Lampe KF, McCann MA. *AMA Handbook of Poisonous and Injurious Plants*. Chicago, IL: AMA, 1985.

[12] Tyler VE. *The Honest Herbal*. Philadelphia, PA: G.F. Stickley Co., 1981.

[13] Katz M, et al. *J Clin Gastroenterol*. 1990;12:203.

[14] Chaparral-induced toxic hepatitis-California and Texas 1992. *MMWR Morb Mortal Wkly Rep*. 1992;41:812-814.

Chaste Tree

SCIENTIFIC NAME(S): *Vitex agnus-castus* L. Family: Verbenaceae

COMMON NAME(S): Chaste tree, chasteberry, monk's pepper

✿✿✿✿ PATIENT INFORMATION ✿✿✿✿

Uses: Chaste tree has been used by women to balance progesterone and estrogen production and regulate menstruation. It has been used for breast pain, ovarian insufficiency, uterine bleeding, and to increase breast milk production.

Side Effects: Minor side effects include GI reactions, itching, rash, headaches, and increased menstrual flow.

Dosing: Daily doses of chaste tree are typically 30 to 40 mg of crushed fruit or 1.6 to 4.2 mg of dried extract. Chaste tree fruit is available in several different standardized extracts, with casticin content used for standardization. *Agncaston* is standardized to 1% casticin, while *PreMens* contains 0.6% casticin. Other products include *Agnolyt* (3.5 to 4.2 mg extract/pill), *Femicur* (Schaper & Brummer) (1.6 to 3 mg extract corresponding to 20 mg drug), *Strotan*, *Mastodynan*, and *Ze 440*. Fluid extracts and tinctures are among the most common dosage forms for this product.[1-4]

BOTANY: The chaste tree is a shrub that grows in moist river banks in southern Europe and the Mediterranean region.[5] It can grow to 660 cm in height and blooms in summer, developing light purple flowers and palm-shaped leaves. The dark brown-to-black fruits are the size of a peppercorn. Collected in autumn, the fruits have a pepperish aroma and flavor.[6,7]

HISTORY: The dried, ripe fruit is used in traditional medicine. The plant has been recognized since antiquity and described in works by Hippocrates, Dioscorides, and Theophrastus.[6] In Homer's epic, *The Iliad*, the plant was featured as a "symbol of chastity, capable of warding off evil."[7] Early physicians recognized its effect on the female reproductive system, suggesting its use in controlling hemorrhages and expelling the placenta after birth. The English name "chaste tree" derives from the belief that the plant reduces unwanted libido. Monks have chewed its parts to decrease sexual desire.[6,7] At least one report is available discussing the chaste tree's use in ancient medicine to the present.[8]

PHARMACOLOGY: Chaste tree berries are thought to be antiandrogenic, inhibiting male hormonal actions. In females, the berries exert progesterogenic effects, balancing progesterone and estrogen production from the ovaries and regulating menstrual cycles.[7] A preparation of chaste tree (0.2% w/w) has been available in Germany since the 1950s and is used in treatment of breast pain, ovarian insufficiency (some cases resulting in pregnancy), and uterine bleeding.[9] Crude herb, alcoholic, or aqueous extracts of pulverized fruit are used in commercial preparations.[10]

When studied in 52 women with luteal phase defects caused by latent hyperprolactinemia, a chaste tree preparation reduced prolactin release, normalized luteal phases, and eliminated deficits in luteal progesterone without side effects.[11] Chaste tree extract contains an active principle that binds to dopamine (D_2) receptor sites, inhibiting prolactin release. This suggests therapeutic usefulness of the plant for treatment of premenstrual breast pain associated with prolactin hypersecretion.[12]

A case report in a female patient evaluated chaste tree therapy in multiple follicular development. Hormone levels after administration of the herb became "disordered;" thus, the authors concluded that chaste tree should not be used to promote normal ovarian function.[13]

Chaste tree is reportedly effective in treating endocrine abnormalities such as menstrual neuroses and dermatoses. It has also been used to treat acne.[9]

In lactating women, extracts of the plant have also been used to increase milk production.[6] When analyzed chemically, the breast milk revealed no compositional changes after chaste tree use.[9]

TOXICOLOGY: Chaste tree administration has not been associated with significant adverse events. In one large German market surveillance study, 17 of 1542 women discontinued treatment because of an adverse event.[6] Minor side effects include GI reactions, allergic reactions (eg, itching, rash), headaches, and menstrual flow increase.[6,9] The safety of the plant has not been determined in children.

[1] Lauritzen C, et al. Treatment of premenstrual tension syndrome with *Vitex agnus castus*. Controlled, double-blind study versus pyridoxine. *Phytomed.* 1997;4:183-189.

[2] Christie S, et al. *Vitex agnus-castus* L.; a review of its traditional and modern therapeutic use and current use from a survey of practitioners. *Eur J Herbal Med.* 1998;3:29-45.

[3] Loch EG, Selle E, Boblitz N. Treatment of premenstrual syndrome with a phytopharmaceutical formulation containing *Vitex agnus castus*. *J Womens Health Gend Based Med.* 2000;9:315-320.

[4] Schellenberg R. *BMJ.* 2001;322:134-137.

[5] Mabberley DJ. *The Plant-Book: A Portable Dictionary of the Higher Plants.* Cambridge: Cambridge University Press, 1987.

[6] Brown DJ. *Quarterly Rev Nat Med.* 1994;Summer:111.

[7] Chevallier A. *Encyclopedia of Medicinal Plants.* New York, NY: DK Publishing 1996;149.

[8] Newall C, et al. *Herbal Medicines.* London, England: Pharmaceutical Press 1996;19-20.

[9] Houghton P. *Pharm J.* 1994 Nov 19;253:720-721.

[10] Leung, AY. *Encyclopedia of Common Natural Ingredients.* New York, NY: John J. Wiley and Sons 1996;151.

[11] Milewicz A, et al. *Arzneimittelforschung.* 1993;43(7):752-756.

[12] Jarry H, et al. *Exp Clin Endocrinol.* 1994;102(6):448-454.

[13] Cahill D, et al. *Hum Reprod.* 1994;9(8):1469-1470.

Chondroitin

SCIENTIFIC NAME(S): Chondroitin sulfate, chondroitin sulfuric acid, chonsurid, structum

COMMON NAME(S): Chondroitin

≈≈≈ PATIENT INFORMATION ≈≈≈

Uses: Chondroitin has been used to treat arthritis. It has also been studied for use in drug delivery and antithrombotic and extravasation therapy.

Side Effects: There is little information on chondroitin's long-term effects. Most reports conclude that it is not harmful.

Dosing: Chondroitin sulfate has been administered orally for treatment of arthritis at a dose of 800 to 1200 mg/day. Positive results often require several months to manifest, and a posttreatment effect has been observed.[1-8]

SOURCE: Chondroitin is a biological polymer that acts as the flexible connecting matrix between the protein filaments in cartilage.[9] Chondroitin can come from natural sources (eg, shark or bovine cartilage) or can be manufactured in the lab using different methods.[10] Danaparoid sodium, a mixture of heparin sulfate, dermatan sulfate, and chondroitin sulfate (21:3:1), is derived from porcine intestinal mucosa.[11]

HISTORY: Chondroitin sulfates were first extracted and purified in 1960. Studies suggested that if enough chondroitin sulfate was available to cells manufacturing proteoglycan, stimulation of matrix synthesis could occur, leading to an accelerated healing process.[12]

PHARMACOLOGY: One report evaluated half-lives of distribution and elimination, volumes of distribution, excretion values, urine and blood levels, and bioavailablity.[13] Another report concludes that oral chondroitin sulfate B (dermatan sulfate) reaches significant plasma levels, with 7% bioavailability.[14] In 22 patients with renal failure, chondroitin sulfate half-life was prolonged, but it could be administered for clot prevention during hemodialysis in this population.[15]

There is considerable controversy regarding absorption of chondroitin. Absorption of glucosamine is 90% to 98%, but chondroitin absorption is only 0% to 13% because of molecule size. Chondroitin is 50 to 300 times larger than glucosamine. Chondroitin may be too large to be delivered to cartilage cells. In addition, there also may be purification and identification problems with some chondroitin products, some of which have tested subpotent.[12]

Chondroitin's role in treating arthritis has gained popularity. Articular cartilage is found between joints (eg, finger, knee, hip) allowing for easy, painless movement. It contains 65% to 80% water, collagen, and proteoglycans. Chondrocytes are also found within this matrix to produce new collagen and proteoglycans from building blocks, including chondroitin sulfate, a glycosaminoglycan (GAG). Glucosamine, another of the beneficial substances in this area, stimulates chondrocyte activity. It is also the critical building block of proteoglycans and other matrix components.[12] Both chondroitin and glucosamine play vital roles in joint maintenance, which is the reason the combination of the two are found in many arthritic nutritional supplements.

In inflammation and repeated wear of the joint, chondrocyte function is disturbed, altering the matrix and causing breakdown.[16] Proper supplementation with glycosaminoglycans (eg, chondroitin sulfate) may enable chondrocytes to replace proteoglycans, offering "chondroprotection."[17] Cartilage contains the biological resources to enhance repair of degenerative injuries and inflammation. It has been proposed that a certain chondroitin sulfate sequence, released from cartilage proteoglycans, can inhibit elastase, regulating the matrix.[18]

Several studies in finger, knee, and hip joint therapy indicate beneficial results in osteoarthritis treatment.[19] An overview of chondroitin sulfate in another report concluded the product has no clear value in osteoarthritis treatment.[20]

Chondroitin sulfate has been used as a drug delivery system for diclofenac and flurbiprofen.[21] The polymer also has been used as a stabilization agent for iron injection hyperalimentation.[22]

Chondroitin sulfate B (dermatan sulfate) has potential as an antithrombolytic agent, as it inhibits venous thrombi, with less effect upon bleeding than heparin. It is an effective anticoagulant in hemodialysis.[23] Dermatan sulfate's efficacy, compared with heparin, has been determined in acute leukemia patients.[24]

Chondroitin sulfate has been used to treat extravasation after ifosfamide therapy, decreasing pain and inflammation.[25] It has also been used to treat extravasation from vindesine,[26] doxorubicin, and vincristine[27] and an etoposide needlestick injury in a health care worker.[28] Levels of chondroitin sulfate increase 10 to 100 times in tumors compared with normal tissue. In one report, all 44 cancer patients analyzed showed the structural anomaly of the urinary chondroitin sulfate. This may provide a potential new marker for diagnosis and follow-up of cancer therapy.[29] General reviews are available on chondroitin sulfate and chondroitin sulfate B.[30,31]

TOXICOLOGY: Little information about long-term toxic effects of chondroitin sulfate is available. Because the drug is concentrated in cartilage, the theory is that it produces no toxic or teratogenic effects.[19] Long-term clinical trials with larger populations are needed to fully determine toxicity.[32]

[1] Morreale P, Manopulo R, Galati M, Boccanera L, Saponati G, Bocchi L. *J Rheumatol.* 1996;23:1385-1391.

[2] Mazieres B, Combe B, Phan Van A, Tondut J, Grynfeltt M. *J Rheumatol.* 2001;28:173-181.

[3] Uebelhart D, Thonar EJ, Delmas PD, Chantraine A, Vignon E. *Osteoarthritis Cartilage.* 1998;6(suppl A):39-46.

[4] Verbruggen G, Goemaere S, Veys EM. *Osteoarthritis Cartilage.* 1998;6(suppl A):37-38.

[5] Bucsi L, Poor G. *Osteoarthritis Cartilage.* 1998;6(suppl A):31-36.

[6] Bourgeois P, Chales G, Dehais G, Delcambre B, Kuntz JL, Rozenberg S. *Osteoarthritis Cartilage.* 1998;6(suppl A):25-30.

[7] Das A Jr, et al. *Osteoarthritis Cartilage.* 2000;8:343-350.

[8] Conrozier T. *Presse Med.* 1998;27:1862-1865.

[9] Budavari S, et al, eds. *The Merck Index.* 11th ed. Rahway: Merck and Co., 1989.

[10] Ma S, et al. *Chin Pharm J.* 1993 Dec 28;741-743.

[11] Reynolds J, ed. *Martindale, the Extra Pharmacopoeia.* 13th ed. London: Royal Pharmaceutial Society, 1996.

[12] Benedikt H. *Nat Pharm.* 1997;1(8):1,22.

[13] Conte A, et al. *Arzneimittelforschung.* 1991;41(7):768-772.

[14] Dawes J, et al. *Br J Clin Pharm.* 1991 Sep;32:361-366.

[15] Gianese F, et al. *Br J Clin Pharm.* 1993 Mar;35:335-339.

[16] Krane S, et al. *Eur J Rheumatol Inflamm.* 1990;10(1):4-9.

[17] Pipitone V. *Drugs Exp Clin Res.* 1991;17(1):3-7.

[18] Paroli E. *Int J Clin Pharmacol Res.* 1993;13 Suppl:1-9.

[19] Leeb B, et al. *Wien Med Wochenschr.* 1996;146(24):609-614.

[20] Anonymous. *Prescrire Int.* 1995;4(20):165-167.

Guide to Popular Natural Products

21 Murata Y, et al. *J Controlled Release.* 1996 Feb;38:101-108.

22 Yamaji A, et al. *J Nippon Hosp Pharm Assoc.* 1979 Jan;5:30-35.

23 Lane D, et al. *Lancet.* 1992 Feb 8;339:334-335.

24 Cofrancesco E. *Lancet.* 1992 May 9;339:1177-1178.

25 Mateu J, et al. *Ann Pharmacother.* 1994 Nov;28:1243-1244.

26 Mateu J, et al. *Ann Pharmacother.* 1994 Jul-Aug;28:967-968.

27 Comas D, et al. *Ann Pharmacother.* 1996 Mar;30:244-246.

28 Mateu J, et al. *Am J Health Syst Pharm.* 1996 May 1;53:1068,1071.

29 Dietrich C, et al. *Lab Invest.* 1993;68(4):439-445.

30 Dosa E, et al. *Acta Pharm Hungarica.* 1977 May;47:102-112.

31 Tamagnone G, et al. *Drugs of the Future.* 1994 Jul;19:638-640.

32 American College of Rheumatology Patient Information. http://www.rheumatology.org/patient/970127.htm.

SCIENTIFIC NAME(S): *Tussilago farfara* (L. Family: Compositae)

COMMON NAME(S): Coltsfoot, coughwort, feuilles de tussilage (Fr.), horse-hoof, huflattichblätter (Ger.), kuandong hua

---

ᶻᵃᶻᵃᶻᵃ PATIENT INFORMATION ᶻᵃᶻᵃᶻᵃ

Uses: Coltsfoot has been used to treat sore throats, asthma, and some related conditions such as bronchitis, laryngitis, pertussis, influenza, and lung congestion.

Side Effects: Allergic reactions may occur. Coltsfoot has an "undefined safety" classification by the FDA. Avoid prolonged use of the plant; it may increase blood pressure and pose a risk of carcinogenicity, hepatotoxicity, or mutagenicity.

Dosing: Because of the content of hepatotoxic pyrrolizidine alkaloids, coltsfoot is not recommended for internal use. Historical use of 4.5 to 6 g/day of crude herb has been documented.[1]

BOTANY: Coltsfoot is a low-growing perennial (up to 30 cm high) with fleshy, woolly leaves. In early spring, the plant produces a stem with a single golden-yellow, narrow, ligulate flower head that blooms from April to June. As the stem dies, the hoof-shaped leaves appear. The plant is native to Europe, but also grows widely in sandy places throughout the US and Canada.[2] Coltsfoot is collected widely from wild plants in the Balkans, Eastern Europe, and Italy.[3] It has also been a part of Chinese folk medicine for centuries. The morphology and anatomy of coltsfoot have been described in detail, including the plant's underground parts.[4] A later report on leaf differentiation is also available.[5]

HISTORY: As part of its Latin name *Tussilago* implies, coltsfoot is reputed as an antitussive.[6] The buds, flowers, and leaves of coltsfoot have long been used in traditional medicine for dry cough and throat irritation. The plant has found particular use in Chinese herbal medicine for the treatment of respiratory diseases, including cough, asthma, and acute and chronic bronchitis. It is also a component of numerous European commercial herbal prepara-

tions for the treatment of respiratory disorders. A mixture containing coltsfoot has been smoked for the management of coughs and wheezes, but the smoke is potentially irritating. Its silky seeds were once used as a stuffing for mattresses and pillows.[7] Extracts of coltsfoot had once been used as flavorings for candies. All early references emphasize the usefulness of coltsfoot's mucilage for soothing throat and mouth irritation.[3]

PHARMACOLOGY: Coltsfoot preparations have long been used to soothe sore throats. The mucilage is most likely responsible for the demulcent effect of the plant. The mucilage is destroyed by burning; smoking the plant or inhaling vapors of the leaves steeped in water would not be expected to provide any degree of symptomatic relief. Instead, the smoke may exacerbate existing respiratory conditions. However, one source mentions coltsfoot in the form of a medicinal cigarette to help relieve asthma.[11] Coltsfoot components have been found to increase the cilia activity in the frog esophagus, and this action may contribute to the plant's expectorant effect.[12] Related conditions for which coltsfoot has been used include bronchitis, laryngitis, pertussis, influenza, and lung congestion.[6-8] It is one of the most popular European remedies to treat chest ailments.[11] Coltsfoot, in a mixture of Chinese herbs, has been evaluated in 66 cases of convalescent asthmatics and found useful in decreasing airway obstruction.[13]

Coltsfoot polysaccharides and flavonoids have anti-inflammatory actions.[11] This effect was similar to that of indomethacin in one report.[14] Weak anti-inflammatory actions have also been observed when tested against induced rat paw edema.[8]

A compound designated L-652,469, was isolated from coltsfoot buds. This compound has been found to be a platelet-activating factor (PAF) inhibitor and a calcium channel blocker. PAF is known to be an integral component of the complex cascade mechanism involved in both acute and chronic asthma, and a number of naturally occurring PAF antagonists are being clinically evaluated for the treatment of this and other inflammatory diseases. The isolation of PAF antagonists from coltsfoot indicates that the traditional uses of the plant in the management of certain inflammatory respiratory diseases may be verifiable.[15]

L-652,469 is also a competitive inhibitor of the calcium channel in the rat aorta, but the clinical importance of this finding has not been explored.

Tussilagone is a potent cardiovascular stimulant. When administered intravenously (0.02 to 0.3 mg/kg), it produced a rapid and dose-dependent pressor effect in dogs. This increase in blood pressure was similar to that observed following the administration of the cardiac stimulant dopamine. The increase in blood pressure was short-lived, lasting about 5 minutes. Tussilagone also increased the rate of respiration. The cardiovascular effects appear to be peripherally mediated, while the site of respiratory stimulation is central.[9]

Aqueous leaf extracts and phenolic components have been found to have in vitro antibacterial activity generally limited to gram-negative bacteria.[16] Some of these organisms include *Staphylococcus aureus, Bordetella pertussis, Pseudomonas aeruginosa*, and *Proteus vulgaris*.[8]

A report discusses coltsfoot's historical, traditional, and modern medical uses, along with the plant's pharmacology and toxicity.[17]

TOXICOLOGY: The use of teas prepared from coltsfoot has not generally been associated with acute toxicity. Several members of this family of plants (eg, chamomile, ragweed) cause common allergies, and some people may exhibit a cross-sensitivity to coltsfoot.[18] While coltsfoot is only a weak topical sensitizer in guinea pigs, other members of the family are strong sensitizers (blessed thistle, dwarf sunflower), and cross-sensitivity may exist.[19]

Several reports have noted the presence of hepatotoxic pyrrolizidine alkaloids in coltsfoot. Pre-blooming flowers have been reported to contain the highest concentration of these alkaloids, although considerable loss of both senkirkine and senecionine occurs upon prolonged storage of the plant.[8] In one long-term safety study, the alkaloid senkirkine (0.015% by weight in dried flowers) was incorporated into rat diets in concentrations of up to 8% of the diet for 2 years. Among the rats fed the 8% meal, two-thirds developed cancerous tumors of the liver characteristic of pyrrolizidine toxicity.[10] This alkaloid is also present in the leaves.[20] The acute intravenous LD-50 of tussilagone is 28.9 mg/kg.[7] These pyrrolizidine alkaloids have well documented toxicities in humans as well, presenting as anorexia, lethargy, abdominal pain and swelling, and liver changes. The alkaloids destroy the liver's hepatocytes and damage small branches of the hepatic vein. In Germany, consumption of more than 1 mg of pyrrolizidine alkaloids per day is prohibited.[21]

Of interest is a case of reversible hepatic veno-occlusive disease in an infant after consumption of coltsfoot, later found to be *Adenostyles alliariae* (these two plants can be easily confused, especially after the time of flowering.) Seneciphylline and related hepatotoxins were identified via thin-layer chromatography, mass spectrometry, and NMR spectroscopy.[22]

Coltsfoot has been classified by the FDA as an herb of "undefined safety."[23] However, although the pyrrolizidine alkaloids of coltsfoot are hepatotoxic, mutagenic, and carcinogenic, there is little danger of acute poisoning when it is used as prescribed (as an occasional tea or cough preparation).[3] The *German Commission E Monographs* recommend a limit of 10 micrograms per day of pyrrolizidine alkaloids with the 1,2-unsaturated necine structure, including their N-oxides.[24]

Excessive consumption of coltsfoot may interfere with preexisting antihypertensive or cardiovascular therapy. Prolonged ingestion of the plant should be avoided. Duration of administration should not exceed 4 to 6 weeks per year.[24]

Because the plant may be an abortifacient, it should not be taken during pregnancy or lactation.[8] The flowers of coltsfoot should not be used. The plant is subject to legal restrictions in some countries.[11]

[1] Gruenwald J, ed. *PDR for Herbal Medicines.* 2nd ed. Montvale, NJ: Thomson Medical Economics; 2000: 209-211.

[2] Tyler, VE. *The New Honest Herbal.* Philadelphia: GF Stickley Co., 1987.

[3] Bisset NG. *Herbal Drugs and Phytopharmaceuticals.* Stuttgart: Medpharm Scientific Publishers, 1994.

[4] Engalycheva E, et al. *Farmatsiia.* 1981;30(3):21-26.

[5] Saukel J. *Scientia Pharmaceutica.* 1991(Dec 31);59:307-319.

[6] Bruneton J. *Pharmacognosy, Phytochemistry, Medicinal Plants, Technique and Documentation.* Paris, France, 1995.

[7] Duke J. *CRC Handbook or Medicinal Herbs.* Boca Raton, FL: CRC Press Inc. 1989;493-494.

[8] Newall C, et al. *Herbal Medicines.* London, England: Pharmaceutical Press, 1996;85–86.

[9] Li Y, et al. *Gen Pharmacol.* 1988;19(2):261-263.

[10] Roder E, et al. *Planta Medica.* 1981(Sep);43:99-102.

[11] Chevallier A. *Encyclopedia of Medicinal Plants.* New York: DK Publishing, 1996;277.

[12] Muller-Limmroth W, et al. *Fortshr Med.* 1980;98(3):95-101.

[13] Fu JX. *Chung Hsi I Chieh Ho Tsa Chih.* 1989;9(11):658.

[14] Engalycheva E, et al. *Farmatsiia.* 1982;31:37-40.

[15] Hwang S, et al. *Eur J Pharmacol.* 1987;141(2):269-281.

[16] Didry N, et al. *Annales Pharmaceutiques Francaises.* 1982;40(1):75-80.

[17] Salvador R. *Canadian Pharmaceutical Journal.* 1996(Jul-Aug);129:48-50.

[18] Toxic Reactions to Plant Products Sold in Health Food Stores. *Med Lett.* 1979;21(7):29.

[19] Zeller W, et al. *Arch Dermatol Res.* 1985;227(1):28.

[20] Smith LW, et al. *J Nat Prod.* 1981;44:129.

[21] Schulz V, et al. *Rational Phytotherapy — A Physician's Guide to Herbal Medicine.* 3rd ed. Berlin, Germany: Springer-Verlag, 1998;34.

[22] Sperl W, et al. *Eur J Pediatr.* 1995;154(2):112-116.

[23] DerMarderosian AH, Liberti LE. *Natural Products Medicine.* Philadelphia: GF Stickley Co., 1988.

[24] Blumenthal M, ed. *The Complete German Commission E Monographs.* Austin, TX: American Botanical Council; Boston: Integrative Medicine Communications, 1998.

SCIENTIFIC NAME(S): *Symphytum officinale* L., *S. asperum* Lepechin, *S. tuberosum*, *Symphytum × uplandicum* Nyman (Russian comfrey) is a hybrid of *S. officinale* and *S. asperum*. Family: Boraginaceae

COMMON NAME(S): Comfrey, Russian comfrey, knitbone, bruisewort, blackwort, slippery root

---

ꜣꜣꜣꜣ PATIENT INFORMATION ꜣꜣꜣꜣ

Uses: Comfrey has been used as a vegetable, as topical treatment for bruises, burns, and sprains, and as internal medicine.

Side Effects: Evidence indicates that comfrey is unsafe in any form and potentially fatal.

Dosing: Because of the content of hepatotoxic pyrrolizidine alkaloids, comfrey is not recommended for internal use. Historically, use of 5 to 10 g of root has been documented.[1]

BOTANY: A perennial that grows to about 90 cm in moist grasslands, comfrey has lanceolate leaves and bell-shaped purple or yellow-white flowers.

HISTORY: Comfrey has been cultivated in Japan as a green vegetable and used in American herbal medicine.[2] Its old name, knitbone, derives from the external use of poultices of the leaves and roots to heal burns, sprains, swelling, and bruises. Comfrey has been claimed to heal gastric ulcers, hemorrhoids, and to suppress bronchial congestion and inflammation.[2] Its use has spanned over 2000 years.[3]

PHARMACOLOGY: Ointments containing comfrey have been found to possess anti-inflammatory activity, which appears to be related to the presence of allantoin and rosmarinic acid[4] or to another hydrocolloid polysaccharide.[5] Lithospermic acid, isolated from the root, appears to have antigonadotropic activity.[6]

TOXICOLOGY: Despite its common use, the long-term ingestion of comfrey may pose a health hazard. Several members of the family Boraginaceae contain related alkaloids reported to cause liver toxicity in animals and humans. Some

of these compounds predispose hepatic tumor development.

Similarly, the alkaloids of Russian comfrey caused chronic liver damage and pancreatic islet cell tumors after 2 years of use in animal models. Eight alkaloids have been isolated from *Symphytum × uplandicum*.[7] Alkaloid levels range from 0.003% to 0.115% with highest concentrations in small young leaves.[8] An indirect estimate of alkaloid ingestion determined the consumption of toxic alkaloids to be 2 mg/700 g of flour. Based on this value, Roitman's calculation of 8 to 26 mg of toxic alkaloids per cup of comfrey root tea (4 to 13 times as great as the episode above) suggests that comfrey ingestion poses a significant health risk.[9] Herbal teas and similar preparations of *Symphytum* contain the pyrrolizidine alkaloid that has been shown to cause blockage of hepatic veins and lead to hepatonecrosis.[10] Veno-occlusive disease has been reported in a woman who ingested a comfrey-pepsin preparation for 4 months;[9] 1 woman died following the ingestion of large quantities of yerba mate tea.[11] A woman who consumed large amounts of comfrey preparations developed ascites-caused veno-occlusive disease,[12] and 4 Chinese women who self-medicated with an herbal preparation that contained pyrrolizidine alkaloids from an unknown plant source also developed the disease.[13] One man presented portal hypertension with hepatic veno-occlusive disease and later died of liver failure. It was discovered that he used comfrey in his vegetarian diet.[14] Oral ingestion of pyrrolizidine-containing plants, such as comfrey, poses the greatest risk since the alkaloids are converted to toxic pyrrole-like derivatives following ingestion;[15] however, the alkaloids of comfrey applied to the skin of rats were detected in the urine, and lactating rats excrete pyrrolizidine alkaloids into breast milk.[16] If animals consume plants containing pyrrolizidine alkaloids, they could pass these alkaloids on to humans via milk.[17]

[1] Gruenwald J, ed. *PDR for Herbal Medicines.* 2nd ed. Montvale, NJ: Thomson Medical Economics; 2000: 212-214.

[2] Bianchi F, Corbetta F. *Health Plants of the World.* New York: Newsweek Books 1975.

[3] Castlemen M. *Herb Quarterly.* 1989;44:18.

[4] Andres R, et al. *Planta Med.* 1989;55:643.

[5] Franz G. *Planta Med.* 1989;55:493.

[6] Wagner H, et al. *Arzneimittelforschung.* 1970;20(5):705.

[7] Culvenor CCJ, et al. *Experientia.* 1980;36:377.

[8] Mattocks, AR. *Lancet.* 1980;2:1136.

[9] Ridker PM, et al. *Gastroenterology.* 1985;88:1050.

[10] Larrey D. *Presse Med.* 1994;23(15):691.

[11] McGee J, et al. *J Clin Pathol.* 1976;29:799.

[12] Bach N, et al. *JAMA.* 1989;87:97.

[13] Kumana CR, et al. *Lancet.* 1983;ii:1360.

[14] Yeong ML, et al. *J Gastroenterol Hepatol.* 1990;5(2):211.

[15] Mattocks AR. *Nature.* 1986;217:724.

[16] Schoenta R. *Toxicol Lett.* 1982;10:323.

[17] Panter KE, James LF. *J Animal Sci.* 1990;68(3):892.

Cramp Bark

SCIENTIFIC NAME(S): *Viburnum opulus* L.; *V. opulus* var. *americanum* (Miller) Ait. Caprifoliaceae (honeysuckle family)

COMMON NAME(S): Cramp bark, guelder rose, snowball, squaw bush, cranberry tree, highbush cranberry, pimbina

---

⋆⋆⋆ PATIENT INFORMATION ⋆⋆⋆

Uses: Cramp bark has been used for painful menstruation and to prevent miscarriage. However, no clinical trials in humans have been performed.

Side Effects: No studies have been performed.

Dosing: 3 to 4 g/day.

BOTANY: *Viburnum opulus* is a large bush that is often grown ornamentally for its attractive white flowers. It is native to northern Asia and Europe. The American variety of *V. opulus* (also known as *V. trilobatum*) has edible red berries while the European variety bears bitter fruit. An extensive study of *Viburnum* botany and pharmacognosy was published in 1932.[1] The trunk and root bark are the commonly used drug products.

HISTORY: The American variety was used by the Iroquois for prolapsed uterus after childbirth,[2] and other tribes recognized its use as a diuretic.[1] The Eclectic medical movement in the 19th century adopted cramp bark for dysmenorrhea and to prevent miscarriage. It was believed to be a stronger antispasmodic than the related *Viburnum* species *V. prunifolium* (black haw).[2] The bark was made official in the *U.S. Pharmacopeia*

in 1894 and was included in the *National Formulary* in 1916. Widespread adulteration by mountain maple (*Acer spicatum*) and other *Viburnum* species led to confusion about the correct source plant. A later review surveyed the botanical, chemical, and pharmacological differences between black haw and cramp bark.[3]

PHARMACOLOGY: Early pharmacologic studies of cramp bark and black haw did not demonstrate activity in uterine preparations. Both scopoletin[4] and viopudial[5] have been determined to be responsible for the uterine relaxant activity of *V. opulus*. However, viopudial has not been found in black haw bark, which may account for its reputation for weaker activity. No clinical studies examining efficacy in humans have been performed.

TOXICOLOGY: There are no studies of the toxicology of cramp bark.

[1] Youngken HW. *J Am Pharm Assoc.* 1932;21:444-462.

[2] Brinker F. *J Naturopathic Med.* 1998;7:11-26.

[3] Hörhammer L, Wagner H, Reinhardt H. *Botan Mag* (Tokyo). 1966;79:510-525.

[4] Jarboe CH, Zirvi KA, Nicholson JA, Schmidt CM. *J Med Chem.* 1967;10:488-489.

[5] Nicholson JA, Darby TD, Jarboe CH. *Proc Soc Exp Biol Med.* 1972;140:457-461.

SCIENTIFIC NAME(S): *Vaccinium macrocarpon* Ait. (cranberry, trailing swamp cranberry), *V. oxycoccos* L. (small cranberry), *V. erythrocarpum* Michx. (Southern mountain cranberry), *V. vitis* (lowbush cranberry), *V. edule* (highbush cranberry). Family: Ericaceae

---

༶༅༅ PATIENT INFORMATION ༶༅༅

Uses: Cranberries and cranberry juice appear to combat urinary tract infections. The acids lower urine pH levels sufficiently to minimize the ammoniated odor in incontinent patients.

Side Effects: Extremely large doses can produce GI symptoms such as diarrhea. Contact your health care provider before taking cranberry products if you are prone to kidney stones.

Dosing: Cranberry juice, juice concentrate, and dried extract have been studied in urinary tract infections. Doses of juice studied have ranged from 120 to 4000 mL/day; 400 mg of cranberry extract daily has been given in an effort to avoid the large volumes that seem to be required for efficacy.[1-10]

BOTANY: A number of related cranberries are found in areas ranging from damp bogs to mountain forests. These plants grow from Alaska to Tennessee as small, trailing evergreen shrubs. Their flowers vary from pink to purple and bloom from May to August depending on the species. The *Vaccinium* genus also includes the blueberry (*V. angustifolium* Ait.), deerberry (*V. stamineum* L.), the bilberry (*V. myrtillus*), and the cowberry (*V. vitis-idaea* L.). They are not to be confused with another highbush cranberry, *Viburnum opulus* L. (family: Caprifoliaceae).[11]

HISTORY: During the mid-1800s, German physicians observed that the urinary excretion of hippuric acid increased after the ingestion of cranberries. It was believed that cranberries, prunes, and plums contained benzoic acid or another compound that the body metabolized and excreted as hippuric acid (a bacteriostatic agent in high concentrations). This hypothesis has always been disputed because the amounts of benzoic acid present in these fruits (approximately 0.1% by weight) could not account for the excretion of the larger amounts of hippuric acid.

Despite a general lack of scientific evidence to indicate that cranberries or their juice are effective urinary acidifiers, interest persists among the public in the medicinal use of cranberries. Cranberries are used in eastern European cultures because of their folkloric role in the treatment of cancers and to reduce fever. Cranberries make flavorful jams and preserves.

PHARMACOLOGY: The discovery of cranberries' ability to acidify urine was based on an early experiment with 2 healthy subjects.[12] Following a basal diet, 1 subject was given 305 g of cooked cranberries and the other, an unspecified amount of prunes. In the first subject, urinary pH decreased from 6.4 to 5.3 with a concomitant increase in the excretion of total acids. Hippuric acid excretion increased from 0.77 to 4.74 g. Presumably, urinary hippurate resulted from the slow biotransformation of quinic and benzoic acids or from a glucoside that hydrolyzed to quinic acid. Since mammalian tissues cannot convert quinic to hippuric acid, intestinal bacteria may play a role in this conversion.[13]

Despite these early observations, the value of cranberries in treating urinary tract infections continues to be controversial. In 1 study, 3 of 4 subjects given 1.5 to 4 L per day of cranberry cocktail (⅓ juice mixed with water and sugar) showed only transient changes in urinary pH.[1] The maximum tolerated amounts of cranberry juice (about 4 L per day) rarely result in enough hippuric acid excretion to achieve urinary concentrations that are bacteriostatic at the optimum activity level of pH 5. The antibiotic activity of hippuric acid decreases about 5-fold at pH 5.6.[14] When 5 subjects were given 1.2 to 4 L per day of cranberry juice, urinary pH decreased only 0.2 to 0.5 units after 4 days of treatment; no urinary pH was ever lowered to pH 5.[14] A placebo-controlled study assessed the value of drinking 300 mL per day of cranberry juice on bacteria and white blood cell counts in the urine of 153 elderly women.[2] The chances of having bacteria or white blood cells in the urine were significantly lower in the group of women who ingested cranberry juice and their odds of remaining bacteria-free from one month to the next were only 27% of the controls. This is one of the largest studies of its kind and suggests that there may be a microbiologic basis for cranberry's activity. Questions have been raised about the study design and specimens used.[15-19]

A study of 9 elderly men and 29 elderly women suggested that drinking cranberry juice reduces the frequency of bacteriuria in the elderly.[20]

Reduced symptomatic urinary tract infections were seen in women residing in a long-term care facility after ingestion of cranberry juice or concentrated cranberry capsules in another study ($P = 0.01$).[21] In a randomized, double-blind, crossover study of 10 young women with recurrent urinary tract infections, it was found that daily treatment with 400 mg of cranberry concentrate resulted in significantly fewer urinary tract infections than in the control group.[3]

In a case-control study of 86 sexually active college students, a 50% reduction in the likelihood of first-time urinary tract infections was related to regular ingestion of cranberry juice.[22]

Two studies in children with neurogenic bladder receiving intermittent catheterization, showed no significant difference in the acidification of urine or frequency of bacteriuria with ingestion of cranberry concentrate.[4,23]

Two reviews assessing the validity of using cranberries for the prevention and treatment of urinary tract infections concluded, on the basis of the available evidence, that cranberry juice cannot be recommended for the prevention nor treatment of urinary tract infections.[24,25] Because of questions that arose from the study, which included 153 elderly women, and these reviews, it was concluded that well-designed, placebo-controlled trials with significant outcomes are still needed.[26]

It is therefore likely that the juice does not exert a direct antibacterial effect via a compound such as hippuric acid, but that an alternate mechanism accounts for the anti-infective activity.[27] This is supported by the observation that cranberry and blueberry juices contain a high molecular weight compound (identified as condensed tannins or proanthocyanidins)[28] that inhibits the common urinary pathogen *Escherichia coli* from adhering to infection sites within the urinary tract, thereby limiting the ability of the bacteria to initiate and spread infections.[29,30] Preliminary data suggest that concentrated cranberry juice has some antibacterial activity, but whether sufficient urinary concentrations of the active ingredients can be achieved needs further investigation.[31]

One promising use for the juice is as a "urinary deodorant." The malodor of fermenting urine from incontinent patients is a persistent, demoralizing problem in hospitals and long-term care facilities. Cranberry juice appears to lower urinary pH sufficiently to retard the degradation of urine by *E. coli*, limiting the generation of the pungent ammoniacal odor.[32-34]

Using the juice in combination with antibiotics has been suggested for the long-term suppressive therapy of urinary tract infections.[5,35] Anecdotal reports have described the benefits of drinking 6 oz of juice twice daily to relieve symptoms of chronic pyelonephritis and to decrease the recurrence of urinary stones.[35]

TOXICOLOGY: There have been no reports of toxicity with the use of cranberry juice. The ingestion of large amounts (greater than 3 to 4 L per day) of the juice often results in diarrhea and other GI symptoms. A case of nephrolithiasis in a 47-year-old man was attributed to his ingestion of cranberry concentrate tablets. As calcium oxalate is the most common type of urinary stone, the oxalate content of the cranberry concentrate tablets contributed to the formation of urinary tract stones.[36] One 450 mg tablet of cranberry concentrate is equivalent to 2880 mL of cranberry concentrate, and 500 mL of cranberry juice contains 22 mg of oxalate.[37]

[1] Kahn HD, Panariello VA, Saeli J, Sampson JR, Schwartz E. *J Am Diet Assoc.* 1967;51:251-254.

[2] Avorn J, Monane M, Gurwitz JH, Glynn RJ, Choodnovskiy I, Lipsitz LA. *JAMA.* 1994;271:751-754.

[3] Walker EB, Barney DP, Mickelsen JN, Walton RJ, Mickelsen RA Jr. *J Fam Pract.* 1997;45:167-168.

[4] Schlager TA, Anderson S, Trudell J, Hendley JO. *J Pediatr.* 1999;135:698-702.

[5] Papas PN, et al. *Southwest Med.* 1966;47:17-20.

[6] Gibson L, et al. *J Naturopathic Med.* 1991;2:45-47.

[7] Pedersen CB, Kyle J, Jenkinson AM, Gardner PT, McPhail DB, Duthie GG. *Eur J Clin Nutr.* 2000;54:405-408.

[8] Schultz A. *J Community Health Nurs.* 1984;1:159-169.

[9] Sobota AE. *J Urol.* 1984;131:1013-1016.

[10] Moen DV. *Wisconsin Med J.* 1962;May:282-283.

[11] Dobelis I. *Magic and Medicine of Plants.* Pleasantville, NY: Reader's Digest Association, 1986.

[12] Blatherwick N, et al. *J Biol Chem.* 1923;57:815.

[13] DerMarderosian A. *Drug Ther.* 1977;7:151.

[14] Bodel P, et al. *J Lab Clin Med.* 1959;54:881.

[15] Hopkins WS, et al. *JAMA.* 1994;272(8):588-590.

[16] Hamilton-Miller JM. *JAMA.* 1994;272:588-590.

[17] Goodfriend R. *JAMA.* 1994;272:588-590. Letter.

[18] Avorn J, et al. *JAMA.* 1994;272:588-590. Letter.

[19] Katz LM. *JAMA.* 1994;272(8):589. Letter.

[20] Haverkorn MJ, et al. *JAMA.* 1994;272(8):590.

[21] Dignam R, et al. *J Am Geriatr Soc.* 1997;45(9):S53.

[22] Foxman B, et al. *Epidemiology.* 1995;6:162-168.

[23] Foda M, et al. *Can J Urol.* 1995;2(1):98-102

[24] Jepson RG, et al. Cranberries for preventing urinary tract infections. *Cochrane Database Syst Rev.* 2001;2.

[25] Jepson R, et al. Cranberries for treating urinary tract infections. *Cochrane Database Syst Rev.* 2001;2.

[26] Lowe F, et al. *Urology.* 2001;57(3):407-13

[27] Tyler V. *The Honest Herbal: A Sensible Guide to the Use of Herbs and Related Remedies.* Binghamtom, NY: The Haworth Press, 1993.

[28] Howell AB, et al. *N Engl J Med.* 1998;339:1085-1086.

[29] Ofek I, et al. *N Engl J Med.* 1991;324:1599.

[30] Ahuja S, et al. *J Urol.* 1998;159:559-662.

[31] Lee YL, et al. *JAMA.* 2000;283:1691.

[32] Kraemer R. *Southwest Med.* 1964;45:211.

[33] Dugan C, et al. *J Psychiatr Nurs.* 1966;8:467.

[34] Walsh BA. *J ET Nurs.* 1992;19:110-113.

[35] Zinsser HH, et al. *NY State J Med.* 1968;68:301-310.

[36] Terris MK, et al. *Urology.* 2001;57:26-29.

[37] Brinkley L, et al. *Urology.* 1981;17:534-538.

Cucurbita

SCIENTIFIC NAME(S): *Cucurbita pepo* L. (pumpkin or pepo), *C. maxima Duchesne* (autumn squash), *C. moschata* Poir. (crookneck squash) Family: Cucurbitaceae

---

ᴥᴥᴥ PATIENT INFORMATION ᴥᴥᴥ

Uses: Squashes, pumpkins, and other fruits of this family are consumed throughout the world. Flowers and seeds of some species are eaten. Seeds of some species are a traditional vermifuge. Also, components of some seeds may be useful in treating prostatic disorders.

Side Effects: Severe toxicity has not been reported with the use of cucurbita extracts.

BOTANY: The members of this genus are plants that develop long vine-like stems that produce large edible fruits. The large, yellow flowers are eaten in some Mediterranean cultures; whereas, the fruits are eaten worldwide. Many cultivated varieties can be found throughout the world.

HISTORY: The seeds of several species of cucurbita have been used in traditional medicine for centuries. They have been used to immobilize and aid in the expulsion of intestinal worms and parasites. Traditionally, the seeds of *Cucurbita* species are ingested after grinding or as a tea. The amount of seeds that can exert a pharmacologic effect appears to vary by species, from as few as 50 g to more than 500 g. These are usually taken in several divided doses. Some cultures suggest eating small amounts of the seeds on a daily basis as a prophylactic against worm infections. The seeds also have been used in the treatment of prostate gland disorders.[1]

PHARMACOLOGY: Characteristics[2] and nutritional aspects[3] of cucurbita have been addressed. Studies on antilipolytic activity of *C. maxima* also have been performed.[4]

The influence of *C. maxima* on age-associated impairments has been reported.[5]

In a randomized, 3-month, double-blind study, a preparation of *C. pepo* (curbicin) improved certain parameters of benign prostatic hyperplasia including urinary flow, micturition time, residual urine, and urinary frequency vs placebo.[6]

Related species *C. ficifolia* exhibits hypoglycemic actions in rabbits.[7,8]

TOXICOLOGY: Severe toxicity has not been reported with the use of cucurbita extracts. In a 53-patient, randomized, double-blind trial, no side effects from *C. pepo* were noted.[6] Ingestion of *C. maxima* seeds by rats and pigs over a 4-week period resulted in no changes in glucose, urea, creatinine, liver enzymes, blood counts, and others.[9] One report on *C. moschata* describes dermatitis.[10]

---

[1] Tyler V. *The New Honest Herbal*. 2nd ed. Philadelphia: G.F. Stickley Co., 1987.

[2] Basaran A, et al. *Acta Pharmaceutica Turcica*. 1998;40(1):17-19.

[3] Jaroniewska D, et al. *Farmacja Polska*. 1997;53(3):134-135.

[4] Wong C, et al. *J Ethnopharmacol*. 1985;13:313-321.

[5] Wichtl M. *Dtsch Apoth Ztg*. 1992;132:1569-1576.

[6] Carbin B, et al. *Brit J Urol*. 1990;66(6):639-641.

[7] Roman-Ramos R, et al. *Arch Med Res*. 1992;23(3):105-109.

[8] Roman-Ramos R, et al. *J Ethnopharmacol*. 1995;48(1):25-32.

[9] Dequeiroz-Neto A, et al. *J Ethnopharmacol*. 1994;43(1):45-51.

[10] Potter T, et al. *Contact Dermatitis*. 1994;30(2):123.

SCIENTIFIC NAME(S): *Taraxacum officinale* Weber, also referred to as *Leontodon taraxacum* L. Family: Compositae

COMMON NAME(S): Dandelion, lion's tooth

ꙮꙮ PATIENT INFORMATION ꙮꙮ

Uses: Dandelion has been used for its nutritional value in addition to other uses including diuresis, regulation of blood glucose, liver and gall bladder disorders, as an appetite stimulant, and for dyspeptic complaints.

Side effects: Contact dermatitis and gastric discomfort have been reported.

Dosing: Dandelion root has been used as a tonic for digestive complaints in doses of 9 to 12 g/day, prepared as a tea.[1]

BOTANY: The dandelion is a weedy compositae plant with a rosette of leaves radiating from its base. The stem is smooth, hollow, and bears a solitary yellow head consisting solely of ray flowers, which produces a cluster of numerous tiny, tufted, single-seed fruits. The plant has a deep taproot. The leaves may be nearly smooth-edged, toothed, or deeply cut; the toothed appearance gives rise to the plant's name.[2] This perennial plant can reach 50 cm in height. It grows wild in most parts of the world and is cultivated in France and Germany.[3]

HISTORY: The dandelion was used in the 10th century by Arab physicians for medicinal purposes.[4] The plant was also recommended in an herbal written in the 13th century by the physicians of Myddfai in Wales.[5] It is native to Europe and Asia, but was naturalized in North America and now grows as a weed in nearly all temperate climates. It is cultivated by some European growers and more than 100 specialized varieties have been developed. The bitter greens are used raw in salads, in wine-making, or cooked like spinach. The root is roasted and used to brew a coffee-like beverage said to lack the stimulant properties of coffee. Dandelions have long been used in herbal remedies for diabetes and disorders of the liver and as a laxative and tonic. The juice of the leaves has been used to treat skin diseases, loss of appetite, and stimulate the flow of bile.[4]

PHARMACOLOGY: Dandelion has been classified as a hepatic, mild laxative, cholegogue, diaphoretic, analgesic, stimulant, tonic, and a regulator of blood glucose.[5-11] The roots have been used as a laxative, diuretic, tonic, hepatic, and for spleen ailments.[6,8,10] Root and leaves have been used for heartburn, bruises, chronic rheumatism, gout, diabetes, eczema, and other skin problems, as well as for cancers.[8,10]

Its diuretic effect, likely a result of sesquiterpene lactone activity and high potassium content,[7] has been used to treat high blood pressure.[3,7] A later report observed no significant diuretic activity from the plant.[12] These same sesquiterpene lactones may contribute to dandelion's mild anti-inflammatory activity.[5,8]

It is effective as a detoxifying herb, working primarily on the liver and gallbladder to remove waste. It may aid in gallbladder ailments and help dissolve gallstones.[3] However, dandelion should only be used for gallstones under a physician's direction; it is generally contraindicated in bile duct obstruction, empyema, or ileus.[5,7-9] Increases of bile secretion in rats (at least 40%) have been attributed to activity of bitter sesquiterpene lactones in the root.[8] These lactones also increase gastric secretions that can cause gastric discomfort.[7,8] Use for dyspeptic disorders may be attributed to the anti-ulcer and gastric antisecretory activity of taraxerol, one of the terpenoid alcohols also found in the root.[13] Dandelion is also considered an appetite-stimulating bitter.[7,13] The bitter principles, previously known as taraxacin, that have recently been identified as eudesmanolides, are contained in the leaves and appear to be unique to dandelion.[7]

Hypoglycemic effects have been demonstrated in healthy, nondiabetic rabbits with a maximum decrease in blood glucose achieved at a dose of 2 g/kg.[5] The maximum effect of dandelion was reported to be 65% of the effect produced by tolbutamide 500 mg/kg.[5] Another report found no effect on glucose homeostasis in mice.[14] Inulin, reported to have antidiabetic activity, may contribute to dandelion's glucose regulating properties.[10,15]

In vitro antitumor activity with a mechanism similar to that of lentinan (a tumor polysaccharide) has been reported.[5]

TOXICOLOGY: Like many plants in this family, dandelions are known to cause contact dermatitis in sensitive individuals.[16,17] A case report of a 9-year-old boy describes positive patch test reactions to dandelion and other compositae-plant oleo resins.[18] Two out of 7 patients, each with histories of dandelion dermatitis, reacted not only to dandelion extracts, but to a sesquiterpene mix.[19] These sesquiterpene lactones are believed to be the allergenic principles in dandelion.[3] Taraxinic acid 1'-O-beta-D-glucopyranoside has also been identified as an allergenic component.[20]

Acute toxicity of dandelion is low. LD_{50} values in mice for the root are 36.8 g/kg and for herb are 28.8 g/kg.[3] A case report describes toxicity in a patient taking an herbal combination tablet that included dandelion. It was unclear as to which constituents were responsible.[21] Dandelion may be potentially toxic because of the high content of potassium, magnesium, and other minerals.[22]

[1] Gruenwald J, ed. *PDR for Herbal Medicines.* 2nd ed. Montvale, NJ: Thomson Medical Economics; 2000:245-246.

[2] Seymour ELD. *The Garden Encyclopedia.* 1936.

[3] Chevallier A. *Encyclopedia of Medicinal Plants.* New York, NY: DK Publishing, 1996;140.

[4] Loewenfeld C, Back P. *The Complete Book of Herbs and Spices.* David E. Charles. London: Seymour, 1974.

[5] Newall C, et al. *Herbal Medicines.* London, England: Pharmaceutical Press, 1996;96-97.

[6] Duke J. *CRC Handbook of Medicinal Herbs.* Boca Raton, FL: CRC Press Inc., 1989;476-477.

[7] Bisset Ng, ed. Max Wichtl. *Herbal Drugs and Phytopharmaceuticals.* Boca Raton, FL: CRC Press Inc., 1994;486-489.

[8] Leung AY; Fosters. *Encyclopedia of Common Natural Ingredients.* New York: John Wiley and Sons, Inc., 1996;205-207.

[9] Brooks S. *Prot J Bot Med.* 1998;2(3):268.

[10] Brooks S. *Prot J Bot Med.* 1996;1(3):163.

[11] Brooks S. *Prot J Bot Med.* 1995;1(1):70.

[12] Hook I, et al. *Int J Pharmacognosy.* 1993;31(1):29-34.

[13] Brooks S. *Prot J Bot Med.* 1996;1(4):231.

[14] Swanston-Flatt S, et al. *Diabetes Res.* 1989;10(2):69-73.

[15] Duke JA. *Handbook of Biologically Active Phytochemicals and Their Activities.* Boca Raton, FL: CRC Press, Inc., 1992;86.

[16] Larregue M, et al. *Ann Dermatol Venerol.* 1978;105:547.

[17] Hausen BM, et al. *Derm Beruf Umwelt.* 1978;26:198.

[18] Guin J, et al. *Arch Dermatol.* 1987;123(4):500-502.

[19] Lovell C, et al. *Contact Dermatitis.* 1991;25(3):135-188.

[20] Hausen BM. *Derm Beruf Umwelt.* 1982;30:51.

[21] DeSmet P, et al. *BMJ.* 1996 Jul 13;313:92.

[22] Hamlin T. *Can J Hosp Pharm.* 1991;44(1):39-40.

SCIENTIFIC NAME(S): *Salvia miltiorrhiza* Bunge, Family: Labiatae

COMMON NAME(S): Danshen, Tan-Shen, Tzu Tan-Ken (roots of purple sage), Hung Ken (red roots), Shu-Wei Ts'ao (rat-tail grass), Ch'ih Shen (scarlet sage), Pin-Ma Ts'ao (horse-racing grass)

ᴥᴥᴥ PATIENT INFORMATION ᴥᴥᴥ

Uses: Danshen has been used for circulation improvement. Danshen has also been used to alleviate menstrual irregularity, abdominal pains, and insomnia.

Drug Interactions: Adverse effects of warfarin are exaggerated when danshen and warfarin are coadministered.

Side Effects: Severe clotting abnormalities and an interaction between danshen and methylsalicylate medicated oil have been reported.

Dosing: The recommended dose of danshen root is 9 to 15 g/day. Exercise caution because of the potential drug interaction with warfarin.[1-4]

BOTANY: Danshen is a perennial herb found mainly on sunny hillsides and stream edges. Violet-blue flowers bloom in the summer. The leaves are oval, with finely serrated edges. The fruit is an oval brown nut. Danshen's roots, from which many of the common names are derived, are a vivid scarlet red.[5] Danshen is related to common sage, the culinary herb.

HISTORY: The herb has been used for menstrual irregularity, to "invigorate" the blood, and for other ailments such as abdominal pain and insomnia.[5]

PHARMACOLOGY: Danshen has been used in improving circulation. Its ability to "invigorate" the blood is proven in many Chinese studies. Danshen has been used for menstrual problems and to relieve bruising.[5]

In animal studies, a combination of danshen with chuanxiong excelled in preventing capillary contraction, thus improving circulation in a hypoxic, high-altitude environment.[6] However, this same combination was not satisfactory to prevent cardiopulmonary changes caused by high altitudes in humans.[7]

Another danshen combination, this time with foshousan, may offer protection to erythrocytes, improving blood flow to the placenta and increasing fetal birth weight in pregnant rats exposed to cigarette smoke.[8]

Danshen use in ischemic stroke has been reported.[9]

Antithrombotic actions of danshen have also been reported.[10] Acetylsalvionolic acid A was found to exert suppressive effects on collagen-induced platelet 5-HT release while inhibiting aggregation in vitro.[11] The rosmarinic acid isolated from danshen also displayed antithrombotic effects when injected into rats. This was because of platelet aggregation and promotion of fibrinolytic activity as well.[12]

Danshen use results in possible dilation of blood vessels, increase in portal blood flow, and prevention of coagulation to improve tissue ischemia. This accelerates repair and enhances nutrition in hepatic cells.[13]

More than 70% of chronic hepatitis patients responded to danshen therapy in relief of symptoms such as nausea, malaise, liver pain, and abdominal distention.[13] Another report confirms danshen's therapeutic effects in chronic active hepatitis as well.[14]

Other effects of danshen include the following: cytotoxic activities (of tanshinone analogs) against certain carcinoma cell lines, many of which were effective at concentrations less than 1 mcg/mL;[15] marked protective action against gastric ulceration;[16] and CNS effects[17] including neurasthenia and insomnia treatments.[5]

TOXICOLOGY: Coadministration of danshen and warfarin results in exaggerated warfarin adverse effects. Both pharmacodynamic and pharmacokinetic parameters were affected when studied in rats. Observed interactions such as increased warfarin bioavailability, decreased warfarin clearance, and prolonged prothrombin times are all indicative of clinically important interactions if danshen and warfarin are taken together.[18,19] Severe clotting abnormalities have been reported in a case where danshen induces overcoagulation in a patient with rheumatic heart disease.[1] Another case report is available describing an interaction between danshen and methylsalicylate medicated oil.[2]

[1] Yu C, et al. *J Intern Med.* 1997;241(4):337–339.

[2] Tam L, et al. *Aust N Z J Med.* 1995;25(3):258.

[3] Gruenwald J, ed. *PDR for Herbal Medicines.* 2nd ed. Montvale, NJ: Thomson Medical Economics; 2000: 636-639.

[4] Izzat MB, Yim AP, El-Zufari MH. *Ann Thor Surg.* 1998;66:941-942.

[5] *A Barefoot Doctor's Manual (The American Translation of the Official Chinese Paramedical Manual).* Philadelphia, PA: Running Press, 1997;657.

[6] Feng S, et al. *Chung Hsi I Chieh Ho Tsa Chih.* 1989;9(11):650-652.

[7] Han Q, et al. *J Tongji Med Univ.* 1995;15(2):120-124.

[8] Anon. *Chin Med J.* 1977;3(4):224-226.

[9] Zhou W, et al. *Am J Chin Med.* 1990;18(1-2):19-24.

[10] Yu W, et al. *Yao Hsueh Hsueh Pao.* 1994;29(6):412-416.

[11] Chang H, et al, ed. *Advances in Chinese Medical Materials Research Symposium.* 1984;217, 559-580.

[12] Zou Z, et al. *Yao Hsueh Hsueh Pao.* 1993;28(4):241-245.

[13] Zhang Z, et al. *Chung Kuo Chung Yao Tsa Chih.* 1990;15(3):177-181.

[14] Bai Y. *Chung Hsi I Chieh Ho Tsa Chih.* 1984;4(2):86-87.

[15] Wu W, et al. *Am J Chin Med.* 1991;19(3-4):207-216.

[16] Gu J. *Chung Hua I Hsueh Tsa Chih.* (Taipei) 1991;71(6):630-632.

[17] Liao J, et al. *Proc Natl Sci Counc Repub China B.* 1995;19(3):151-58.

[18] Lo A, et al. *Eur J Drug Metab Pharmacokinet.* 1992;17(4):257-62.

[19] Chan K, et al. *J Pharm Pharmacol.* 1995;47(5):402-6.

SCIENTIFIC NAME(S): *Angelica sinensis* (Oliv.) Diels, synonymous with *A. polymorpha* var. *sinensis* Oliv. Family: Apiaceae (carrot family)

COMMON NAME(S): Dong quai, danggui, tang-kuei, Chinese angelica

---

⭐⭐⭐ PATIENT INFORMATION ⭐⭐⭐

Uses: Traditionally used as an analgesic for rheumatism, an allergy suppressant, and in the treatment of menstrual disorders, dong quai has been shown to possess antiasthmatic, antispasmodic, anti-inflammatory, and anticoagulant properties. It has also been used to flavor liqueurs and confections.

Drug Interactions: The possibility of dong quai interactions with warfarin has been postulated and is supported by at least 1 report. Possible synergism with calcium channel blockers may occur.

Side Effects: No reported side effects have occurred with authentic dong quai, but with *A. gigas*, *A. dahurica*, and *A. pubescens*, there is a very reasonable risk of phototoxicity. *Angelica archangelica* L. is reported to be an abortifacient and to affect the menstrual cycle. *A. sinensis* has uterine stimulant activity.

Dosing: Crude dong quai root has been given in doses ranging from 0.75 g/day to as much as 30 g/day. More typical doses are around 4.5 g/day.[1,2]

BOTANY: Three species of *Angelica* are monographed separately in the Chinese Pharmacopeia: Dong quai, the root of *Angelica sinensis*; Bai zi, the root of *Angelica dahurica* (Fisch.) Benth. et. Hook. f. or *A. dahurica* var. *formosana* (Boiss.) Shan et Yuan; and Du huo, the root of *A. pubescens* Maxim. *f. biserrata* Shan et Yuan.[3] In Korea, *A. gigas* Nakai is used medicinally, while in Japan, *A. acutiloba* Kitagawa is used. The European *A. archangelic* L. is used to flavor liqueurs and confections. While botanically related, do not confuse the various species of *Angelica*, which differ in chemistry, pharmacology, and toxicology. A molecular biology study of *A. acutiloba* may lead to efficient methods for distinguishing raw materials.[4]

HISTORY: Dong quai is widely used in traditional Chinese medicine and continues to be popular in China and elsewhere. It is used to treat menstrual disorders, as an analgesic in rheumatism, and in suppressing allergy symptoms. It is promoted for similar uses in the American herb market.

PHARMACOLOGY:

Antiallergy effects: A water extract of *A. sinensis* inhibited IgE-antibody production in a mouse model of atopic allergy. The extract was active orally and the activity was retained on dialysis, indicating that it was caused by high molecular weight components of the extract.[5]

Antispasmodic effects: The simple lactone ligustilide is thought to be a major bioactive principle of dong quai. Its antiasthmatic action was studied in guinea pigs.[6] Ligustilide and the related butylidenephthalide and butylphthalide were found to have antispasmodic activity against rat uterine contractions and in other smooth muscle systems. The compounds were characterized as nonspecific antispasmodics with a mechanism different from papaverine.[7] The ligustilide and butylidenephthalide constituents of Japanese angelica root were found to reverse the decrease in pentobarbital sleep induced by either isolation stress or yohimbine, implicating central noradrenergic or GABA systems in their actions.[8]

Anticoagulant effects: The coumarins of *Angelica* species have been associated with both bioactivity and toxicity of the plants; however, the low coumarin content of *A. sinensis* minimizes its importance in dong quai pharmacology. In other species of *Angelica*, coumarins clearly play an important role. Simple coumarins often have anticoagulant effects, while the linear furocoumarins are well known as photosensitizing agents.[9]

Anti-inflammatory effects: The simple prenylcoumarin, osthole, is a major constituent of *A. pubescens* (Du huo).[10] Osthole showed anti-inflammatory activity in carageenan-induced rat paw edema and acetic acid-induced writhing in mice.[10] Osthole also caused relaxation of rat thoracic aorta preparations[11] and inhibited proliferation of rat vascular smooth muscle cells.[12] Another study found that osthole inhibited the second phase of edema caused by formalin in the rat.[13] An inhibitory effect was also seen for osthole on 5-lipoxygenase and cyclooxygenase.[14] The related prenylcoumarin angelols were shown to inhibit platelet aggregation.[15]

The linear furocoumarin phellopterin was found to bind with high affinity to benzodiazepine receptors in vitro; however, other closely related furocoumarins were weaker or inactive.[16] Phellopterin was characterized as a competitive partial agonist of central benzodiazepine receptors by GABA and TBPS shift assays.[17] No in vivo experiments were reported. Other furocoumarins from

A. dahurica inhibited histamine release in a mouse peritoneal cavity assay,[18] while isoimperatorin was analgesic; columbianadin, columbianetin acetate, and bergapten were anti-inflammatory and analgesic.[13] Finally, the action of various coumarins from *A. dahurica* on lipolysis in fat cells of rats were examined, with some coumarins activating lipolysis and other coumarins inhibiting lipolysis.[19]

Menopause: Dong quai is widely used in the US to treat hot flashes and other symptoms of menopause. A randomized, double-blind, placebo-controlled trial of *A. sinensis* as a single agent found no effect on vasomotor flushes, endometrial thickness, or on the level of estradiol or estrone. The study material was standardized for ferulic acid content.[1] A polyherbal preparation including dong quai was shown to reduce menopausal symptoms in a much smaller clinical trial.[2]

TOXICOLOGY: Coumarins are the focus of toxicology in *Angelica*. Furanocoumarins such as bergapten and psoralen have been widely studied for their photoactivated toxicity; however, only *A. gigas* (Korean angelica) has been demonstrated to cause photodermatitis.[20] Clearly the risk of phototoxicity should be correlated with the content of specific toxic furocoumarins. In the case of *A. sinensis*, there appears to be little risk, but with *A. gigas*, *A. dahurica*, and *A. pubescens*, there is a very reasonable cause for caution. Possible synergism with calcium channel blockers may occur. *Angelica archangelica* L. is reported to be an abortifacient and to affect the menstrual cycle. *A. sinensis* has uterine stimulant activity.

[1] Hirata J, et al. *Fertil Steril.* 1997;68:981-986.
[2] Hudson T, et al. *J Naturopathic Med.* 1998;7:73.

[3] Tang W, et al. Chinese Drugs of Plant Origin: Chemistry, Pharmacology, and Use in Traditional and Modern Medicine. Berlin: Springer-Verlag, 1992:113-125.

[4] Mizukami H. *Biol Pharm Bull*. 1995;18:1299-1301.

[5] Sung C, et al. *J Nat Prod*. 1982;45:398-406.

[6] Tao J, et al. *Yao Hsueh Hsueh Pao*. 1984;19:561-565. Chinese.

[7] Ko W. *Jpn J Pharmacol*. 1980;30:85-91.

[8] Matsumoto K, et al. *Life Sci*. 1998;62:2073-2082.

[9] Hoult J, et al. *Gen Pharmacol*. 1996;27:713-722. Review.

[10] Kosuge T, et al. *Chem Pharm Bull*. 1985;33:5351-5354.

[11] Ko F, et al. *Eur J Pharmacol*. 1992;219:29-34.

[12] Guh J, et al. *Eur J Pharmacol*. 1996;298:191-197.

[13] Chen Y, et al. *Planta Med*. 1995;61:2-8.

[14] Liu J, et al. *Planta Med*. 1998;64:525-529.

[15] Liu J, et al. *Phytochemistry*. 1989;39:1099.

[16] Bergendorff O, et al. *Phytochemistry*. 1997;44:1121-1124.

[17] Dekermendjian K, et al. *Neurosci Lett*. 1996;219:151.

[18] Kimura Y, et al. *J Nat Prod*. 1997;60:249-251.

[19] Kimura Y, et al. *Planta Med*. 1982;45:183-187.

[20] Hann S, et al. *Photodermatol Photoimmunol Photomed*. 1991;8:84-85.

Echinacea

SCIENTIFIC NAME(S): *Echinacea angustifolia* DC. The related species *E. purpurea* (L.) Moench and *E. pallida* (Nutt.) Britton have also been used in traditional medicine. Family: Compositae

COMMON NAME(S): American coneflower, black susans, comb flower, echinacea, hedgehog, Indian head, Kansas snakeroot, narrow-leaved purple coneflower, purple coneflower, scurvy root, snakeroot

---

⋟⋟⋞⋞ PATIENT INFORMATION ⋟⋟⋞⋞

Uses: There is some evidence that echinacea (*purpurea* and *pallida* species) is effective in shortening the duration of symptoms of upper respiratory tract infections (URIs), including the common cold, but it has not been shown to be effective as a preventative. The variation in available products makes specific recommendations difficult to determine.

Side Effects: Side effects are rare. Patients with allergies, specifically allergies to daisy-type plants (Asteraceae/Compositae family) might be more susceptible to reactions. Nausea and other mild GI effects have been reported in clinical trials.

Dose: Variable doses and preparations were used in the studies that make specific dosing recommendations difficult. The dosing range for *E. pallida* root is 6 to 9 mL/day and *E. purpurea* leaf is approximately 900 mg/day. Because echinacea may be an immunostimulant, it should not be taken for more than 8 consecutive weeks. Usually 7 to 14 days is sufficient. However, there is no data to support or refute this theory.

BOTANY: There are at least 9 species of echinacea. The ones most commonly studied are *E. purpurea*, *E. pallida*, and *E. angustifolia*.[1]

Echinacea is native to Kansas, Nebraska, and Missouri. There has been confusion regarding the identification of echinacea. Because of this confusion, it should be recognized that much of the early research conducted on this plant (in particular with European *E. angustifolia*) was probably conducted on *E. pallida*.[2] At least 6 synonyms have been documented for these plants.

E. angustifolia is a perennial herb with narrow leaves and a stout stem that grows to 90 cm in height. The plant terminates in a single, colorful flower head. The plant imparts a pungent, acrid taste when chewed and causes tingling of the lips and tongue.

Echinacea products have been found to be adulterated with another member of the family Compositae, *Parthenium integrifolium* L. This plant has no pharmacologic activity.

HISTORY: Echinacea is a popular herbal remedy in the central US, an area to which it is indigenous. The plant was used in traditional medicine by the American Indians and quickly adopted by the settlers. During the 1800s, claims for the curative properties of the plant ranged from a blood purifier to a treatment for dizziness and rattlesnake bites.[3] During the early part of the 20th century, extracts of the plant were used as anti-infectives; however, the use of these products fell out of favor after the discovery of modern antibiotics.

The plant and its extracts continue to be used topically for wound-healing action and internally to stimulate the immune system. Most of the research during the past 10 years has focused on the immunostimulant properties of this plant.

PHARMACOLOGY: A small but growing body of evidence is developing to support the traditional uses of echinacea as a wound-healing agent and immunostimulant.

Most studies have indicated that the lipophilic fraction of the root and leaves contains the most potent immunostimulating components. Although a number of pharmacologically active components have been isolated, no single type of compound appears to be responsible for the plant's activity. Polyunsaturated alkamides from *E. angustifolia* have been shown to inhibit in vitro the activity of sheep cyclooxygenase and porcine 5-lipoxygenase assays.[4]

Treatment of the common cold: Nineteen German controlled clinical trials examined the efficacy of 7 different echinacea preparations, alone or in combination, for the prevention or treatment of URIs including the common cold. The authors rated the overall quality of the studies, with a median score of 37% and a range of 7% to 70%.[5] These results correspond to the average scores (38.5%) found for other clinical trials in journals from 1990.[5] The authors of this review determined that the studies available as of 1993 revealed that echinacea may have an effect on the immune system, but that there is insufficient evidence to provide specific recommendations.[6]

Barrett and colleagues published an evidence-based clinical review of echinacea in 1999. They examined 13 trials, 9 of which were reviewed by Melchart in 1994, and 4 additional studies (1 unpublished report). Barrett et al, found conclusions similar to those of Melchart in that there is some evidence that echinacea is effective for treatment, but not for the prevention of URIs, there is still a lack of definitive information to provide specific recommendations.[7] Brinkeborn and colleagues reported that patients receiving a commercially available echinacea product in Germany with 6.78 mg, 95% herb, and 5% root or a concentrate with 48.27 mg of the same crude extract, had a 50% reduction in 12 cold symptoms as judged by the patient and 60% as judged by physicians compared with placebo. In addition, approximately 70% of physicians and 80% of patients judged the treatment to be effective. There was no information on whether echinacea decreased the duration of a cold. The authors did not speculate as to why it was effective while the fresh plant preparation was not.[8] Degenring provided information concerning an open-label, "adjunctive treatment" trial in 77 patients receiving echinacea. Results showed that 72% of patients became symptom-free within 14 days. However, without a placebo-control, it is impossible to determine if patients would have improved without treatment.[9] Dorn and colleagues used an unidentified *E. pallida radix* extract 900 mg/day in an unspecified divided dose regimen for 8 to 10 days to determine its effect on both viral and bacterial infections compared with a placebo. *E. pallida* decreased the length of the illness from 13 to 9.8 days compared with placebo for bacterial infections and 12.9 days to 9.1 days for viral infections ($P < 0.0001$).[10]

Another study used a commercially available echinacea product in Germany. Results showed a direct correlation to time of administration with patients taking the medication during the early phase ("...identified by the course of an indicator symptom during the first three days of observation") showing faster improvement than those who started echinacea later. In the treatment group, 55.3% had greater than or equal to 50% improvement in global score compared with 27.3% in the placebo group.[11] Hoheisel and colleagues demonstrated that another commercially available product in Germany was more effective in shortening the duration of a cold and required treatment of a cold than placebo using subjective measures such as "Did you have a 'real cold'?" (fully expressed symptoms of acute respiratory tract infection). Although more patients experienced a "real cold" with placebo than echinacea, the severity of symptoms were similar in the 2 groups.[12] Thom and colleagues used a commercially available *E. pallida* root extract combination product (Kanjang mixture) in Scandinavia. Compared to placebo, the Kanjang mixture caused a decrease in subjective symptoms such as degree and frequency of cough, quality of sleep, efficacy of mucus discharge, nasal congestion, and global evaluation compared with placebo. These improvements were noted as early as 2 days after initiation of treatment and were more prominent at day 4. Patients took the echinacea treatment for an average of 5.2 days vs 9.2 days for placebo. No side effects were reported in either group; however, 2 patients discontinued the active treatment because they could not tolerate the taste of the medication.[13]

Prevention of the common cold: Three clinical trials, 2 were randomized, double-blind, placebo-controlled English-language trials, and 1 placebo-controlled have been conducted that examined the effectiveness of echinacea in the prevention of the common cold and other URIs. None of the studies found echinacea to be effective. However, 1 study did not calculate power (ie, the ability of a study to find a significant difference, if, in fact, one exists). One calculated the study power at only 20% and the other 75%, suggesting that neither study probably enrolled enough subjects.[14-16] Melchart and colleagues commented that echinacea may cause a 10% to 20% relative risk reduction for the occurrence of a

cold; however, larger patient populations than those used would be required to prove this theory.[14] As with the treatment trials, 2 of the studies determined whether the placebo was a true placebo.[14,16] The other study questioned whether patients thought they were receiving a placebo, and the investigators found no significant difference between groups. However, the dosage form used in this study was not described. Only 1 of the studies tested the products for quality.[15] However, the study did not list the species they used or if the product contained the desired components. None of the studies standardized their products prior to initiation of the study.[17] Melchart and colleagues reported that 45% of the subjects had tried echinacea before, which could have affected the results. This study also used an echinacea species (*angustifolia*) and plant parts (*purpurea* root) that are not approved by The German Commission E because they lack documentation of efficacy.[14]

Several caffeoyl conjugates have been isolated from *E. angustifolia* that demonstrate antihyaluronidase activity; these include chicoric acid, cynarine, chlorogenic acid, and caftaric acid.[18] The inhibition of this enzyme is believed to limit the progression of certain degenerative inflammatory diseases.

One study found the administration of echinacea extracts to humans stimulated cell-mediated immunity following a single dose, but that repeated daily doses suppressed the immune response.[20] In a more recent German study conducted in a small number of patients (15) with advanced metastasized colorectal cancer, echinacin (a component of the plant) was added to treatment consisting of cyclophosphamide and thymostimulin; the mean survival time was 4 months, and 2 patients survived for more than 8 months, suggesting that this form of immunotherapy may have some value in treating these ill patients.[21]

Although the results are encouraging, they are too preliminary to draw conclusions about the appropriate therapeutic uses of echinacea extracts. Similarly, there are no well-controlled studies that have evaluated the effects of OTC echinacea supplements. Consequently, dosages are not well defined.

Photodamage prevention/treatment: An in vitro study demonstrated that typical constituents of echinacea species applied topically were effective in prevention/treatment of photodamage of the skin caused by UV/UVB radiation.[22]

TOXICOLOGY: Little is known about the toxicity of echinacea despite its widespread use in many countries. It has been documented in American traditional medicine for more than a century and generally has not been associated with acute or chronic toxicity. Purified echinacea polysaccharide is relatively nontoxic. Acute toxicity studies found that doses of arabinogalactan as high as 4 g/kg injected intraperitoneally or IV were essentially devoid of toxic effects.[19]

Side effects: According to The German Commission E, *Echinacea purpurea* and *pallida*, when taken orally, do not cause any side effects.[23] Parnham and colleagues reported results from an unpublished practice study to determine adverse effects and safety of the squeezed sap of *E. purpurea*. A total of 1231 patients with relapsing respiratory and urinary infections given echinacea for 4 to 6 weeks demonstrated the following side effects: Unpleasant taste (1.7%); nausea or vomiting (0.48%); abdominal pain, diarrhea,

sore throat (0.24%). The authors reported that 90% of patients took the medication as directed. Parenteral administration was associated with immunostimulating-type reactions such as shivering, fever, and muscle weakness.[24] Degenring reported that 1 out of 77 patients who received the 6.78 mg, 95% herb, and 5% root formulation experienced nausea, restlessness, and aggravation of cold symptoms 4 days after starting the medication.[9] The symptoms were severe enough to require discontinuation of therapy. Other side effects reported in clinical trials were primarily GI in nature, such as mild nausea.[8,9,11,16] At the American Academy of Allergy, Asthma and Immunology 2000 annual meeting, 23 unpublished cases (2 "certain," 10 "probable," and 11 "possible") of allergic reaction to echinacea consistent with IgE-mediated hypersensitivity were reported. Of the 23 cases, 34% were atopic, 13% were nonatopic, and 44% did not provide this information. Of another 100 atopic patients who had never taken echinacea, 20% had positive skin test reactions to echinacea, indicating a hypersensitivity without prior exposure to echinacea.[25] There was also a case of anaphylaxis caused by a combination echinacea product (*E. angustifolia* and *E. purpurea*) with other dietary supplements. The amount of echinacea product consumed was approximately double that recommended by the manufacturer. The patient had a high incidence of allergies to other substances. Of an additional 84 patients with asthma or allergic rhinitis, 16 subjects (19%) reacted to an echinacea skin prick. Only 2 patients had prior exposure to echinacea.[26]

[1] Chavez M, et al. *Hosp Pharm*. 1998;33:180-188.

[2] Bauer R, et al. *Planta Med*. 1988;54:426.

[3] Tyler V. *The New Honest Herbal*. Philadelphia: GF Stickley Co., 1987.

[4] Muller-Jakic B, et al. *Planta Med*. 1994;60(1):37-40.

[5] Melchart D, et al. *Phytomedicine*. 1994;1:245-254.

[6] Rochon P, et al. *JAMA*. 1994;272:108-113.

[7] Barrett B, et al. *J Fam Pract*. 1999;48:628-635. Review.

[8] Brinkeborn R, et al. *Phytomedicine*. 1999;6:1-5.

[9] Degenring F. *Schweiz Zschr Ganzheits Medizin*. 1995;2:88-94.

[10] Dorn M. *Complement Ther Med*. 1997;5:40-42.

[11] Henneicke-von Zepelin H, et al. *Curr Med Res Opin*. 1999;15(3):214-227.

[12] Hoheisel O, et al. *Eur J Clin Res*. 1997;9:261-268.

[13] Thom E, et al. *Phytother Res*. 1997;11:207-210.

[14] Melchart D, et al. *Arch Fam Med*. 1998;7:541-545.

[15] Turner R, et al. *Antimicrob Agents Chemother*. 2000;44(6):1708-1709.

[16] Grimm W, et al. *Am J Med*. 1999;106:138-143.

[17] Awang D, et al. *Can Pharm J*. 1991;124:512-516.

[18] Facino R, et al. *Farmaco*. 1993;48(10):1447-1461.

[19] Luettig B, et al. *J Nat Cancer Inst*. 1989;81(9):669-675.

[20] Coeugniet E, et al. *Onkologie*. 1987;10(suppl 3):27-33.

[21] Lersch C, et al. *Cancer Invest*. 1992;10(5):343–348.

[22] Facino R, et al. *Planta Med*. 1995;61:510-514.

[23] Blumenthal M, et al. (ed.) *The Complete German Commission E Monographs: Therapeutic Guide to Herbal Medicines*. Boston: American Botanical Council, 1998.

[24] Parnham M. *Phytomedicine*. 1996;3:95-102.

[25] www.aaaai.org/media/pressreleases/2000/03/000307.html.

[26] Mullins R. *Med J Aust*. 1998;168:170-171.

c

SCIENTIFIC NAME(S): *Sambucus canadensis* L. (American elder) and *Sambucus nigra* L. (European elder). Family: Caprifoliaceae

COMMON NAME(S): Sweet elder, common elder, elderberry, sambucus[1]

❧❧❧ PATIENT INFORMATION ❧❧❧

Uses: Elder flowers and berries have been used in flavorings and are considered to have diuretic and laxative properties.

Side Effects: There have been reports of toxicity, particularly involving the stems and leaves.

Dosing: A tea made from elder flowers has been used for coughs and colds, with a daily dosage of 10 to 15 g.[2]

BOTANY: The American elder is a tall shrub that grows to 3.6 m. It is native to North America. The European elder grows to approximately 9 m, and while native to Europe, it has been naturalized to the US.

HISTORY: Elder flowers and berries have been used in traditional medicine and as flavorings for centuries. In folk medicine, the flowers have been used for their diuretic and laxative properties and as an astringent. Various parts of the elder have been used to treat cancer and a host of other unrelated disorders.[3] Distilled elder flower water has been used as a scented vehicle for topical preparations and extracts are used to flavor foods, including alcoholic beverages. The fruits have been used to prepare elderberry wine.

PHARMACOLOGY: Elder flowers are considered to have diuretic and laxative properties; however, the specific compounds responsible for these activities have not been well established. The compound sambuculin A and a mixture of alpha- and beta-amyrin palmitate have been found to exhibit strong anti-hepatotoxic activity against liver damage induced experimentally by carbon tetrachloride.[4]

TOXICOLOGY: Because of the cyanogenic potential of the leaves, extracts of the plant may be used in foods, provided HCN levels do not exceed 25 ppm in the flavor. Toxicity in children who used pea shooters made from elderberry stems has been reported.[2]

One report of severe illness following the ingestion of juice prepared from elderberries has been recorded by the Centers for Disease Control.[5] People attending a picnic, who ingested several glasses of juice made from berries picked the day before, reported nausea, vomiting, weakness, dizziness, numbness, and stupor. One person who consumed 5 glasses of juice was hospitalized for stupor; all recovered. Although cyanide levels were not reported, there remains the possibility of cyanide-induced toxicity in these patients. While elderberries are safe to consume, particularly when cooked (uncooked berries may produce nausea), leaves and stems should not be crushed when making elderberry juice.

[1] Leung AY. *Encyclopedia of Common Natural Ingredients Used in Food, Drugs, and Cosmetics.* New York, NY: John Wiley and Sons, 1980.

[2] Gruenwald J, ed. *PDR for Herbal Medicines.* 2nd ed. Montvale, NJ: Thomson Medical Economics; 2000:288-289.

[3] Duke JA. *Handbook of Medicinal Herbs.* Boca Raton, FL: CRC Press, 1985.

[4] Lin C-N, Tome W-P. *Planta Med.* 1988;54(3):223.

[5] Anonymous. *MMWR.* 1984;33(13):173.

Eleutherococcus

SCIENTIFIC NAME(S): *Eleutherococcus senticosus* Maxim. *Acanthopanax senticosus* Rupr. et Maxim. *Hedera senticosa*. Family: Araliaceae

COMMON NAME(S): Devil's shrub, eleutheroccoc, shigoka, Siberian ginseng, touch-me-not, wild pepper

---

·:·:· PATIENT INFORMATION ·:·:·

Uses: Eleutherococcus is similar to ginseng in its properties and alleged effects. It has been used as a hypotensive, immunostimulant, energy enhancer, and aphrodisiac. Extracts of the roots have been used for a wide variety of therapeutic purposes in which they are said to have an adaptogenic effect. Although preparations from *E. senticosus* have been found to be effective against a variety of somatic disorders, the labels on OTC preparations do not supply adequate directions for taking the product or clarify the ingredients. In addition, standardization of the active ingredients is not clear. The German Commission E recommends limiting use to 3 months.

Side Effects: Although side effects appear to be rare, eleutherococcus should not be used by patients in febrile states, hypertensive crisis, or those with MI. Use is contraindicated in hypertensive patients. In some individuals it may produce drowsiness or nervousness.

Interactions: Possible assay interference with digoxin may occur; concomitant therapy increased digoxin level to greater than 5 mg/mL without symptoms of toxicity.

Dosing: As an adaptogen, eleutherococcus has been given as the powdered root in doses of 1 to 4 g/day. Extracts of *E. senticosus* are recommended at less than 1 g/day.[1,2]

BOTANY: *E. senticosus* belongs to the same family (Araliceae) as *Panax ginseng*. The geographical distribution of eleutherococcus coincides with the borders of the distribution of *P. ginseng*. Eleutherococcus is found in forests of broadleaf trees, broadleafs with spruce, and broadleafs with cedar. It grows at elevations of up to 800 m or more above sea level. The plant is a shrub, commonly attaining a height of 2 to 3 m or, less commonly, 5 to 7 m. It possesses gray or grayish-brown bark and numerous thin thorns. The leaves are long-stalked and palmate. Eleutherococcus has male and female forms with globular umbrella-shaped flowers. Male plants produce violet flowers, while female plants have yellowish flowers; the fruit takes the form of black, oval berries. Most commonly, the root is used in herbal medicine; however, it was found that leaves and berries also produce pharmacologically active metabolites. Because it is more abundant than Panox, it has become a popular substitute for ginseng.[3]

HISTORY: Eleutherococcus has been studied extensively in Russia. It is used as a health food in China, but Asian folk medicine has largely ignored eleutherococcus in favor of its relative, ginseng. As with ginseng, root extracts of the plant have been promoted as "adaptogens" that aid the body in responding to external (eg, environmental) and internal (eg, a disease) stress. The plant extracts have been used to normalize high or low blood pressure, to stimulate the immune system, and to increase work capacity. Reputed effects include increasing body energy levels, protection from motion sickness and against toxins, control of alloxan-induced diabetes, reduction of tumors, and control of atherosclerosis.[3,4]

PHARMACOLOGY:

Eleutherococcus extracts, like those of *P. ginseng*, bind to progestin, mineralocorticoid, and glucocorticoid receptors. In addition, eleutherococcus extracts bind to estrogen receptors. This may explain the observed glucocorticoid-like activity of the extracts.[5]

There is evidence of therapeutic benefits of eleutherococcus in humans. In 1 study of 36 healthy volunteers, a 3-times-daily injection of an ethanolic extract for 4 weeks produced increases in the absolute numbers of immunocompetent cells, particularly T-cells. The increase was most marked for helper/inducer cells, although cytotoxic and natural killer cells also increased in number. A general enhancement of the activation state of T-cells was evident.[6]

In hypotensive children between 7 and 10 years of age, an eleutherococcus extract improved subjective signs, significantly raised systolic and diastolic blood pressures, and increased total peripheral resistance.[7]

Other studies have described the wide range of eleutherococcus properties, including the effects on the human physical working capacity,[8] the immune systems of cancer patients,[9] the heart structure in MI,[10] malignant arrhythmias,[11] myocarditis and other coronary heart diseases,[12] radiation recovery,[13] diabetes,[14] hyperlipemia,[15] its antimicrobial actions,[16] prenatal prevention of congenital developmental anomalies in rats,[17] and enhanced proliferation of human lymphocytes.[18] Although preparations from *E. senticosus* have been found to be effective against a variety of somatic disorders, the labels on OTC preparations do not supply adequate directions for taking the product or clarify the ingredients.[19-21]

TOXICOLOGY:

There are possible estrogenic effects in females. Side effects, toxicity, contraindications, and warnings similar to those for *Panax* species (see ginseng) apply. Experience suggests that this product should not be used for people under the age of 40 and that only low doses be taken on a daily basis. Patients are advised to abstain from alcohol, sexual activity, bitter substances, and spicy foods. Avoid use during pregnancy and lactation. High doses of eleutherococcus are associated with irritability, insomnia, and anxiety. Other adverse effects include skin eruptions, headache, diarrhea, hypertension, and pericardial pain in rheumatic heart patients. Use of eleutherococcus extract has been associated with little or no toxicity. No pathologic, cytotoxic, or histologic changes were noted in mice that ingested infusions of the plant for up to 96 days.[22] In 1 human study, there were no side effects during the 6 months of follow-up.[6] However, use is not recommended for patients in febrile states, hypertensive crisis, or those with MI. Use is contraindicated in hypertensive patients. Rare reported side effects have included slight languor or drowsiness immediately after administration; this may be the result of a hypoglycemic effect of the extract.[4]

Most of the reviewed literature on eleutherococcus suggests that the plant preparations bear minimal toxicity and are fairly safe to use. There was a case in which an eleutherococcus preparation caused severe side effects, but it was later discovered that the preparation did not include eleutherococcus but rather another related species.[3,23,24]

[1] Asano K, et al. *Planta Med.* 1986;48:175-177.

[2] Dowling EA, et al. *Med Sci Sports Exerc.* 1996;28:482-489.

[3] Brekhman I, et al. *Man and Biologically Active Substances: The Effects of Drugs, Diet, and Pollution on Health.* Oxford: Pergamon Press, 1980.

[4] Brekhman I, et al. *Farmatsiia.* 1991;40(1):39.

[5] Pearce P, et al. *Endocrinol Jpn.* 1982;29(5):567-573.

[6] Bohn B, et al. *Arzneimittelforschung.* 1987;37(10):1193.

[7] Kaloeva, Z. *Farmakol Toksikol.* 1986;49(5):73.

[8] Asano K, et al. *Planta Med.* 1986;48(3):175.

[9] Kupin V, et al. *Vopr Onkol.* 1986;32(7):21.

[10] Afanas'eva T, et al. *Bull Eksper Bio Med.* 1987;103(2):212.

[11] Tian B, et al. *Chung Kuo Chun Yao Tsa Chih.* 1989;14(8):493-495.

[12] Shang Y, et al. *Chung Hsi i Chih Ho Tsa Chih.* 1991;11(5):280.

[13] Minkova M, et al. *Acta Physiol Pharmacol Bulg.* 1987;13(4):66-70.

[14] Molokovskii D, et al. *Probl Endokrinol.* 1989;35(6):82.

[15] Shi Z, et al. *Chung Hsi i Chieh Ho Tsa Chih.* 1990;10(3):155.

[16] Tarle D, et al. *Farma Glasnik.* 1993;49:161.

[17] Godeichuk T, et al *Ontogenez.* 1993;24(1):48.

[18] Borchers A, et al. *Int J Immunother.* 1998;14(3):143-52.

[19] http://www.19nordiol.com/nutrionline/ginseng51.html.

[20] http://www.enrich.com/us/prod_cat_eng/preprint_0251.html.

[21] http://www.tfnutrition.com/sportsnutrition/sibgin60.html.

[22] Lewis W, et al. *J Ethnopharmacol.* 1983;8(2):209.

[23] Wagner H, et al. *Phytomedicine.* 1994;1:63-76.

[24] Wagner H, et al. *Dtsch Apoth Ztg.* 1977;117:743.

Emblica

SCIENTIFIC NAME(S): *Phyllanthius emblica* (L.), *Emblica officinalis* Gaertn. Family: Euphorbiaceae

COMMON NAME(S): Indian gooseberry, Amla (Hindi), Amalaki (Sanskrit), Emblic Myrobalan (English)

ᴥᴥᴥ PATIENT INFORMATION ᴥᴥᴥ

Uses: Emblica has cholesterol-lowering, antimicrobial, anticancer, and anti-inflammatory effects.

Side Effects: No major toxicities have been reported.

Dosing: Emblic fruits often are taken in doses from 0.25 to 3 g/day as a source of vitamin C. There are no published clinical studies to support this dosage; however, it is a reasonable dose given the high vitamin C content of emblic fruits.

BOTANY: Emblica is a deciduous tree native to India and the Middle East. The round greenish-yellow fruits are commonly used in the Indian diet. Its leaves are feather-like with pale green flowers and are very high in vitamin C.[1]

HISTORY: Emblica is mentioned in an Ayurvedic text dating back to the 7th century.[1]

PHARMACOLOGY: Emblica has documented effects on cholesterol levels. In a clinical trial, normal and hypercholesterolemic men (35 to 55 years of age) given emblica supplementation experienced a decrease in serum cholesterol levels, which was reversible upon discontinuation of the drug.[2] The plant also has inhibited lipid peroxidation in biological membranes[3] and has displayed a protective effect in myocardial necrosis in rats.[4]

Ayurvedic medicine also employs emblica, in the form of fruit juice, as therapy for diabetic patients to strengthen the pancreas.[1] Current investigation in this area studied dogs with acute pancreatitis. The treated group showed less cell damage and marked inflammatory score decreases confirmed by microscopic examination.[5]

Emblica has also been studied for its anticancer and antimicrobial effects. It has inhibited induced mutagenesis in *Salmonella* strains.[6] In another study, the plant significantly inhibited dose-dependent hepatocarcinogenesis as measured by parameters such as tumor incidence, enzyme measurements, and other liver injury markers.[7] Alcoholic extracts of emblica showed activity against a number of test bacteria in another report.[8] In addition, the plant was effective against certain dermatophytes in another study.[9]

Other reported effects of emblica include the following: anti-inflammatory (in water fraction of methanol leaf extract),[10] dyspepsia treatment,[11] organ restoration, and treatment for eye problems, joint pain, diarrhea, and dysentery.[1]

TOXICOLOGY: No major reported toxicities have been associated with the fruit.

[1] Chevallier A. *Encyclopedia of Medicinal Plants.* New York, NY: DK Publishing 1996;202.

[2] Jacob A, et al. *Eur J Clin Nutr.* 1988;42(11):939-944.

[3] Kumar K, et al. *J Ethnopharmacol.* 1999;64(2):135-139.

[4] Tariq M, et al. *Indian J Exp Biol.* 1977;15(6):485-486.

[5] Thorat S, et al. *HPB Surg.* 1995;9(1):25-30.

[6] Grover I, et al. *Indian J Exp Biol.* 1989;27(3):207-209.

[7] Jeena K, et al. *Cancer Lett.* 1999;136(1):11-16.

[8] Nandi P, et al. *Br J Cancer.* 1997;76(10):1279-1283.

[9] Menon L, et al. *J Exp Clin Cancer Res.* 1997;16(4):365-368.

[10] Ahmad I, et al. *J Ethnopharmacol.* 1998;62(2):183-193.

[11] Dutta B, et al. *Mycoses.* 1998;41(11-12):535-536.

SCIENTIFIC NAME(S): *Oenothera biennis* L. Family: Onagraceae

COMMON NAME(S): Evening primrose, EPO, OEP

⚉⚉ PATIENT INFORMATION ⚉⚉

Uses: EPO has been used to treat cardiovascular disease, breast disorders, premenstrual syndrome, mastalgia, rheumatoid arthritis, multiple sclerosis, atopic eczema, dermatological disorders, and other illnesses.

Side effects: No adverse effects have been attributed to EPO.

Dosing: EPO has been administered orally in clinical trials for arthritis, atopic dermatitis, premenstrual syndrome (PMS), and diabetic neuropathy at doses between 3 and 6 g/day. The typical content of gamma-linolenic acid is 8% to 10% in the oil.[1-3]

BOTANY: The evening primrose is a large, delicate wildflower native to North America and is not a true primrose. The blooms usually last 1 evening. Primrose is an annual or biennial and can grow in height from 1 to 3 m. The flowers are yellow and the fruit is a dry pod about 5 cm long, which contains many small seeds.[4] The small seeds contain an oil characterized by its high content of gamma-linolenic acid (GLA).[5] Wild varieties of *O. biennis* contain variable amounts of linoleic acid and GLA; however, extensive cross-breeding has produced a commercial variety that consistently yields an oil with 72% cis-linoleic acid and 9% GLA. This is perhaps the richest plant source of GLA, although a commercially grown fungus has been reported to produce an oil containing 20% GLA and newer strains may produce even greater yields.[6]

PHARMACOLOGY: Essential fatty acids (EFAs) are important cellular structural elements and precursors of prostaglandins, which regulate metabolic functions.[4] EFAs are the biologically active parts of polyunsaturated fats. EFA ingestion is believed to help reduce the incidences of cardiovascular disease and obesity. EFAs cannot be manufactured by the body and must be provided by the diet in relatively large amounts. It has been recommended that

1% to 3% of total daily caloric intake be EFAs.[7] The World Health Organization recommends an increased level of 5% for children and pregnant or lactating women.[8]

Animal studies have shown that dietary EFA deprivation can lead to eczema-like lesions, hair loss, a generalized defect in connective tissue synthesis with poor wound healing, failure to respond immunologically to infection, infertility (especially in males), fatty degeneration of the liver, renal lesions with a lack of normal water balance, and atrophy of lacrimal and salivary exocrine glands. This suggests that human illnesses with similar symptoms may result in part from poor EFA metabolism or insufficient dietary EFA. Because EPO represents a rich source of EFAs, particularly GLA, its use has been suggested in the treatment of these deficiency syndromes. It has been postulated that GLA, DGLA (the prostaglandin precursor dl-homo-GLA), and arachidonic acid are present in human milk for an important and specific purpose.[9,10] It is believed that the conversion of linoleic acid to GLA in humans is a rate-limiting metabolic step,[11] with only a relatively small amount of dietary linoleic acid (LA) being converted to GLA and to other metabolites.[12] The delta-6-desaturase enzyme is required for this conversion.

Factors interfering with this GLA production include aging, diabetes, high alcohol intake, high fat diets, certain vitamin deficiencies, hormones, high cholesterol levels, and viral infections.[8] The essential fatty acids beyond this rate-limiting step are crucial for proper development of many body tissues, especially in the brain. The brain contains approximately 20% of 6-desaturated EFAs by weight. Infants cannot form an adequate amount of EFAs if linoleic acid is the only dietary source of n-6-EFA; this may be why preformed GLA, DGLA, and arachidonic acid are present in human milk. Studies have compared fatty acids in the phospholipids of red blood cells from infants fed human milk with those from infants fed commercial milk formulas. Infants fed commercial formulas showed phospholipids containing higher levels of linoleic acid and significantly lower levels of DGLA and arachidonic acid. Dietary supplementation to pregnant women with EPO results in an increase of total fat and EFA content in breast milk.[13] The presence of linoleic acid metabolites in human milk can affect the composition of red blood cell membranes.[14]

Taking large amounts (30 to 40 g/day) of linoleic acid has little effect on DGLA or arachidonic acid blood levels.[15-17] However, taking less than 500 mg GLA/day can produce a significant increase in DGLA concentration and a smaller increase in arachidonic acid in plasma phospholipids.[12] These elevated levels do not exceed normal amounts found in the US diet.[18] Therefore, GLA, not linoleic acid, is capable of elevating the levels of linoleic acid metabolites in human blood. Below-normal plasma or adipose-tissue concentrations of GLA, DGLA, or arachidonic acid may occur in the following: healthy middle-aged men who will later develop heart disease;[19-22] healthy middle-aged people who will later suffer stroke;[23] diabetic patients;[24,25] patients with atopic dermatitis;[25-27] heavy drinkers;[28,29] females with premenstrual syndrome;[30] and older people.[31,32]

Cardiovascular disease: Linoleic acid can reduce elevated serum cholesterol levels, but GLA has cholesterol-lowering activity about 170 times greater than the parent compound.[33] In 79 patients who took 4 g *Efamol*/day in a placebo controlled study, a significant ($P < 0.001$) decrease of approximately 32% in serum cholesterol was noted after 3 months of treatment. A nonsignificant (NS) decrease was observed in the placebo group.[34] In some studies, GLA has lowered plasma cholesterol and triglycerides and inhibited in vivo platelet aggregation.[35] Elevated plasma lipids and in vivo platelet aggregation are risk factors for heart disease and stroke, and GLA lowers both of these.[36] In a report of 20 hyperlipidemic patients, 2.4 to 7.2 mL/day of primrose oil (containing 9% GLA) was administered. There were no changes in serum cholesterol, HDL cholesterol, or triglyceride levels.[37]

Breast cancer and related disorders: Improvement in serum fatty acid levels by EPO supplementation in women with benign breast disorders has not been associated with a clinical response.[38] In women with proven recurrent breast cysts, EPO treatment for 1 year resulted in a slightly lower (NS) recurrence rate compared with placebo.[39]

PMS and mastalgia: Clinical studies investigating EPO use in these conditions have had positive results. It has been suggested that an abnormal sensitivity to prolactin or a deficiency of PGE1 (thought to attenuate the biologic activity of prolactin) may contribute to PMS. Levels of GLA and subsequent metabolites were lower in women with PMS than in controls, indicating a possible defect in the conversion of linoleic acid to GLA. This may result in an exceptional sensitivity to normal changes in prolactin levels.[40] In 19 PMS patients receiving evening primrose oil each morning and evening during the last 14 days before menstruation for 5 consecutive cycles, PMS symptoms were decreased. The greatest effect was seen during the fifth cycle.[41]

PMS and breast pain are common with high fat intake. Women with breast pain may be unable to convert LA to GLA.[8] In some studies, PMS and premenstrual breast pain (cyclic mastalgia) have been relieved by GLA to a significantly greater degree than with placebo.[42] However, a placebo-controlled evaluation of EPO found the oil to have no effect and that the effects observed in women with moderate PMS were solely due to a placebo effect.[43]

A number of clinical studies have evaluated the effect of EPO in women with nodular or polycystic breast disease. Treatments with agents such as bromocriptine, danazol, or EPO have been associated with improvement in breast pain in up to 77% of patients with cyclical mastalgia and 44% of those with noncyclical mastalgia.[44]

Rheumatoid arthritis: A double-blind, placebo-controlled study investigated the effects of altering dietary EFAs on requirements for nonsteroidal anti-inflammatory drugs (NSAIDs) in patients with rheumatoid arthritis. The major aim was to determine whether EPO or EPO/fish oil could replace NSAIDs. An initial 1-year treatment period was followed by 3 months of placebo. At 1 year, EPO and EPO/fish oil produced significant subjective improvement compared with placebo. Furthermore, by 1 year, the patients taking EPO or EPO/fish oil had significantly reduced their use of NSAIDs. Following 3 months of placebo, those receiving initial NSAID treatment had relapsed. Despite decreased NSAID use, measures of disease activity did not worsen. However, there was no evidence that EPO and EPO/fish oil acted as disease-modifying agents.[45] EPO therapy for rheumatoid arthritis requires longer than 3 months for any beneficial effects.[8] A study of EPO vs olive oil found that EPO use resulted in a significant reduction in morning stiffness after 3 months.[46]

Multiple sclerosis (MS): In MS there is abnormality in EFA metabolism and lymphocytic function. Several studies have shown slight but variable improvement in patients fed diets high in linoleic acid. In an open trial of EPO, 3 of 8 patients with MS showed improvement in the manual dexterity test, but no improvement was noted in grip strength. When the oil was given with colchicine, 4 of 6 patients improved in their general physical tone.[47] Others have noted similar improvement with GLA therapy.[48-50]

Atopic dermatitis and dermatologic disorders: In atopic dermatitis, GLA was more effective than placebo in improving skin condition, providing relief from pruritus, and allowing reduced reliance on corticosteroid medication.[51,52] Other reports exist (most double-blind, crossover, randomized, or placebo-controlled) that evaluate EPO in atopic dermatitis treatment. All reports suggest improvement in atopic eczema, regarding factors such as itch, scaling, disease severity, grade of inflammation, percent of body surface area involvement, dryness, erythema, and surface damage.[51-56] Women with "premenstrual flare" of eczema reported improvement in their condition.[56] A meta-analysis involving 311 patients (1 to 60 years of age) in 9 randomized, double-blind, placebo-controlled studies determined EPO to be more effective than placebo.[57]

A defect in the function of delta-6-desaturase, the enzyme responsible for the conversion of linoleic acid to GLA, has been found in patients with atopic dermatitis.[58] Forty-eight children (2 to 8 years of age) administered 0.5 g/kg/day of EPO showed significant improvement in disease severity independent of whether the patients had IgE-mediated allergy manifestations. EPO also increased content of n-6 fatty acids in red blood cell membranes, without affecting membrane microviscosity.[59] EPO doses of 6 g/day in a double-blind, placebo-controlled study of 102 patients improved the lipid profile of the epidermis in patients with atopic dermatitis[60] but it was not effective in treatment of the disease itself.[1]

Other diseases: In diabetic patients, GLA reversed neurological damage.[61] GLA supplementation to children with Type 1 diabetes mellitus (insulin-dependent diabetes mellitus) indicated that favorable and statistically significant increases in serum essential fatty acid levels and decreases in PGE2 levels occurred, which may provide a therapeutic benefit.[62] One study demonstrated that GLA accelerated recovery of liver function in alcoholics and reduced the severity of withdrawal symptoms.[29]

EPO has been tested for use in diagnosis and symptom relief of myalgic encephalomyelitis (Tapanui flu).[63] EPO may prevent or slow the development of hypertension in pregnancy by its pressor response to angiotensin II.[64] In combination therapy, 3 patients with Crohn disease remained in relapse-free remission after EPO administration.[65]

The value of a drug that is effective in a wide variety of EFA-deficiency disorders cannot be overstated. The treatment of several unique medical conditions with EPO has been undertaken, often with excellent results. Many of the published studies have been open trials that require confirmation through double-blind testing; however, these studies generally have been well designed and their results adequately analyzed. The disorders treated include autoimmune diseases, childhood hyperactivity, chronic inflammation, ethanol-induced toxicity and acute alcohol withdrawal syndrome, ichthyosis vulgaris, scleroderma, Sjogren syndrome, and Sicca syndrome, brittle nails, mastalgia, psychiatric syndromes, tardive dyskinesia, ulcerative colitis, and migraine headaches. GLA has shown in vitro antitumor activity against primary liver cancer cells, but this effect was not demonstrated in a clinical trial.[66] Reviews of evening primrose oil are listed in the bibliography.[67-77]

TOXICOLOGY: As a nutritional supplement, the maximum label-recommended daily dose of EPO is approximately 4 g. This dose contains 300 to 360 mg GLA, which contributes: (1) 6 to 7 mg GLA/kg/day likely to be produced from linoleic acid in the healthy adult female, (2) 23 to 65 mg GLA/kg/day consumed by a breastfed baby, or (3) 70 to 400 mg/kg/day of all the metabolites of linoleic acid consumed by a breastfed infant. According to these estimates, the amounts of GLA in the recommended doses of EPO are in the same range as the amounts of GLA and other related EFAs present in widely consumed foods. Thus, there is little concern about the safety of EPO as a dietary supplement in the recommended dosage range. In toxicological studies carried out for 1 year, EPO at doses up to 2.5 mL/kg/day in rats and 5 mL/kg/day in dogs was found to possess no toxic properties. Similar results were obtained in 2-year carcinogenicity and teratological investigations. With about 1000 tons of EPO sold in several countries as a nutritional supplement since the 1970s, there have been no complaints concerning the safety of the product.

[1] Blumenthal M, et al. *Popular Herbs in the U.S. Market. Therapeutic Monographs.* American Botanical Council, 1997.

[2] Budeiri D, et al. *Control Clin Trials.* 1996;17:60-68.

[3] Berth-Jones J. *Lancet.* 1993;341(Jun 19):1557-1560.

[4] Leung A. *Encyclopedia of Common Natural Ingredients.* 2nd ed. New York, NY: John Wiley, 1996.

[5] DerMarderosian A, et al. *Natural Product Medicine.* Philadelphia, PA: George F. Stickley Co., 1988.

[6] *Market Letter.* 1986;Aug 4:21.

[7] Horrobin DF. *Holistic Med.* 1981;3:118.

[8] Winther M. *Nat Pharm.* 1996;(Oct/Nov):8-9,27.

[9] Clandinin M, et al. *Lipid Res.* 1982;20:901.

[10] Crawford MA. *Progr Food Nutr Sci.* 1980;4:755.7

[11] Brenner RR. *Progr Lipid Res.* 1982;20:41.

[12] Manku MS, et al. *Eur J Clin Nutr.* 1988;42:55.

[13] Cant A, et al. *J Nutr Sci Vitaminol.* 1991;37:573.

[14] Putnam JC, et al. *Am J Clin Nutr.* 1982;36:106.

[15] Dayton S, et al. *J Lipid Res.* 1966;7:103.

[16] Lasserre M, et al. *Lipids.* 1983;20:227.

[17] Singer P, et al. *Prostaglandins Leukotr Med.* 1984;15(2):159.

[18] Holman RT. *Am J Clin Nutr.* 1979;32:2390.

[19] Horrobin DF, Huang YR. *Intl J Cardiol.* 1987;17:241.

[20] Miettinen TA, et al. *Br Med J.* 1982;285:993.

[21] Salonen JT, et al. *Am J Cardiol.* 1985;58:226.

[22] Wood DA, et al. *Lancet.* 1984;2:117.

[23] Miettinen TA. *Monogr Atheroscler.* 1986;4:19.

[24] Jones DB, et al. *Br Med J.* 1983;286:178.

[25] Mercuri O, et al. *Biochem Biophys Acta.* 1988;116:407.

[26] Manku MS, et al. *Br J Dermatol.* 1984;110:643.

[27] Strannegard IL, et al. *Intl Arch Allergy Appl Immunol.* 1987;82:423.

[28] Glen L, et al. *Clin Exp Res.* 1987;11:37.

[29] Nervi AM, et al. *Lipids.* 1980;15:263.

[30] Bruch MG, et al. *Am J Obstet Gynecol.* 1984;150:363.

[31] Darcet P, et al. *Ann Nutr Alim.* 1980;34:277.

[32] Horrobin DF. *Rev Pure Appl Pharmacol Sci.* 1983;4:339.

[33] Horrobin DF, Manku MS. *Lipids.* 1983;18:558.

[34] Horrobin DF, Manku MS. Intern conference on oils, fats, and waxes 1983, Auckland, New Zealand.

[35] van Doormal JJ, et al. *Diabetologia.* 1986;29:A603.

[36] Puolaka J, et al. *J Reprod Med.* 1985;30:149.

[37] Viikari J, et al. *Int J Clin Pharmacol Ther Toxicol.* 1986;24(Dec):668-670.

[38] Gateley CA, et al. *Br J Surg.* 1992;79:407.

[39] Mansel RE, et al. *Ann NY Acad Sci.* 1990;586:288.

[40] Horrobin DF. Abstract, Int. Symposium on Premenstrual Tension and Dysmenorrhea (1983), Charleston, SC.

[41] Larsson B, et al. *Curr Ther Res.* 1989;46(Jul):58-63.

[42] Pye J, et al. *Lancet.* 1985;2(Aug 17):373-377.

[43] Khoo S, et al. *Med J Aust.* 1990;153(Aug 20):189-192.

[44] Gateley CA, Mansel RE. *Br Med Bull.* 1991;47:284.

[45] Belch JJF, et al. *Ann Rheum Dis.* 1988;47:96.

[46] Brzeski M, et al. *Br J Rheumatol.* 1991;30:370.

[47] Horrobin DF. *Med Hypoth.* 1979;5:365.

[48] Field EF. *Lancet.* 1978;1:780

[49] Millar JHD, et al. *Br Med J.* 1973;1:765.

[50] Field EF, Joyce G. *Eur Neurol.* 1983;22:78.

[51] Schalin-Karrila M. *Br J Dermatol.* 1987;117:11.

[52] Wright S, Burton JL. *Lancet.* 1982;2:1120.

[53] Lovell C, et al. *Lancet.* 1981;1(Jan 31):278.

[54] Bordoni A, et al. *Drugs Exp Clin Res.* 1988;14(4):291-297.

[55] Biagli P, et al. *Drugs Exp Clin Res.* 1988;14(4):285-290.

[56] Humphreys F, et al. *Eur J Dermatol.* 1994;4(8):598-603.

[57] Morse P, et al. *Br J Dermatol.* 1989;121(Jul):75-90.

[58] Kerscher MJ, Horting HC. *Clin Investig.* 1992;70:167.

[59] Biagli P, et al. *Drugs Exp Clin Res.* 1994;20(2):77-84.

[60] Schafer L, Kragballe K. *Lipids.* 1991;26:557.

[61] Jamal GA. *Lancet.* 1986;1:1098.

[62] Arisaka M, et al. *Prostaglandins Leukot Essent Fatty Acids.* 1991;43:197.

[63] Simpson L. *N Z Pharm.* 1985;5(Jan):14.

[64] O'Brien P, et al. *Br J Clin Pharmacol.* 1985;19(Mar):335-342.

[65] Novak E. *Can Med Assoc J.* 1988;139(Jul 1):14.

[66] van der Merwe CF, et al. *Prostaglandins Leukot Essent Fatty Acids.* 1990;40:199.

[67] Ballentine C, et al. *FDA Consumer.* 1987;21(Nov):34-35.

[68] Sinclair B. *N Z Pharm.* 1988;8(Jan):28-29,31.

[69] Barber A. *Pharm J.* 1988;240(Jun 4):723-725.

[70] Anonymous. *S Afr Pharm J.* 1989;56(Feb):55-75.

[71] Barber A. *Ir Pharm Union Rev.* 1989;14(Apr):121-122,124.

[72] Kleijnen J. *Pharm Weekbl.* 1989;124(Jun 9):418-423.

[73] Po A. *Pharm J.* 1991;246(Jun 1):676-678.

[74] Pittit J. *Ir Pharm Union Rev.* 1991;16(Oct):248,250-251, 253-256,258-259.

[75] Anonymous. *Ir Pharm Union Rev.* 1992;17(Sep):199,201.

[76] Docherty M. *Aust J Pharm.* 1994;75(Jan):48-53.

[77] Kleijnen J. *Br Med J.* 1994;309(Oct 1):824-825.

SCIENTIFIC NAME(S): *Chamaelirium luteum* (L.) Gray, Family: Liliaceae (Lilies)

COMMON NAME(S): False unicorn, helonias root, devil's bit, blazing star, drooping starwort, rattlesnake, fairy-wand

---

❧❧❧ PATIENT INFORMATION ❧❧❧

Uses: Historically, false unicorn has been used as a uterine tonic for treatment of amenorrhea and morning sickness, as an appetite stimulant, diuretic, vermifuge, emetic, and insecticide.

Side effects: False unicorn can be emetic at high doses. Safety has not been established during pregnancy.

Dosing: Traditional doses of false unicorn root are 2 g as a uterine tonic or diuretic; however, no clinical studies have been performed to support a particular dose.

BOTANY: *Chamaelirium luteum* is a native lily of the eastern US. It is considered a threatened species because of a loss of habitat and effects of collection from the wild for herbal use. Cultivation is considered possible, but has not yet become commercially important. The root is collected in autumn. *C. luteum* is a dioecious species (ie, the male and female flowers are borne on separate plants). The plant has been confused with the lilies *Helonias bullata* and *Aletris farinosa* (true unicorn root), because of several shared common names.[1-3]

HISTORY: False unicorn root was used by the Eclectic medical movement of the late 19th and early 20th centuries. Its chief use for female complaints or as a uterine tonic in the treatment of amenorrhea or morning sickness. It has also been used for appetite stimulation and as a diuretic, vermifuge, emetic, and insecticide.[2-6]

PHARMACOLOGY: The fluid extract of false unicorn root was examined for its effects on isolated guinea pig uterus; however, no stimulant or relaxant effect was detected.[7,8,9] Similar experiments in the intact dog were also negative.[10] One observation suggests that false unicorn root may act through increasing human chorionic gonadotropin.[11] Nevertheless, a water extract did not block gonadotropin release in the rat.[12] The notion that the occurrence of diosgenin might be responsible for hormonal effects is incorrect because the parent saponin is unlikely to be hydrolyzed to a free sterol in vivo. An understanding of false unicorn root's effects must await additional studies.

TOXICOLOGY: False unicorn root is emetic at high doses. Cattle have died from consumption of the plant.[4] The safety of the plant for use in pregnancy has not been established.

[1] Clause E. *Pharmacognosy,* 3d ed. Philadelphia, PA: Lea & Febiger, 1956.

[2] Foster S. *Herbs for Health.* 1999 Jan/Feb;22.

[3] Grieve M. *A Modern Herbal.* London, England: Jonathan Cape, 1931.

[4] Meyer C. *The Herbalist,* 3rd ed. 1976.

[5] Harding Ar. *Ginseng and Other Medicinal Plants.* Columbus, OH: A.R. Harding Publishing Co., 1908.

[6] Brinker FA. *J Naturopathic Med.* 1997;7(1):11.

[7] Pilcher JD. *J Am Med Assoc.* 1916;67:490.

[8] Pilcher JD, et al. *Arch Intern Med.* 1916;18:557.

[9] Pilcher JD. *J Pharmacol.* 1916;8:110.

[10] Pilcher JD, et al. *Surg Gynecol Obstet.* 1918;27:97.

[11] Brandt D. A clinician's view. *HerbalGram.* 1996;36:75.

[12] Graham RCB, et al. *Endocrinology.* 1955;56:239.

Fennel

SCIENTIFIC NAME(S): *Foeniculum vulgare* Mill. syn. F. *officinale* All. and *Anethum foeniculum.* Family: Apiaceae (Umbelliferae). A number of subspecies have been identified and their names add to the potential confusion surrounding the terminology of these plants.

COMMON NAME(S): Common, sweet or bitter fennel, carosella, Florence fennel, finocchio, garden fennel, large fennel, wild fennel[1,2]

❧❧❧❧ PATIENT INFORMATION ❧❧❧❧

Uses: Fennel has been used as a flavoring, scent, insect repellent, herbal remedy for poisoning and Gastrointestinal conditions, and as a stimulant to promote lactation and menstruation.

Side Effects: Fennel may cause photodermatitis, contact dermatitis, and cross reactions. The oil may induce hallucinations and seizures. Poison hemlock is sometimes mistaken for fennel.

Dosing: Fennel seed and fennel seed oil have been used as stimulant and carminative agents in doses of 5 to 7 g and 0.1 to 0.6 mL, respectively.[3]

BOTANY: Fennel is an herb native to southern Europe and Asia Minor. It is cultivated in the US, Great Britain, and temperate areas of Eurasia. All parts of the plant are aromatic. When cultivated, fennel stalks grow to a height of approximately 90 cm. Plants have finely divided leaves composed of many linear or awl-shaped segments. Grayish, compound umbels bear small, yellowish flowers. The fruits or seeds are oblong ovals approximately 6 mm long and greenish or yellowish brown; they have 5 prominent dorsal ridges. The seeds have a taste resembling that of anise. Besides *F. vulgare*, *F. dulce* ("carosella") is grown for its stalks, while *F. vulgare* var *azoricum* Thell. ("finocchio") is grown for its bulbous stalk bases.

HISTORY: According to Greek legend, man received knowledge from Mount Olympus as a fiery coal enclosed in a stalk of fennel. The herb was known to the ancient Chinese, Indian, Egyptian, and Greek civilizations, and Pliny recommended it for improving the eyesight. The name *foeniculum* is from the Latin word for "fragrant hay." Fennel was in great demand during the Middle Ages. The rich added the seed to fish and vegetable dishes, while the poor reserved it as an appetite suppressant. The plant was introduced to North America by Spanish priests and the English brought it to their early settlements in Virginia.[4] All parts of the plant have been used for flavorings, and the stalks eaten as a vegetable. The seeds serve as a traditional carminative. Fennel has been used to flavor candies, liqueurs, medicines, and food, especially pastries, sweet pickles, and fish. The oil can be used to protect stored fruits and vegetables against infection by pathogenic fungi.[5] Beekeepers have grown it as a honey plant.[4] Health claims have included its use as a purported antidote to poisonous herbs, mushrooms, and snakebites,[6] and for the treatment of gastroenteritis, indigestion, to stimulate lactation, and as an expectorant and emmenagogue.[1] Tea made from crushed fennel seeds has been used as an eyewash.[4] Powdered fennel is said to drive fleas away from kennels and stables.[5]

PHARMACOLOGY: As an herbal medicine, fennel is reputed to increase milk secretion, promote menstruation, facilitate birth, ease the male climacteric, and increase the libido. These supposed properties led to research on fennel for the development of synthetic estrogens during the 1930s. The principal estrogenic component of fennel was originally thought to be anethole, but it is now believed to be a polymer of anethole, such as dianethole or photoanethole.[7] The volatile oil of fennel increases the phasic contraction of ileal and tracheal smooth muscle in the guinea pig. The effect was generally greater with ileal muscle.[8]

TOXICOLOGY: Administration of the volatile oil to rats has exacerbated experimentally-induced liver damage.[9] Ingestion of the volatile oil may induce nausea, vomiting, seizures, and pulmonary edema.[10] Its therapeutic use in Morocco has occasionally induced epileptiform madness and hallucinations.[5] The principal hazards with fennel itself are photodermatitis and contact dermatitis. Some individuals exhibit cross-reactivity to several species of Apiaceae, characteristic of the so-called celery-carrot-mugwort-condiment syndrome.[11] Rare allergic reactions have been reported following the ingestion of fennel.

Fennel oil was found to be genotoxic in the *Bacillus subtilis* DNA-repair test.[12] Estragole, present in the volatile oil, has been shown to cause tumors in animals.

A survey of fennel samples in Italy found viable aerobic bacteria, including coliforms, fecal streptococci, and *Salmonella* species, suggesting the plant may serve as a vector of infectious GI diseases.[13]

A serious hazard associated with fennel is that poison hemlock can easily be mistaken for the herb. Hemlock contains highly narcotic coniine, and a small amount of hemlock juice can cause vomiting, paralysis, and death.[6]

[1] Locock RA. *CPJ/RPC*. 93/94;12/1:503.

[2] Meyer JE. *The Herbalist*. Hammond, IN: Hammond Book Co., 1934.

[3] Blumenthal M, eds. *Herbal Medicine: Expanded Commission E Monographs*. Newton, MA: Integrative Medicine Communications; 2000.

[4] Dobelis IN, ed. *Magic and Medicine of Plants*. Pleasantville, NY: Reader's Digest Assoc., 1986.

[5] Duke JA. *Handbook of Medicinal Herbs*. Boca Raton, FL: CRC Press, 1985.4

[6] Loewenfeld C, et al. *The Complete Book of Herbs and Spices*. London: David E. Charles, 1974.

[7] Albert-Puleo M. *J Ethnopharmacol*. 1980;2:337.

[8] Reiter M, et al. *Arzneimittelforsch*. 1985;35(1A):408.

[9] Gershbein LL. *Food Cosmet Toxicol*. 1977;15:173.

[10] Marcus C, et al. *J Agric Food Chem*. 1979;27:1217.

[11] Wuthrich B, et al. *Dtsch Med Wochenschr*. 1984;109:981.

[12] Sekizawa J, et al. *Mutat Res*. 1982;101:127.

[13] Ercolani GL. *Appl Environ Microbiol*. 1976;31:847.

Feverfew

SCIENTIFIC NAME(S): *Tanacetum parthenium* Schulz-Bip. synonymous with *Chrysanthemum parthenium* L. Bernh., *Leucanthemum parthenium* (L.) Gren and Godron, and *Pyrethrum parthenium* (L.) Sm.[1] Alternately described as a member of the genus *Matricaria*. Family: Asteraceae/Compositae

COMMON NAME(S): Feverfew, featherfew, altamisa, bachelor's button, featherfoil, febrifuge plant, midsummer daisy, nosebleed, Santa Maria, wild chamomile, wild quinine[2-5]

➹➹➹ PATIENT INFORMATION ➹➹➹

Uses: Traditionally an antipyretic, feverfew has been used in recent times to avert migraines and relieve menstrual pain, asthma, dermatitis, and arthritis.

Drug Interactions: Possible interaction with anticoagulants.

Side Effects: Patients withdrawn from feverfew experienced a syndrome of ill effects. Most adverse effects of treatment with feverfew are mild, although some patients experience increased heart rate. Feverfew should not be used by pregnant or lactating women or children under 2 years of age.

Dosing: Feverfew generally is given for migraine at a daily dose of 50 to 150 mg of dried leaves. While some products have been standardized for parthenolide content (0.2 to 0.6 mg/dose), this compound has not been confirmed as a major active principle for migraine.[6-9]

BOTANY: A short bushy perennial that grows from 15 to 60 cm tall along fields and roadsides, the feverfew's yellow-green leaves and yellow flowers resemble those of chamomile (*Matricaria chamomilla*). The flowers bloom from July to October.

HISTORY: The herb feverfew has had a long history of use in traditional and folk medicine, especially among Greek and early European herbalists. However, during the last few hundred years feverfew had fallen into general disuse, until recently.[10] It has now become popular as a prophylactic treatment for migraine headaches and its extracts have been claimed to relieve menstrual pain, asthma, dermatitis, and arthritis. Traditionally, the herb has been used as an antipyretic, from which its common name is derived. The leaves are ingested, fresh or dried, with a typical daily dose of 2 to 3 leaves. These are bitter and are often sweetened before ingestion. It has also been planted around houses to purify the air because of its strong, lasting odor. A tincture of its blossoms doubles as an insect repellant and balm for insect bites.[3] It was once used as an antidote for overindulgence in opium.[2]

PHARMACOLOGY: Feverfew extracts affect a wide variety of physiologic pathways.

In vitro: Feverfew may inhibit prostaglandin synthesis. Extracts of the aboveground portions of the plant suppress prostaglandin production; leaf extracts inhibit prostaglandin production; however, this effect is not moderated by cyclooxygenase.[11]

Aqueous extracts prevent the release of arachidonic acid and inhibit in vitro aggregation of platelets stimulated by adenosine diphosphate (ADP) or thrombin.[12] It is controversial whether these extracts block the synthesis of thromboxane, a prostaglandin involved in platelet aggregation.[13,14] Data suggest that feverfew's mechanism of prostaglandin synthesis inhibition differs from that of the salicylates. Extracts may inhibit platelet behavior via effects on platelet sulfhydryl groups.[15,16]

Feverfew extracts are potent inhibitors of serotonin release from platelets and polymorphonuclear leucocyte granules, providing a plausible connection between the claimed benefit of feverfew in migraines and arthritis. Feverfew may produce an antimigraine effect similar to methysergide maleate (*Sansert*), a known serotonin antagonist.[17,18] Extracts of the plant also inhibit the release of enzymes from white cells found in inflamed joints (a similar antiinflammatory effect may occur in the skin) providing a rationale for the use of feverfew in psoriasis.

In addition, feverfew extracts inhibit phagocytosis, the deposition of platelets on collagen surfaces, and mast cell release of histamine,[19] exhibit antithrombotic potential and cytotoxic activity,[20] and have in vitro antibacterial activity. Monoterpenes in the plant may exert insecticidal activity, and alpha-pinene derivatives may possess sedative and mild tranquilizing effects.

Clinical Uses: Much interest has been focused on the activity of feverfew in the treatment and prevention of migraine headaches.[21] The first account of its use as a preventative for migraine appeared in 1978 about a woman who had suffered from severe migraine since 16 years of age. At the age of 68, she began using 3 leaves of feverfew daily, and after 10 months her headaches ceased altogether. This case prompted studies by Dr. E. Stewart Johnson.[10]

A study in 8 feverfew-treated patients and 9 placebo-controlled patients found that fewer headaches were reported by patients taking feverfew for up to 6 months of treatment. Patients in both groups had self-medicated with feverfew for several years before enrolling in the study. The incidence of headaches remained constant in those patients taking feverfew but increased almost 3-fold in those switched to placebo during the trial ($P < 0.02$).[6] Abrupt discontinuation of feverfew in patients switched to placebo caused incapacitating headaches in some patients. Nausea and vomiting were reduced in patients taking feverfew. The statistical analysis has been questioned but the results provide a unique insight into the activity of feverfew.[22] These results were confirmed in a more recent placebo-controlled study[7] It was predicted that feverfew will be useful not only for the classical migraine and cluster headache, but for premenstrual, menstrual, and other headaches as well.[23]

However, some studies found that the experimental observations may not be clinically relevant to migraine patients taking feverfew.[24] Ten patients who had taken extracts of the plant for up to 8 years to control migraine headaches were evaluated for physiologic changes. The platelets of all treated patients aggregated characteristically to ADP and thrombin and similarly to those of control patients. However, aggregation in response to serotonin was greatly attenuated in the feverfew users.

Canada's Health Protection Branch has granted a Drug Identification Number (DIN) for a British feverfew (*Tanacetum parthenium*) product. This allows the manufacturer, Herbal Laboratories, Ltd., to claim, as a nonprescription drug, the product's effectiveness in the prevention of migraine headache. Canada's Health Protection Branch recommends a daily dosage of 125 mg of a dried feverfew leaf preparation, from authenticated *Tanacetum parthenium* containing at least 0.2% parthenolide for the prevention of migraine.[25]

TOXICOLOGY: In one study, patients received 50 mg/day, roughly equivalent to 2 leaves.[6] Adverse effects during

6 months of continued feverfew treatment were mild and did not result in discontinuation. Four of the 8 patients taking the plant had no adverse effects. Heart rate increased by up to 26 beats/min in 2 treated patients. There were no differences between treatment groups in laboratory test results.

Patients who were switched to placebo after taking feverfew for several years experienced a cluster of nervous system reactions (rebound of migraine symptoms, anxiety, poor sleep patterns) along with muscle and joint stiffness, which was referred to as "postfeverfew syndrome."

In a larger series of feverfew users, 18% reported adverse effects, the most troublesome being mouth ulceration (11%). Feverfew can induce more widespread inflammation of the oral mucosa and tongue, often with lip swelling and loss of taste.[6] Dermatitis has been associated with this plant.[19,26]

The leaves of the plant have been shown to possess potential emmenagogue activity and is not recommended for pregnant or lactating mothers or children younger than 2 years of age.[25] Although an interaction with anticoagulants is undocumented, this may be clinically important in sensitive patients.

Analysis of the frequency of chromosomal aberrations and sister chromatid exchanges in circulating lymphocytes from patients who ingested feverfew for 11 months did not find any aberrations, which suggested that the plant does not induce chromosomal abnormalities.[27]

[1] Awang DVC. *Can Pharm J.* 1989;122:266.

[2] Duke JA. *Handbook of Medicinal Herbs.* Boca Raton, FL: CRC Press, 1985.

[3] Dobelis IN, ed. *Magic and Medicine of Plants.* Pleasantville, NY: Reader's Digest Assoc., 1986.

[4] Meyer JE. *The Herbalist.* Hammond, IN: Hammond Book Co., 1934.4

[5] Castleman M. *The Healing Herbs.* Emmaus, PA: Rodale Press, 1991.

[6] Johnson ES, et al. *BMJ.* 1985;291:569.

[7] Murphy JJ, et al. *Lancet.* 1988;2:189.

[8] Pattrick M, et al. *Ann Rheum Dis.* 1989;48:547-549.

[9] Palevitch D, et al. *Phytother Res.* 1997;11:508-511.

[10] Hobbs C. *National Headache Foundation Newsletter.* Winter 1990:11.

[11] Collier HOJ, et al. *Lancet.* 1980;2:922.

[12] Loecshe EW, et al. *Folia Haematol.* 1988;115:181.

[13] Makheja AN, et al. *Lancet.* 1981;2:1054.

[14] Heptinstall S, et al. *Lancet.* 1985;1:1071.

[15] Heptinstall S, et al. *J Pharm Pharmacol.* 1987;39:459.

[16] Voyno-Yesenetskaya TA, et al. *J Pharm Pharmacol.* 1988;40:501.

[17] Tyler VE. *The New Honest Herbal.* Philadelphia, PA: GF Stickley Co., 1987.

[18] Olin BR, Hebel SK, eds. *Drug Facts and Comparisons.* St. Louis: Facts and Comparisons, 1991(Oct):257.

[19] Hayes NA, et al. *J Pharm Pharmacol.* 1987;39:466.

[20] Hobbs C. *HerbalGram.* 1989;20:26.

[21] *Lancet.* 1985;1:1084.

[22] Waller PC, et al. *BMJ.* 1985;291:1128.

[23] Hobbs C. *National Headache Foundation Newsletter.* Winter 1990:10.

[24] Biggs, et al. *Lancet.* 1982;2:776.

[25] Awang DVC. *HerbalGram.* 1993;29:34.

[26] Vickers HR. *BMJ.* 1985;291:827.

[27] Anderson D, et al. *Human Toxicol.* 1988;7:145.

SCIENTIFIC NAME(S): *Linum usitatissimum* L. Family: Linaceae

COMMON NAME(S): Flax, flaxseed, linseed, lint bells,[1] linum

---

♨♨♨ PATIENT INFORMATION ♨♨♨

Uses: Linseed oil, derived from flaxseed, has been used as a topical demulcent and emollient, laxative, and as treatment for coughs, colds, and urinary tract infections. Although there are no clinical trials to support these uses, flaxseed cakes have been used as cattle feed. Limited research suggests dietary flaxseed may improve blood lipid profile.

Side Effects: Ingestion of large amounts may be harmful. Many workers exposed to flax show immunologically positive antigens.

Dosing: Flax seed has been given in clinical trials for serum lipid control and other indications at doses from 5 to 50 g/day. Flax seed oil has been given at doses of 3 to 6 g/day.[2-6]

BOTANY: The flax plant grows as a slender annual and reaches 30 to 90 cm in height. It branches at the top and has small, pale green alternate leaves that grow on the stems and branches. Flax was introduced to the North American continent from Europe and grows in Canada and the northwestern US. Each branch is tipped with 1 or 2 delicate blue flowers that bloom from February through September.[7]

HISTORY: Flax has been used for more than 10,000 years as a source of fiber for weaving.[7] It was one of the earliest plants recognized for purposes other than as food. Flax is prepared from the fibers in the stem of the plant.[8] Linseed oil, derived from the flaxseed, has been used as a topical demulcent and emollient and as a laxative, particularly for animals. Linseed oil is used in paints and varnishes as a waterproofing agent. Flaxseed cakes have been used as cattle feed.

Traditional medicinal uses of the plant have varied. One text notes that the seeds have been used to remove foreign material from the eye. A moistened seed would be placed under the closed eyelid for a few moments allowing the material to adhere to the seed, thereby facilitating removal.[9] Other uses include the treatment of coughs and colds, constipation, and urinary tract infections.[7] The related *L. catharticum* yields a purgative decoction.[9]

PHARMACOLOGY: Considerable interest has centered on the ability of diets rich in flax to improve the blood lipid profile. Preliminary work indicated that egg yolk was enriched with alpha-linolenic acid by feeding hens diets containing flax. Furthermore, the cholesterol content of the liver tissue of the chicks born to the flax-fed hens was lower ($P > 0.05$) than in chicks hatched from control hens.[10]

More recent evidence indicates that flax-supplemented diets reduce atherogenic risk factors. When hyperlipemic subjects ate 3 slices of bread containing flaxseed plus 15 g of ground flaxseed daily for 3 months, serum total and low-density lipoprotein cholesterol levels were reduced. However, high-density lipoprotein cholesterol levels did not change. In addition, thrombin-stimulated platelet aggregation decreased with the flax supplement. These changes suggest beneficial improvement in plasma lipid and related cardiovascular risk factors.[2]

When healthy female volunteers supplemented their diet with 50 g/day of ground flaxseed for 4 weeks, the diet raised alpha-linolenic acid levels in both plasma and erythrocytes; serum total cholesterol decreased by 9% and low-density lipoprotein cholesterol dropped by 18%. Similar results were obtained when either flaxseed oil or flour was used, suggesting high bioavailability of the alpha-linolenic acid from ground flaxseed. No cyanogenic glucosides were detected in baked flax muffins.[11]

Flax contains lignans (phytochemicals shown to have weakly estrogenic and antiestrogenic properties). When healthy women ingested flaxseed powder for 3 menstrual cycles, the ovulatory cycles had a longer luteal phase. There were no differences between control and flax in estradiol or estrone levels, although the luteal phase progesterone/estradiol

ratios were higher with flax. These findings suggest a specific role for flax lignans in the relationship between diet and sex steroid action, and possibly between diet and the risk of breast and other hormone-dependent cancers.[5]

TOXICOLOGY: The cyanogenic properties of some of the constituents of flax suggest that ingestion of large amounts of the plant may be harmful. However, this is primarily a veterinary problem encountered in grazing animals.

In 1 survey, approximately 50% of the workers exposed to flax at their jobs demonstrated immunologically positive antigen tests.[12] No other clinically important toxicity has been associated with dietary levels of flax.

[1] Meyer JE. *The Herbalist*. Hammond, IN: Hammond Book Co., 1934.

[2] Bierenbaum ML, et al. *J Am Coll Nutr*. 1993;12:501.

[3] Haggans CJ, et al. *Nutr Cancer*. 1999;69:188-195.

[4] Jenkins DJ, et al. *Am J Clin Nutr*. 1999;69:395-402.

[5] Phipps WR, et al. *J Clin Endocrinol Metab*. 1993;77:1215.

[6] Arjmandi BH, et al. *Nutrition Res*. 1998;18:1203-1214.

[7] Dobelis IN. *Magic and Medicine of Plants*. Pleasantville, NY: Reader's Digest Association, 1986.

[8] Lewis WH, Elvin-Lewis MPF. *Medical Botany: Plants Affecting Man's Health*. New York: John Wiley & Sons, 1977.

[9] Evans WC. *Trease and Evans' Pharmacognosy*. 13th ed. London: Balliere Tindall, 1989.

[10] Cherian G, Sim JS. *Lipids*. 1992;27:706.

[11] Cunnane SC, et al. *Br J Nutr*. 1993;69:443.

[12] Zuskin E, et al. *Environ Res*. 1992;59:350.

SCIENTIFIC NAME(S): *Polygonum multiflorum* Thunb. (Polygonaceae)

COMMON NAME(S): He shou wu, flowery knotweed, climbing knotweed, Chinese cornbind. This plant should not be confused with the commercial product *Fo-ti Tieng*, which does not contain fo-ti.

♦♦♦♦ PATIENT INFORMATION ♦♦♦♦

Uses: Fo-ti has been used in China for its rejuvenating and toning properties, to increase liver and kidney function, and to cleanse the blood. It is also used for insomnia, weak bones, constipation, and atherosclerosis. It can increase fertility and blood sugar levels, relieve muscle aches, and exhibit antimicrobial properties against tuberculosis bacillus and malaria.

Side Effects: Little information exists on fo-ti's side effects. Discourage use in pregnant women.

Dosing: Fo-ti is used at daily doses of 9 to 15 g of raw herb; however, there do not appear to be any clinical studies supporting this dosage.

BOTANY: Fo-ti is native to central and southern China and distributed in Japan and Taiwan. It is a perennial climbing herb, which can grow to 9 m in height. The plant has red stems, heart-shaped leaves, and white or pink flowers. The roots of 3- to 4-year-old plants are dried in autumn. The stems and leaves are also used.[1,2]

HISTORY: Fo-ti is a popular Chinese tonic herb, dating back to 713 ad.[1] It is considered one of the country's great four herbal tonics (along with angelica, lycium, and panax).[3] Regarded as a rejuvenating plant, fo-ti has been thought to prevent aging and promote longevity.[1]

PHARMACOLOGY: In China, fo-ti is used for its rejuvenating and toning properties. It is used to increase liver and kidney function and cleanse the blood. The plant is also prescribed for symptoms of premature aging such as gray hair.[1] It is also indicated for insomnia, weak bones, constipation, and atherosclerosis.[2]

Fo-ti has been shown to reduce blood cholesterol levels in animals.[1] The root portion of the plant has exhibited an inhibitory effect on triglyceride accumulation and reduced enlargement of mice livers.[4] In a human clinical trial, fo-ti had similar cholesterol-lowering effects.[1]

Fo-ti exhibits antimicrobial properties against tuberculosis bacillus and malaria.[1] Other uses of the plant include: increasing fertility and blood sugar levels,[1] treating anemia, and relieving muscle aches.[3]

TOXICOLOGY: There is little information in the area of toxicology from fo-ti. However, all plants that contain anthraquinone cathartic compounds should be used cautiously to prevent developing dependence on their laxative effects. One case report describes herb-induced hepatitis in a 31-year-old pregnant Chinese woman from medicine prepared from the plant.[5] The use of these compounds in pregnant women should be discouraged.

[1] Chevallier A. *Encyclopedia of Medicinal Plants*. New York, NY: DK Publishing, 1996;121.

[2] Reid D. *Chinese Herbal Medicine*. Boston, MA: Shambhala Publishing, Inc., 1994;150.

[3] Duke J. *CRC Handbook of Medicinal Herbs*. Boca Raton, FL: CRC Press, Inc., 1989;163-164.

[4] Liu C, et al. *Chung Kuo Chung Yao Tsa Chih*. 1992;17(10):595-596.

[5] Hong, et al. *Am J Chin Med*. 1994;22(1):63-70.

SCIENTIFIC NAME(S): Gamma linolenic acid

COMMON NAME(S): GLA, gamolenic acid[1]

ᴥᴥᴥ PATIENT INFORMATION ᴥᴥᴥ

Uses: A few small clinical studies have found GLA to be of benefit for the treatment and prevention of AD, adjunctive treatment of RA, management of lipid lowering in cardiovascular diseases, and treatment of diabetic neuropathies.

Side Effects: No serious adverse effects have been noted. Pregnant women, hemophiliac patients, and patients taking warfarin should avoid its use.

BOTANY: GLA is found in the seeds and oils of a range of plants including *Onagraceae* (evening primrose), *Saxifragaceae* (borage), and *Rubaceae* (blackcurrant). The richest source of GLA is borage (*Borago officinalis*).[1]

HISTORY: The evening primrose plant is native to North America and was introduced into Europe in the 17th century. American Indians consumed the leaves, roots, and seedpods as food and prepared extracts of the oil for use as a painkiller and asthma treatment. Some of these early therapeutic effects are thought to be because of GLA, which is found in high quantities in the oil.[2]

In the 1930s and 1940s, several investigators found dietary supplementation with essential fatty acids such as GLA to be of therapeutic value in atopic dermatitis (AD).[3] In 1947, the first study was published that suggested a relationship between disturbances in linoleic acid metabolism and the pathogenesis of AD.[4] The advent of topical glucocorticoids brought an end to this form of treatment. However, by the early 1980s, there was a return to using these agents because of the unwanted side effects of glucocorticoids, and they have regained scientific interest.[3] Over the last 2 decades, numerous other indications have been proposed for GLA.

PHARMACOLOGY: Unsaturated fatty acids are essential components of cell membranes and can influence receptors, enzymes, ion channels, and signal transduction pathways. Dihydro-γ-linolenic, arachidonic, and eicosapentaenoic acids are precursors of eicosanoids, which can influence numerous inflammatory and immunological processes. After intake, n-3 unsaturated fatty acids are rapidly incorporated into the cell membranes of immune and inflammatory cells, where they compete with n-6 unsaturated fatty acids as substrates for the cyclooxygenase and lipoxygenase pathways. This results in a diminished production of biologically active leukotrienes and prostaglandins.[5] GLA has been extensively studied, with many reports in the literature demonstrating benefit in a number of diseases. This review provides a summary of those clinically relevant indications for GLA with the most substantial supporting evidence.

Atopic dermatitis (AD): AD usually becomes evident during the first 2 to 3 months of life.[6] It is generally accepted that patients show an increased IgE production. Increased levels of linoleic acid and deficiencies in GLA have been observed in the plasma and epidermis of patients with AD.[7] This is proposed to be because of a defect in the function of the enzyme delta-6-desaturase, which is responsible for conversion of linoleic acid to GLA; GLA is a precursor of eicosanoids.[3]

Supplementation of AD patients with GLA appears to be rational therapy. The beneficial effect of GLA-rich plant oils has been demonstrated in several placebo-controlled studies. Oral GLA therapy has been demonstrated to reduce pruritus, the degree of erythema, and roughness of atopic skin,[6,7] as well as reduce inflammation and overall disease severity.[3] This improvement in severity appears to be dose-related (maximum dose, 7.5 g/day).[8]

A study in 10 children with AD evaluated GLA 3 g/day for 28 days. A gradual improvement in erythema, excoriations, and lichenification was seen.[9] No side effects were recorded.[6,8,9] It should be noted that the placebo effect is remarkably strong in practically all studies, underlying the importance of robust study designs.

Atopic bronchial asthma: Atopic disease in children is often characterized by a change in the clinical picture from dermatitis in early childhood to a later presentation of bronchial asthma. However, there appears to be no biochemical evidence for a defect in the enzyme delta-6-desaturase (see Atopic dermatitis) in children with atopic bronchial asthma and, therefore, there is no rationale for GLA supplementation in atopic patients.[4]

Prevention of atopic diseases: Breastfeeding has been shown to protect against the development of atopic diseases, although infants may develop atopic diseases during exclusive breastfeeding.[10] Breast milk of allergic mothers has been shown to contain less GLA than that of healthy mothers. Similarly, infants with atopic diseases have less GLA than healthy infants. Reduced dietary proportions of GLA may be a risk factor for the development of atopic disease.[10] After maternal supplementation, increased levels of GLA can be present in breast milk.[11] Results support the theory that a defect in the conversion of linoleic acid into its long-chain polyunsaturated metabolites occurs in infants predisposed to atopic dermatitis.[12]

Psoriasis: Although psoriasis does not have an atopic component, use of GLA has been investigated. In a small study (n = 17), patients with psoriasis were fed a low-fat diet supplemented with a combination of n-3 (linoleic acid) and n-6 (GLA) fatty acids or placebo. Some improvement was noted in patients after 4 months of treatment. It was not possible to predict which patients would respond to dietary therapy as the effects were variable and 18% of the patients showed no improvement.[13] Therefore, use of GLA in the treatment of psoriasis is questionable.

Rheumatoid arthritis (RA): Rheumatologic conditions such as arthritis are common, progressive, and disabling disease processes. Although conventional treatment of these conditions generally is considered to have improved in terms of effectiveness, the use of nonsteroidal anti-inflammatory drugs (NSAIDs), second-line therapies, and corticosteroids all have been associated with adverse reactions. For this reason, patients suffering chronic musculoskeletal disorders are likely to seek alternative methods of symptomatic relief, and studies have shown rheumatology patients to be among the highest users of complementary and alternative medicine. The Cochrane Collaboration, an international health care review organization, performed an extensive search of the literature to evaluate which herbal therapies could be used for RA. Seven studies compared GLA with placebo (n = 286). Sources of GLA included evening primrose oil, borage seed oil, and blackcurrant seed oil. These sources provided between 525 mg/day and 2.8 g/day of GLA and were administered for 6 weeks to 12 months. All of the GLA studies found some improvement in clinical outcomes but methodology and study quality were variable. However, other studies suggest potential relief of pain, morning stiffness, and joint tenderness. Benefits appeared to be increased when dosages were greater than 1.4 g/day and were administered for at least 6 months, although it appears that maximum benefit may not be achieved within this time period. The authors suggest that further studies are required to establish optimum dosage and duration of therapy.[14]

Cancer: It has been proposed that linoleic acid and GLA may play important roles in cancer treatment. Oxidation of linoleic acid by lipoxidase increases tumor cell death and GLA inhibits urokinase-type plasminogen activator (uPA) activity. Increased uPA activity is responsible for cancer invasion and metastases and for proteolysis of lipoxidase, which promotes a decrease in cancer cell death. Hence, it has been proposed that the addition of linoleic acid and GLA to available therapeutic regimens may be worth consideration in cancer treatment.[15]

Investigations in this area primarily are performed on transformed cell lines. Such studies have shown GLA to have tumoricidal activity in bladder cancer[16] and to reduce estrogen receptor expression in breast cancer.[17]

A further area of interest is that of gliomas. Intratumoral injection of 1 mg/day of GLA caused regression of cerebral gliomas as evaluated by computerized tomography and improved survival by 1.5 to 2 years.[18]

It should be noted that all of the studies cited were relatively small and it would be beneficial if the proposed effects were investigated further.

Immune system: Lymphocytes are key components of the regulation, amplification, and memory of the cell-mediated immune response. A study was performed with 48 healthy subjects, 55 to 75 years of age, who were randomly allocated to treatment or placebo. The treatment group consumed capsules rich in unsaturated fatty acids (4 g) including GLA. The study found that GLA reduced lymphocyte production by up to 65%. This decrease was partially reversed 4 weeks after stopping the medication.[19]

Cardiovascular protection: The apparent low death rate from coronary heart disease among Eskimos has focused interest on the potential benefits of the n-3 polyunsaturated fatty acids. Several epidemiological studies indicate that populations consuming large amounts of n-3 polyunsaturated fatty acids have relatively low incidences of atherosclerotic cardiovascular disease. In a small study, 12 hyperlipidemic males were randomly allocated to evening primrose oil capsules (containing 240 mg GLA) or placebo. GLA supplementation decreased plasma triglyceride levels by 48% and increased HDL cholesterol concentration by 22%. Total cholesterol and LDL cholesterol were decreased. Additionally, platelet aggregation decreased. These effects suggest that GLA may contribute to cardiovascular protection.[20] However, this is still an area of controversy.

Diabetes mellitus: There are multiple abnormalities of essential fatty acid metabolism in diabetes. Diabetic subjects require higher amounts of these fats than nondiabetic patients. Conversion of linoleic acid to GLA is impaired. There have been several successful attempts to manage diabetic complications by the provision of very high levels of linoleic acid intake. These studies have shown that the development of cataracts, retinopathy, and cardiovascular damage can all be slowed by the administration of large daily doses of essential fatty acids. However, outcomes have been disappointing, largely because most patients are unable to maintain this diet. Therefore, administration of GLA as an alternative to this strict diet has been studied.[21] Diabetic neuropathy is the most common complication of diabetes mellitus. A small study showed possible benefits of GLA for diabetic peripheral neuropathy.[22] This was followed by a multicenter, randomized study of 100 patients where the effect of administration of GLA (480 mg/day) on neuropathies was investigated. The GLA group demonstrated consistent and progressive improvement while the placebo group showed deterioration.[23]

Breast pain and premenstrual syndrome (PMS): PMS involves a wide range of psychological and physical symptoms. Breast pain is one of the common symptoms of PMS. Breast pain and PMS appear to be common when the intake of fat, especially saturated fat, is high. A drastic reduction in fat intake has been shown to relieve breast pain. Experimental investigations have demonstrated that hormone receptors in membranes richer than normal in saturated fats and poorer than normal in essential fatty acids have increased affinity for

their ligands. Therefore, normal levels of hormones will produce an exaggerated peripheral response. In support of these findings, clinical studies have shown that GLA is more effective than placebo at relieving PMS symptoms.[21]

Lower-limb atherosclerosis: The Cochrane Collaboration reviewed the literature on the use of lipid-lowering therapy in patients with lower-limb arterial disease. Nine eligible randomized, controlled trials were located. The reviewers concluded that lipid-lowering therapy may be useful in preventing deterioration of underlying disease and in alleviating symptoms. However, their results could not be used to determine whether one lipid-lowering regimen was superior to another.[24]

TOXICOLOGY: There have been no reports of serious adverse events in those taking GLA supplements. GLA is usually very well tolerated, with no clinically significant adverse effects. GLA should not be used by pregnant women and nursing mothers unless recommended by a physician. Because of possible antithrombotic activity, hemophiliac patients and patients who take warfarin should exercise caution. GLA should not be used before surgery.[1]

[1] http://www.lapinskas.com/pubs/3547.html
[2] Nemecz G. US Pharm. 1998;23:85-94.
[3] Kerscher MJ, Korting HC. Clin Investig. 1992;70:167-171.
[4] Leichsenring M, Kochsiek U, Paul K. Pediatr Allergy Immunol. 1995;6:209-212.
[5] Worm M, Henz BM. Dermatology. 2000;201:191-195.
[6] Andreassi M, Forleo P, Di Lorio A, Masci S, Abate G, Amerio P. J Int Med Res. 1997;25:266-274.
[7] Melnik B, Plewig G. J Am Acad Dermatol. 1991;25(5 pt 1):859-860.
[8] Biagi PL, Bordoni A, Hrelia S, et al. Drugs Exp Clin Res. 1994;20:77-84.
[9] Fiocchi A, Sala M, Signoroni P, Banderali G, Agostoni C, Riva E. J Int Med Res. 1994;22:24-32.
[10] Kankaanpää P, Nurmela K, Erkkilä A, et al. Allergy. 2001;56:633-638.
[11] Cant A, Shay J, Horrobin DF. J Nutr Sci Vitaminol. 1991;37:573-579.
[12] Wright S, Bolton C. Br J Nutr. 1989;62:693-697.
[13] Kragballe K. Acta Derm Venereol. 1989;69:265-268.
[14] Little C, Parsons T. Cochrane Database Syst Rev. 2001;CD002948.
[15] Van Aswegen CH, Du Plessis DJ. Med Hypotheses. 1994;43:415-417.
[16] Solomon LZ, Jennings AM, Foley SJ, Birch BR, Cooper AJ. Br J Urol. 1998;82:122-126.
[17] Kenny FS, Gee JM, Nicholson RI, et al. Int J Cancer. 2001;92:342-347.
[18] Falconer JS, Fearon KC, Ross JA, Carter DC. World Rev Nutr Diet. 1994;76:74-76.

[19] Thies F, Nebe-von-Caron G, Powell JR, Yaqoob P, Newsholme EA, Calder PC. *J Nutr.* 2001;131:1918-1927.

[20] Guivernau M, Meza N, Barja P, Roman O. *Prostaglandins Leukot Essent Fatty Acids.* 1994;51:311-316.

[21] Horrobin DF. *Prog Lipid Res.* 1992;31:163-194.

[22] Jamal GA, Carmichael H. *Diabet Med.* 1990;7:319-323.

[23] Keen H, Payan J, Allawi J, et al. *Diabetes Care.* 1993;16:8-15.

[24] Leng GC, Price JF, Jepson RG. *Cochrane Database Syst Rev.* 2000:CD000123.

SCIENTIFIC NAME(S): *Allium sativum* L. Family: Liliaceae (lilies)

COMMON NAME(S): Garlic, allium, stinking rose, rustic treacle, nectar of the gods, camphor of the poor, poor man's treacle[1]

❧❧❧ PATIENT INFORMATION ❧❧❧

Uses: Clinical evidence suggests that garlic may modestly affect cholesterol and lipids. Among its traditional uses, it has been employed for its antiseptic and antibacterial properties.

Side Effects: Garlic may affect patients being treated with anticoagulants. It may also cause allergic reactions.

Dosing: Garlic dosage is complicated by the volatility and instability of important constituents and by such products as "deodorized garlic," "aged" extracts, and distilled oils. Doses of fresh bulbs studied in clinical trials for hyperlipidemia or atherosclerosis range from 2 to 4 g/day and a daily intake of 2 to 12 mg allicin has been proposed. Because garlic is a widely consumed foodstuff, dosage will remain a matter of personal tolerance.[2-5]

BOTANY: A perennial bulb with a tall, erect flowering stem that grows to 0.7 to 1 m. The plant produces pink to purple flowers that bloom from July to September. The bulb is odiferous.

HISTORY: The name *Allium* comes from the Celtic word *all* meaning burning or smarting. Garlic was valued as an exchange medium in ancient Egypt; its virtues were described in inscriptions on the Great Pyramid of Cheops. The folk uses of garlic have ranged from the treatment of leprosy in humans to managing clotting disorders in horses. Physicians prescribed the herb during the Middle Ages to cure deafness and the American Indians used garlic as a remedy for earaches, flatulence, and scurvy.

PHARMACOLOGY: A number of trials have examined the effects of garlic on lipoproteins and hypercholesterolemia. The exact mechanism for this action is uncertain, but it is thought that the organic disulfides present in garlic oil can reduce the activity of the thiol group found in many enzymes and can oxidize nicotinamide adenine dinucleotide phosphate (NADPH). These compounds can inactivate thiol enzymes such as coenzyme A and HMG-CoA reductase, and can oxidize NADPH, all of which are factors normally required for lipid synthesis.

Individual randomized controlled trials comparing garlic to placebo have provided disparate results. Some studies have suggested that garlic has no effect in adults with mild to moderate hypercholesterolemia.[6-10] Evidence has shown that garlic has no effect on cardiovascular risk factors in pediatric patients with familial hyperlipidemia.[2] However, other studies looking specifically at moderate hypercholesterolemia in males have demonstrated that garlic has beneficial effects on lipid profiles (reduction in total cholesterol and LDL cholesterol).[11,12] Other data have shown that there may be a role for garlic as add-on therapy to traditional medicines (eg, reducing the dose of HMG-CoA reductase inhibitors).[13] Additional trials have demonstrated that allicin (the presumed active ingredient of garlic) may reduce total cholesterol and LDL cholesterol in adults with moderate hypercholesterolemia.[14]

One meta-analysis report on the use of garlic for hypercholesterolemia specifically examined randomized, controlled trials comparing garlic with placebo.[13] The inclusion criteria were patients with a mean total cholesterol level of 5.17 mmol/L (200 mg/dL). Pooling data from 13 trials (including 796 patients) suggested that garlic is superior to placebo in reducing cholesterol levels. However the effect is modest (6% reduction in total cholesterol).

Another meta-analysis of 16 randomized, controlled trials (including 1365 patients) also showed a modest reduction in serum lipids.[15] Overall, a 12% greater reduction was observed with garlic therapy compared with placebo. This meta-analysis, however, consisted of small randomized studies of poor quality and not all patients recruited had hyperlipidemia.[15]

Overall, these effects are generally short-term and whether they are sustainable beyond 3 months is unclear. The evidence for lowering LDL and total cholesterol is still questionable and may not be clinically meaningful.

Researchers demonstrated that allicin increased the levels of 2 important antioxidant enzymes in the blood: catalase and glutathione peroxidase. This discovery confirmed the antioxidant and free-radical scavenging potential of allicin. The clinical utility of antioxidant activity is not clear to researchers. Other researchers studied the sulfur compounds in aged garlic extract (a popular deodorized form of garlic) and found 5 sulfur compounds that inhibited lipid peroxidation in the liver, preventing a reaction that is considered to be one of the main features of aging in liver cells. According to the findings, the sulfur compounds "appear to be approximately 1000 times more potent in antioxidant activity than the crude, aged garlic extract."[16]

Studies on the effects of platelet aggregation have produced inconsistent re-

sults, possibly related to variations in study design and in the garlic preparation used. The proposed mechanism for garlic oil inhibition of platelet function is by interfering with thromboxane synthesis.[17] Researchers isolated a component of garlic oil that inhibits platelet aggregation and identified it as methylallyltrisulphide (MATS). MATS is present in natural oil in a concentration of 4% to 10%. The purified compound inhibits ADP-induced platelet aggregation at a concentration of more than 10 mcmol/L in plasma.[18]

Further studies indicated that the most potent antithrombotic compound in garlic is 4,5,9, trithiadodeca-1,6,11-triene 9-oxide, also known as ajoene. This compound is formed by an acid-catalyzed reaction of 2 allicin molecules followed by rearrangement; the compound can be synthesized commercially. Unlike other antithrombotics now under investigation, ajoene appears to inhibit platelet aggregation regardless of the mechanism of induction.[19]

Scientists demonstrated the effect of ajoene in preventing clot formation caused by vascular damage. The experiment was designed to mimic the conditions of blood flow in small- and medium-sized arteries by varying the velocity of the blood; the compound proved to be effective in both conditions. The authors suggested that the compound may be useful in situations where emergency treatment is needed to prevent clot formation produced by vascular damage.[16] Clinical studies have demonstrated that inhibition of platelet aggregation is also observed in vivo after ingestion of fresh garlic. In 1 study, the platelets from healthy subjects who had eaten garlic cloves (100 to 150 mg/kg) showed complete inhibition to aggregation induced by 5-hydroxytryptamine.[20] Other studies have shown that ingestion of "aged" garlic extract can produce an inhibition of some of the platelet functions important for initiating thromboembolic events in the arterial circulation.[21] The effects of garlic on platelet aggregation may be dependent on the garlic preparation used. Differences appear to be mostly dependent on their content of organo-sulfur compounds, many of which are unstable or capable of interconversion during processing.[22]

Strong evidence for the effect of garlic on blood pressure is lacking. The results of a meta-analysis suggest that garlic supplements of 600 to 900 mg/day for 1 to 3 months are associated with a clinically important reduction in blood pressure.[23] Their meta-analysis included 8 trials consisting of 415 patients. However, the trials were of generally moderate to poor quality and not all patients were hypertensive. A review of the literature suggested that the effects of garlic on blood pressure were insignificant.[24] No firm conclusions should be drawn from these trials.

The effect of garlic on the GI system has been the topic of some debate. Oral administration of the oil (0.1 mL/10 g) in mice reduced the gastric transit time of a charcoal meal by 75% and prevented castor oil-induced diarrhea for up to 3 hours.[25] The investigators concluded that garlic oil can be investigated for its effectiveness in the management of hypermotile intestinal disorders.

An additional role proposed in the literature is that garlic may be used in the treatment of *Helicobacter pylori* infection; however, the evidence does not support this.[26]

The protective effect of garlic against colorectal and stomach cancers was addressed in meta-analyses of 18 studies.[27] It was concluded that high intake of garlic may offer protection. These results should be interpreted with caution because of the heterogeneity of the trials included in the meta-analyses.

Garlic has been suggested to reduce blood glucose levels,[28] increase serum insulin, and improve liver glycogen storage.[29] A review of the literature[30] demonstrated that glucose levels decreased from 89 to 9 mg/dL in healthy volunteers given garlic (800 mg dried powder for 35 days) as compared with placebo group. However, other reviews have shown that, in fact, garlic has no effect on glucose levels.[24] Garlic administration should not be recommended for this indication because of the lack of randomized controlled trials.

The antiseptic and antibacterial properties of garlic have been known for centuries. As recently as World War II, garlic extracts were used to disinfect wounds. During the 1800s, physicians routinely prescribed garlic inhalation for the treatment of tuberculosis. Garlic extracts inhibit the growth of numerous strains of *Mycobacterium*, but at concentrations that may be difficult to achieve in human tissues.[29] Preparations containing garlic extracts are used widely in Russia and Japan. Both gram-positive and gram-negative organisms are inhibited in vitro by garlic extracts. The potency of garlic is such that 1 mg is equivalent to 15 Oxford units of penicillin, making garlic about 1% as active as penicillin.[29]

Garlic extracts have shown antifungal activity when tested in vitro[29] and their use has been suggested in the treatment of oral and vaginal candidiasis. In an attempt to quantitate the in vivo activity of garlic extracts, researchers administered 25 mL of fresh garlic extract orally to volunteers.[31] Serum and urine samples were tested for antifungal activity against 15 species of fungal pathogens. While serum exhibited anticandidal and anticryptococcal activity within 30 minutes after ingestion, no biological activity was found in urine. The findings suggest that while garlic extracts may exhibit some antifungal activity in vivo, they are probably of limited use in the treatment of systemic infections.

Oncology: The antineoplastic activity of garlic has been studied in mice injected with cancer cells that had been pretreated with a garlic extract. No deaths occurred in this treatment group for up to 6 months, while mice injected with untreated cancer cells died within 16 days.[29] It is believed that the reaction of allicin with sulfhydryl groups (the concentration of which increases rapidly in dividing cells) may contribute to this inhibitory effect. Scant data, primarily from case-control studies, suggest that dietary garlic consumption is associated with decreased odds of laryngeal, gastric, colorectal, and endometrial cancer and adenomatous colorectal polyps.[32]

Immunology: Garlic contains the trace elements germanium and selenium, which have been thought to play a role in improving host immunity. One study found that 2 oil-soluble compounds from garlic, diallyl sulfide and diallyl disulfide, when applied topically succeeded in protecting mice against carcinogen-induced skin tumors and increased survival rate.[16]

INTERACTIONS: For potential interactions, refer to the "Potential Herb-Drug Interactions" appendix.

TOXICOLOGY: Although garlic is used extensively for culinary purposes with essentially no ill effects, the safety of the long-term use of concentrated extracts is unclear. Ingestion of a single 25 mL dose of fresh garlic extract has caused burning of the mouth, esophagus, and stomach, nausea, sweating, and lightheadedness; safety of repeated doses of this amount has not been defined. Rarely, ingestion may also cause anaphylaxis.[33]

Topical exposure to crushed, uncooked garlic cloves for 3 to 5 minutes has resulted in toxic contact dermatitis.[34] Additionally, repeated exposure to garlic dust can induce asthmatic reactions.[17] Garlic dust allergy, presenting as coughing, wheezing, chest tightness, difficulty breathing, blocked or runny nose, sneezing, and running or itching eyes is relatively rare. However, an IgE-mediated hypersensitivity reaction has been reported to affect mainly young atopic subjects. Cross-sensitivity to other members of the Liliaceae family may be observed.[35] The degree of cross-reactivity appears to vary among individuals.[36]

There are no studies that evaluate the effect of garlic and its extracts in people who require stringent blood glucose control or in patients being treated with anticoagulants (coumarins), salicylates, or antiplatelet drugs, but the potential for serious interactions should be kept in mind.

[1] Dobelis IN. *Magic and Medicine of Plants*. Pleasantville, NY: The Reader's Digest Association; 1986.

[2] McCrindle BW, Helden E, Conner WT. *Arch Pediatr Adolesc Med*. 1998;152:1089-1094.

[3] Stevinson C, Pittler MH, Ernst E. *Ann Intern Med*. 2000;133:420-429.

[4] Koscielny J, Klussendorf D, Latza R, et al. *Atherosclerosis*. 1999;144:237-249.

[5] Warshafsky S, Kamer RS, Sivak SL. *Ann Intern Med*. 1993;119(7 Pt. 1):599-605.

[6] Simons LA, Balasubramaniam S, von Konigsmark M, et al. *Atherosclerosis*. 1995;113:219-225.

[7] Superko HR, Krauss RM. *J Am Coll Cardiol*. 2000;35:321-326.

[8] Isaacsohn JL, Moser M, Stein EA, et al. *Arch Intern Med*. 1998;158:1189-1194.

[9] Neil HA, Silagy CA, Lancaster T, et al. *J R Coll Physicians Lond*. 1996;30:329-334.

[10] Steiner M, Khan AH, Holbert D, et al. *Am J Clin Nutr*. 1996;64:866-870.

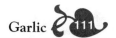

[11] Berthold HK, Sudhop T, von Bergmann K. *JAMA*. 1998;279:1900-1902.

[12] Adler AJ, Holub BJ. *Am J Clin Nutr*. 1997;65:445-450.

[13] Lash JP, Cardoso LR, Mesler PM, et al. *Transplant Proc*. 1998;30:189-191.

[14] Jain AK, Vargas R, Gotzkowsky S, et al. *Am J Med*. 1993;94:632-635.

[15] Silagy C, Neil A. *J R Coll Physicians Lond*. 1994;28:39-45.

[16] McCaleb R. *HerbalGram*. 1993;29:18.

[17] Makheia AN, Vanderhoek JY, Bailey JM. *Lancet*. 1979;1:781. Letter.

[18] Ariga T, et al. *Lancet*. 1981;1:150-151.

[19] *Chem Eng News*. 1985;63:34.

[20] Boullin DJ. *Lancet* 1981;1:776-777. Letter.

[21] Steiner M, Lin RS. *J Cardiovasc Pharmacol*. 1998;31:904-908.

[22] Berthold HK, Sudhop T. *Curr Opin Lipidol*. 1998;9:565-569.

[23] Silagy CA, Neil HAW. *J Hypertens*. 1994;12:463-468.

[24] Ackermann RT, Mulrow CD, Ramirez G, et al. *Arch Intern Med*. 2001;161:813-824.

[25] Joshi DJ, et al. *Phytother Res*. 1987;1:141.

[26] Graham DY, Anderson SY, Lang T. *Am J Gastroenterol*. 1999;94:1200-1202.

[27] Fleischauer AT, Poole C, Arab L. *Am J Clin Nutr*. 2000;72:1047-1052.

[28] Castleman M. *The Healing Herbs*. Emmaus, PA: Rodale Press; 1991.

[29] Pareddy SR, Rosenberg JM. *Hosp Pharm Rep*. 1993;8:27.

[30] Ernst E. *Perfusion*. 1996;9:416-418.

[31] Caporaso N, Smith SM, Eng RH. *Antimicrob Agents Chemother*. 1983;23:700-702.

[32] http://www.ahcpr.gov/clinic/garlicsum.htm

[33] Perez-Pimiento AJ, Moneo I, Santaolalla M, et al. *Allergy*. 1999;54:626-629.

[34] Eming SA, Piontek JO, Hunzelmann N, et al. Br J Dermatol. 1999;141:391-392.

[35] Anibarro B, Fontela JL, De La Hoz F. *J Allergy Clin Immunol*. 1997;100:734-738.

[36] Sanchez-Hernandez MC, Hernandez M, Delgado J, et al. *Allergy*. 2000;55:297-299.

Gentian

SCIENTIFIC NAME(S): *Gentiana lutea* L. Stemless gentian is derived from *G. acaulis* L. Family: Gentianaceae

COMMON NAME(S): Gentian, stemless gentian, yellow gentian, bitter root, pale gentian, gall weed

---

♣♣♣♣ PATIENT INFORMATION ♣♣♣♣

Uses: Gentian is used to stimulate the appetite, improve digestion, and treat gastrointestinal complaints. It has also been used to treat wounds, sore throat, arthritic inflammations, and jaundice.

Side Effects: The extract may cause gastric irritation and not be tolerated by pregnant women or those with hypertension.

Dosing: Gentian root has been used as a bitter digestive tonic in doses from 1 to 4 g/day. There are no clinical studies to substantiate this dose recommendation.

BOTANY: Native to Europe and western Asia, *G. lutea*, a perennial herb with erect stems and oval leaves, grows to 1.8 m in height. The plant produces a cluster of fragrant orange-yellow flowers. *G. acaulis* is a small herb with a basal rosette of lance-shaped leaves and grows to 10 cm in height. It is native to the European Alps at 900 to 1500 m above sea level. The roots and rhizomes are nearly cylindrical, sometimes branched, varying in thickness from 5 to 40 mm. The root and rhizome portions are longitudinally wrinkled. The color of the rhizomes, ranging from dark brown to light tan, appears to be related to its bitter principal content.[1] The roots and rhizome of *G. lutea* are used medicinally, whereas the entire plant of *G. acaulis* is used.

HISTORY: Gentians have been used to stimulate the appetite, improve digestion, and treat gastrointestinal problems.[2,3] Gentian and stemless gentian are approved for food use. Stemless gentian is used as a tea or alcoholic extract such as *Angostura bitters*. Ex-tracts are used in foods, cosmetics, and antismoking products. The plant has been used externally to treat wounds and internally to treat sore throat, arthritic inflammations, and jaundice.

PHARMACOLOGY: Ingestion of bitter substances may improve the appetite and aid in digestion. However, because gentian is most often consumed as an ingredient in an alcoholic beverage, it is difficult to distinguish the effects of gentian from those of alcohol.[4]

TOXICOLOGY: Usually, the extract is taken in small doses that do not cause adverse effects. One author suggested that gentian may not be well tolerated in hypertension or pregnancy.[5] The extract may cause gastric irritation, resulting in nausea and vomiting.

The highly toxic white hellebore (*Veratrum album* L.) often grows in close proximity to gentian. At least 5 cases of acute veratrum alkaloid poisoning have been reported in people preparing homemade gentian wine that is accidentally contaminated by veratrum.[6]

[1] Meyer JE. *The Herbalist*. Hammond, IN: Hammond Book Co., 1934.

[2] Leung AY. *Encyclopedia of Common Natural Ingredients Used in Food, Drugs, and Cosmetics*. New York, NY: John Wiley and Sons, 1980.

[3] DerMarderosian A, et al. *Natural Product Medicine*. Philadelphia, PA: G.F. Stickley Co., 1988.

[4] Tyler VE. *The New Honest Herbal*. Philadelphia, PA: G.F. Stickley Co., 1987.

[5] Tyler VE. *The Honest Herbal*. Philadelphia, PA: G.F. Stickley Co., 1982.

[6] Garnier R, et al. *Ann Med Interne* 1985;136:125.

Ginger

SCIENTIFIC NAME(S): *Zingiber officinale* Roscoe; occasionally *Z. capitatum* Smith.[1]
Family: Zingiberaceae

COMMON NAME(S): Ginger, ginger root, black ginger, zingiberis rhizoma

---

✦✦✦✦ PATIENT INFORMATION ✦✦✦✦

Uses: Ginger and its constituents have antiemetic, cardiotonic, antithrombotic, antibacterial, antioxidant, antitussive, antihepatotoxic, anti-inflammatory, antimutagenic, stimulant, diaphoretic, diuretic, spasmolytic, immunostimulant, carminative, and cholagogue actions. Ginger is used to promote gastric secretions, increase intestinal peristalsis, lower cholesterol levels, raise blood glucose, and stimulate peripheral circulation. Traditionally used to stimulate digestion, its modern uses include prophylaxis for nausea and vomiting (associated with motion sickness, hypermesis gravidarum, and anesthesia), dyspepsia, lack of appetite, anorexia, colic, bronchitis, and rheumatic complaints. Ginger can be used as a flavoring or spice as well as a fungicide and pesticide.

Side Effects: Excessive amounts may cause CNS depression and may interfere with cardiac function or anticoagulant activity.

Dosing: Ginger root has been given for nausea in clinical trials in 1 g doses, repeated as necessary.[2,3]

BOTANY: A native of tropical Asia, this perennial is cultivated in tropical climates such as Australia, Brazil, China, India, Jamaica, West Africa, and parts of the US.[1] The term "root" is actually a misnomer because it is the rhizome that is used medicinally and as a culinary spice. Cultivation with natural manuring is thought to increase the spiciness of the rhizome and is therefore preferred to wild crafting.[1] The rhizome is harvested between 6 and 20 months; taste and pungency increase with maturity.[1] The plant carries a green-purple flower in terminal spikes; the flowers are similar to orchids.[1,4]

HISTORY: Medicinal use of ginger dates back to ancient China and India; references to its use are found in Chinese pharmacopoeias, the Sesruta scriptures of Ayurvedic medicine as well as Sanskrit writings.[1] Once its culinary properties were discovered in the 13th century, use of this herb became widespread throughout Europe. In the Middle Ages, it held a firm place in apothecaries for travel sickness, nausea, hangovers, and flatulence.[1]

Traditionally, ginger is used as an acrid bitter to strengthen and stimulate digestion.[1] Modern uses include prophylaxis for nausea and vomiting (associated with motion sickness, hyperemesis gravidarum, and surgical anesthesia), dyspepsia, lack of appetite, anorexia, colic, bronchitis, and rheumatic complaints.[1,5-7]

Ginger is in the official pharmacopoeias of Austria, China, Egypt, Great Britain, India, Japan, the Netherlands, and Switzerland.[1,6,7] It is approved as a nonprescription drug in Germany and as a dietary supplement in the US.[6] Only scraped or unscraped, unbleached ginger is accepted as a medicinal-grade drug, medicinal grade containing greater than or equal to 1.5% volatile oil.[1] Langner, et al consider Jamaican and Cochin ginger to be the best varieties, and report the Japanese plant to be of inferior quality and do not recommend it for medicinal use.[1] Standards of quality for ginger can be found in *The United States Pharmacopeia National Formulary*.

PHARMACOLOGY: The active constituents of ginger, the gingerols and the related compound shogaol, have been found to possess cardiotonic activity. The gingerols have been found to exert a dose-dependent positive inotropic action at doses as low as 10^{-4} g/mL when applied to isolated atrial tissue.[8] Cardiac workload is further decreased by dilation of blood vessels via stimulation of prostacyclin biosynthesis.[1]

Other ginger constituents, [6]-gingerol, the dehydrogingerdiones, and the gingerdiones are potent inhibitors of prostaglandin biosynthesis through the inhibition of prostaglandin synthetase (cyclooxygenase).[9] Inhibition of thromboxane synthesis results in inhibition of platelet aggregation, but evidence indicates this is dose dependent or may only occur with fresh ginger.[1,10]

Ginger has been reported to have weak fungicidal, strong antibacterial, and anthelmintic properties. Active constituents have been shown to inhibit reproduction of *Escherichia coli*, *Proteus* species, staphylococci, streptococci, and *Salmonella* but to stimulate lactobacilli growth.[1] Activity has also been reported against parasites, such as *Schistosoma* and *Anisakis*.[1]

The cytotoxic compound zerumbone and its epoxide have been isolated from the rhizomes of *Z. zerumbet*. This plant, also a member of the family Zingiberaceae, has been used traditionally in China as an antineoplastic. The isolates inhibited the growth of a hepatoma tissue culture.[11]

Human clinical trials have examined ginger's antiemetic effects related to kinetosis (motion sickness), perioperative anesthesia, and hyperemesis gravi-

darum. However, little is still known regarding its human pharmacology in these settings.

One clinical trial (N = 12) employed gastroduodenal manometry to evaluate prokinetic effects of ginger in fasting and postprandial healthy subjects. A significant increase in antral motility and in corpus motor response with a trend toward increased motor response in all regions was found.[12] However, no effect of ginger on gastric motility using an acetaminophen absorption technique was found in 16 healthy volunteers.[13]

Kinetosis: One double-blind study (N = 36) compared the effect of 940 mg powdered ginger root, 100 mg dimenhydrinate, and placebo (chickweed herb) in the prevention of motion sickness. Preparations were administered 20 to 25 minutes prior to placing blindfolded subjects in a rotating chair. Those receiving ginger root remained in the chair longer (average of 5.5 minutes, compared with 3.5 and 1.5 minutes for the dimenhydrinate and placebo groups, respectively), and 50% remained in the chair for the full 6 minutes of the test; none of the subjects in the other groups completed the test. In general, it took longer for the ginger group to begin feeling sick, but once the vomiting center was activated, sensations of nausea and vomiting progressed at the same rate in all groups.[14]

A double-blind, placebo-controlled study in seasick marine cadets (N = 79) reported significant reductions in symptoms (vomiting and cold sweats) and noticeably suppressed dizziness following administration of 1 g ginger rhizome. Nystagmus was reported as unchanged.[1] A study involving 1741 participants on an ocean sailing tour described the administration of 250 mg ginger prior to departure to be as effective as cinnarizine, scopolamine, dimenhydrinate, meclizine, and cyclizine.[1] Ginger (500 mg every 4 hours) and dimenhydrinate (100 mg every 4 hours) were compared in another double-blind study with similar protective effects, however those receiving ginger reported no side effects.[1]

Other trials have shown no significant differences among ginger, antiemetics, and placebo with regard to gastric as well as nongastric symptoms. Two separate investigations showed no effect of ginger on the CNS impairment caused by kinetosis as subjects retained the ability to perform certain head and eye movements. A scopolamine/d-amphetamine combination proved most effective but resulted in definite side effects.[1]

Another placebo-controlled study evaluated participants' ability to tolerate head movements in a rotating chair while blindfolded.[15] Ginger was compared against scopolamine (0.6 mg orally) in several small groups of test subjects. It was concluded that ginger administered as 500 to 1000 mg powdered root or 1000 mg fresh root provided no protection against motion sickness under various test conditions, while the scopolamine group was able to tolerate a significant increase in number of head movements. In this same study, gastric emptying and gastric electrical activity (via electrogastrogram [EGG]) were evaluated in 2 more small groups of subjects. Ginger partially inhibited and stabilized tachygastria but did not affect EGG amplitude. The authors concluded that symptoms of motion sickness can be dissociated from gastric electrical activity and that the partial tachygastric effects of ginger offer little to relieve the onset or severity of these symptoms.[15]

It has been proposed that, unlike antihistamines that act on the CNS, the aromatic, carminative, and possibly absorbent properties of ginger ameliorate the effects of motion sickness in the GI tract directly.[1,14,16] It may increase gastric motility and block GI reactions and subsequent nausea feedback.[14]

Postoperative nausea and vomiting (PONV): The anti-emetic effects of ginger have been compared with metoclopramide and droperidol in prevention of PONV.[17,18] One prospective, randomized, double-blind trial (n = 120) evaluated 1 g powdered ginger root and 10 mg metoclopramide administered 1 hour prior to anesthesia in women undergoing gynecological laparoscopy; anesthesia was induced with propofol, fentanyl, and atracurium. Findings supported those of previous studies; ginger and metoclopramide were equally effective and were more effective than placebo in reducing the incidence of PONV (21%, 27%, and 41%, respectively). The need for postoperative antiemetics was significantly reduced in those receiving ginger over the placebo group (15% vs 38%, p = 0.006).[17]

In a placebo-controlled comparison against droperidol, no statistically significant difference was found with ginger root or ginger root plus droperidol in the incidence of PONV in 120 women undergoing outpatient gynecological laparoscopy; anesthesia was induced with thiopental, fentanyl, and succinylcholine. Patients were given droperidol (1.25 mg IV), oral ginger root (1 g given 1 hour prior to induction of anesthesia and 1 g given 30 minutes prior to discharge), ginger plus droperidol or placebo. While incidences of postoperative nausea (20%, 22%, 33%, and 32%) and vomiting (13%, 25%, 25%, and 35%) did not reach statistical significance, the figures appear to have potential clinical importance.[18]

A dosage study (randomized, double-blind, placebo-controlled) concluded that 0.5 g and 1 g powdered ginger root were ineffective in reducing the incidence of PONV in 108 patients. However, study methods in this particular trial could be questioned. To allow the identifying aroma of the ginger capsules to dissipate, capsules were removed from their original container and stored in pairs for 2 days in plastic bags until the odor disappeared. It has already been noted that the pungent principles (including the sesquiterpenes lending ginger its characteristic aroma) are responsible for ginger's pharmacological activity.[19]

Hyperemesis gravidarum: Pregnant women suffering from hyperemesis gravidarum received ginger (250 mg 4 times daily) or placebo for 4 days. About 70% of women subjectively preferred ginger treatment, with greater symptomatic relief being observed compared with placebo.[20]

Selective serotonin reuptake inhibitor discontinuation syndrome: One case report describes the successful use of ginger in one female patient with subsequent beneficial use in over 20 additional patients for the amelioration of symptoms (eg, disequilibrium, nausea) associated with abrupt discontinuation or intermittent noncompliance of selective serotonin reuptake inhibitors. Administration of 1100 mg ginger root 3 times daily at the onset of discontinuation-induced symptoms resulted in partial to complete relief of symptoms within 24 to 48 hours; ginger therapy was continued for approximately 2 weeks, the time required for symptoms to usually abate.[21]

TOXICOLOGY: There are no reports of severe toxicity in humans from the ingestion of ginger root. In culinary quantities, the root is generally devoid of activity. Large overdoses carry the potential for causing CNS depression. Inhibition of platelet aggregation has been reported after consumption of large (clinically impractical) amounts of ginger but returned to normal within one week of discontinuation.[10] Reports that ginger extracts may be mutagenic or antimutagenic in experimental test models require confirmation.[1,21]

There is no convincing evidence regarding the safety of ingesting large amounts of ginger by pregnant women. The German Commission E contraindicates ginger for the use of morning sickness, however, data are lacking to support toxic effects in pregnant women.[1,5,6] The FDA considers ginger as a food supplement as generally recognized as safe (GRAS).[22,23]

[1] Langner E, et al. *Adv Ther*. 1998;15(1):25-44.
[2] Ernst E, Pittler MH. *Br J Anaesth*. 2000;84:367-371.
[3] Grontved A, et al. *Acta Otolaryngol*. 1988;105:45-49.
[4] Schauenberg P, et al. *Guide to Medicinal Plants*. New Canaan, CT: Keats Publishing, Inc., 1977.
[5] Blumenthal M, et al. 1997. *German Commission E Monographs: Therapeutic Monographs on Medicinal Plants for Human Use*. Austin, TX: American Botanical Council.
[6] Blumenthal M. 1997. *Popular Herbs in the US Market: Therapeutic Monographs*. Austin, TX:American Botanical Council.
[7] Newall C, et al. 1996. *Herbal Medicines: A Guide for Healthcare Professionals*. London: Pharmaceutical Press.
[8] Shoji N, et al. *J Pharm Sci*. 1982;71(1):1174-1175.
[9] Kiuchi F, et al. *Chem Pharm Bull*. 1982;30(2):754-757.
[10] Lumb A. *Thromb Haemost*. 1994;71(1):110-111.
[11] Matthes H, et al. *Phytochemistry*. 1980;19:2643.
[12] Mackefield G, et al. *Int J Clin Pharmacol Ther*. 1999;37(7):341-346.
[13] Phillips S, et al. *Anaesthesia*. 1993;48(5):393-395.
[14] Mowrey D, et al. *Lancet*. 1982;1(8273):655-657.
[15] Stewart J, et al. *Pharmacology*. 1991;42(2):111-120.
[16] Yang R, et al. *Economic Botany*. 1988;42(3):376.

[17] Phillips S, et al.*Anaesthesia.* 1993;48(8):715-717.

[18] Visalyaputra S, et al. *Anaesthesia.* 1998;53:506-510.

[19] Arfeen Z, et al. *Anaesth Intensive Care.* 1995;23:449-452.

[20] Fischer-Rasmussen W, et al. *Eur J Obstet Gynecol Reprod Biol.* 1991;38(1):19-24.

[21] Schechter J. *J Clin Psychiatry.* 1998;59(8):431-432.

[22] Food and Drug Administration, Department of Health and Human Services. Code of Federal Regulations, 21CFR182.10. Accessed via http://www.access.gpo.gov/nara/cfr/cfr-table-search.html. March 2000.

[23] *Herb safety and drug interactions.* 1998. Boulder, CO: Herb Research Foundation.

SCIENTIFIC NAME(S): *Ginkgo biloba* L. Family: Ginkgoaceae

COMMON NAME(S): Ginkgo, maidenhair tree, kew tree, ginkyo, yinhsing (Silver Apricot-Japanese)

✺✺✺ PATIENT INFORMATION ✺✺✺

Uses: Ginkgo has been used to treat Raynaud disease, cerebral insufficiency, anxiety/stress, tinnitus, dementias, circulatory disorders/asthma. It has positive effects on memory and diseases associated with free radical generation.

Side Effects: Severe side effects are rare; possible effects include headache, dizziness, heart palpitations, and gastrointestinal (GI) and dermatologic reactions. Ginkgo pollen can be strongly allergenic. Contact with the fleshy fruit pulp causes allergic dermatitis, similar to poison ivy.

Dosing: Standardized gingko leaf extracts such as EGb761 (*Tebonin forte*, Schwabe) have been used in clinical trials for dementia, memory, and circulatory disorders at daily doses of 120 to 720 mg of extract. Extracts usually are standardized to 24% flavones and 6% terpene lactones.[1-8]

BOTANY: Ginkgo is the world's oldest living tree species and can be traced back more than 200 million years to fossils of the Permian period. It is the sole survivor of the family Ginkgoaceae. Individual trees may live as long as 1000 years. They grow to a height of approximately 37 m and have fan-shaped leaves. The species is dioecious; male trees more than 20 years old blossom in the spring. Adult female trees produce a plum-like, gray-tan fruit that falls in late autumn. Its fleshy pulp has a foul, offensive odor and causes contact dermatitis. The edible inner seed resembles an almond and is sold in Asian markets.[9]

HISTORY: In China, where the species survived the ice age, ginkgo was cultivated as a sacred tree, and is still found decorating Buddhist temples throughout Asia. It has not been found in the wild. Preparations have been used for medicinal purposes for more than 1000 years. Traditional Chinese physicians used ginkgo leaves to treat asthma and chillblains, which is the swelling of the hands and feet from exposure to damp cold. The ancient Chinese and Japanese ate roasted ginkgo seeds, and considered them a digestive aid and preventive against drunkenness.[10] The flavonoids act as free radical scavengers and the terpenes (ginkgolides) inhibit platelet activating factor.[11] Currently, oral and IV forms are available in Europe, where it is one of the most widely prescribed medications. Neither form has been approved for medical use in the US, where ginkgo is sold as a nutritional supplement.

PHARMACOLOGY: Numerous studies on the pharmacological actions of ginkgo have been reported, including treatment of cerebral insufficiency, dementia, circulatory disorders, and asthma. The plant is also known for its antioxidant and neuroprotective effects.

Cerebral insufficiency: Cerebral insufficiency may cause anxiety and stress; memory, concentration, and mood impairment; and hearing disorders, all of which may benefit from ginkgo therapy. IV injection of ginkgo biloba extract (GBE) increased cerebral blood flow in approximately 70% of the patients evaluated. This increase was age-related: Patients between 30 and 50 years of age had a 20% increase from baseline, compared with 70% in those 50 to 70 years of age. Further, the time to reach peak blood flow was shorter in the elderly.[12] Cerebral insufficiency in 112 patients (average age 70.5 years) treated with ginkgo leaf extract (120 mg) for 1 year, resulted in reduced symptoms such as headache, dizziness, short-term memory, vigilance, and disturbance.[13] Electroencephalographic effects of different preparations of GBE have been measured.[14] A review of 40 clinical trials, most evaluating 120 mg GBE per day for 4 to 6 weeks, reported positive results in treating cerebral insufficiency. Only 8 studies did not have major methodological flaws; the results from these studies were, nevertheless, difficult to interpret. They suggested that long-term treatment (more than 6 weeks) is required and that any effect is similar to that observed following treatment with ergoloids.[15] A meta-analysis of 11 placebo-controlled, randomized, double-blinded studies, concluded GBE (150 mg/day) was superior to placebo in patients with cerebrovascular insufficiency.[16]

Antianxiety/Stress: MAO inhibition in rats produced by extracts of ginkgo (dried and fresh leaves) was detected, suggesting a mechanism by which the plant exerts its antistress actions.[17]

Memory improvement: In elderly men with slight age-related memory loss, ginkgo supplementation reduced the time required to process visual information.[18] Effects of GBE on event-related potentials in 48 patients with age-associated memory impairment have been measured.[19] Significant improvement in memory (as measured by a series of psychological testing), in 8 patients (average age, 32 years) was found one hour after administration of 600 mg GBE vs placebo, again confirming the plant's usefulness in this area.[13]

Tinnitus hearing disorder therapy: Because of the diverse etiology of tinnitus and lack of objective method to measure its symptoms, results using GBE for treatment of this disease are contradictory. GBE may have positive effects in some individuals.[20]

In patients with hearing disorders secondary to vascular insufficiency of the ear, approximately 40% of those treated orally with a leaf extract for 2 to 6 months showed improvement in auditory measurements. The extract was also effective in relieving vertigo associated with vestibular dysfunction.[21]

Dementias: Therapeutic effectiveness of ginkgo biloba in dementia syndromes has been demonstrated.[22,23] One report recommends early GBE therapy in dementias, especially because there are no side effects associated with other dementia drugs.[24]

Effects of 240 mg/day GBE in approximately 200 patients with dementia of Alzheimer type and multi-infarct dementia, have been investigated in a randomized, double-blinded, placebo-controlled, multi-center study. Parameters such as psychopathological assessment, attention, memory, and behavior were monitored, resulting in clinical efficacy of the extract in dementias of both types.[25] In another set of patients with moderate dementias (of Alzheimer, vascular, or mixed type), short-term IV infusion therapy with GBE also had positive results, improving psychopathology and cognitive performance.[26] In a 52-week, randomized, double-blinded, placebo-controlled, multi-center study, mild-to-severe Alzheimer or multi-infarct dementia patients received 120 mg/day GBE vs placebo. Results of this report again confirm improved cognitive performance and social functioning in a number of cases.[27]

Circulatory disorders/asthma: Ginkgolides competitively inhibit the binding of platelet-activating factor (PAF) to its membrane receptor.[13,28] Effects of this mechanism are useful in the treatment of allergic reaction and inflammation (asthma and bronchospasm) and also in circulatory diseases.

In 1 double-blinded, randomized, crossover study in asthma patients, ginkgolides were effective in early and late phases of airway hyperactivity.[13]

A meta-analysis evaluating GBE in peripheral arterial disease, concludes a highly significant therapeutic effect of the extract in this area.[29] Numerous studies are available concerning GBE and circulatory disorders including its ability to protect against cardiac ischemia reperfusion injury,[30] to adjust fibrinolytic activity,[31] and, in combination with aspirin, to treat thrombosis.[32] It also appears useful in management of peripheral vascular disorders such as Raynaud disease, acrocyanosis, and post-phlebitis syndrome.[21] IV injection of 50 to 200 mg of ginkgo extract caused a dose-dependent increase in microcirculation and blood viscoelasticity in patients with pathologic blood flow disorders.[33]

A 6-month, double-blind trial suggested some efficacy in treating obliterative arterial disease of the lower limbs. Patients who received extract showed a clinically and statistically significant improvement in pain-free walking distance, maximum walking distance, and plethysmorgraphic recordings of peripheral blood flow.[34] GBE improved walking performance in 60 patients with intermittent claudication, with good tolerance to the drug.[1] However, another report concluded that GBE 120 mg/day has no effect on walking distance or leg pain in intermittent claudication patients (but found other cognitive functions to be improved).[35] A

review of 10 controlled trials evaluating treatment with the plant for this condition, found poor methodological quality, but did note all the studies to show clinical effectiveness of GBE in treating intermittent claudication.[36]

Antioxidant/neuroprotective effects: GBE is known to improve diseases associated with free radical generation. The ginkgolides may contribute to neuroprotective effects. The flavonoid fraction contains free radical scavengers, both of which are important in areas such as hypoxia, seizure activity, and peripheral nerve damage.[37]

In Chernobyl accident recovery workers, GBE's antioxidant effects were studied. Clastogenic factors (risk factors for development of late effects of irradiation) were successfully reduced by the plant.[38]

A number of potentially beneficial effects have been observed for ginkgo, including its ability to prevent the deterioration of lipid profiles when subjects were challenged with high-cholesterol meals over an extended holiday season,[39] improvement in the symptoms of PMS, particularly breast-related symptoms,[40] use in eye problems,[28] and its scavenging abilities to reduce functional and morphological retina impairments.[41] In addition, GBE has in vitro and in vivo activity against *Pneumocystis carinii*,[42] and has been studied in animals with diabetes[43,44] and human diabetic patients. When GBE extract was given, peripheral blood flow increased by 40% to 45%, compared with an increase of 35% after administration of nicotinic acid.[45] Other reports suggest GBE to be effective in arresting fibrosis development (in 86 chronic hepatitis patients),[46] promoting hair regrowth in mice,[47] and relaxing penile tissue, suggesting a possible use as a drug for impotence.[48] Seed extracts of the plant possess antibacterial and anti-fungal activity.[28]

TOXICOLOGY: Ingestion of the extract has not been associated with severe side effects. Adverse events from clinical trials of up to 160 mg/day for 4 to 6 weeks did not differ from the placebo group. German literature lists ginkgo's possible side effects as headache, dizziness, heart palpitations, and GI and dermatologic reactions. Injectable forms of ginkgo may cause circulatory disturbances, skin allergy, or phlebitis. Willmar Schwabe Co. has withdrawn its parenteral ginkgo product *Tebonin* from the market because of the possible severity of side effects from this form.[28]

A toxic syndrome ("Gin-nan" food poisoning) has been recognized in Asia in children who have ingested ginkgo seeds. Approximately 50 seeds produce tonic/clonic seizures and loss of consciousness.[49] Seventy reports (between 1930 and 1960) found 27% lethality, with infants being most vulnerable. Ginkgotoxin (4-O-methylpyridoxine), found only in the seeds, was responsible for this toxicity.[13,28]

Contact with the fleshy fruit pulp is known to irritate the skin. Constituents alkylbenzoic acid, alkylphenol, and their derivatives cause reactions of this type. Allergic dermatitis such as erythema, edema, blisters, and itching have all been reported.[28] A cross-allergenicity exists between ginkgo fruit pulp and poison ivy. Ginkgolic acid and bilobin are structurally similar to the allergens of poison ivy, mango rind, and cashew nut shell oil. Contact with the fruit pulp causes erythema and edema, with the rapid formation of vesicles accompanied by severe itching. Symptoms last 7 to 10 days. Ingestion of two pieces of pulp has been reported to cause perioral erythema, rectal burning, and painful spasms of the anal sphincter.[9]

Allergans ginkgols and ginkgolic acids can cause contact reactions of mucous membranes, resulting in cheilitis and GI irritation. However, oral ginkgo preparations do not have this ability.[13,28] Ginkgo pollen can be strongly allergenic.[50]

In one report, spontaneous bilateral subdural hematomas have been associated with ingestion of the plant.[51]

Because no human data are available about pregnancy and lactation, ginkgo should be avoided by this population.[5,20]

[1] Blume J, et al. *VASA*. 1996;25(3):265-274.

[2] Peters H, et al. *VASA*. 1998;27:106-110.

[3] Kanowski S, et al. *Phytomed*. 1997;4:3-13.

[4] Hofferberth B. *Human Psychopharmacol*. 1994;9:215-222.

[5] Le Bars PL, et al. *JAMA*. 1997;278:1327-1332.

[6] Hofferberth B. *Arzneimittelforschung*. 1989;39:918-922.

[7] Dubreuil C. *Presse Med*. 1986;15:1559-1561.

[8] Becker LE, et al. *JAMA* 1975;231:1162.

[9] Wettstein A. *Fortschr Med*. 1999;117:48-49.

[10] Castleman M. *The Herb Quarterly*. 1990 Spring:26.

[11] Z'Brun A. *Schweiz Rundsch Med Prax*. 1995;84(1):1-6.

[12] Pistolese GR. *Minerva Med*. 1973;79:4166.

[13] Newall C, et al. *Herbal Medicines*. London, England: Pharmaceutical Press, 1996;138-140.

[14] Kunkel H. *Neuropsychobiology*. 1993;27(1):40-45.

[15] Kleijnen J, et al. *Br J Clin Pharmacol*. 1992;34(4):352-58.

[16] Hopfenmuller W. *Arzneimittelforschung*. 1994;44(9):1005-1013.

[17] White H, et al. *Life Sci*. 1996;58(16):1315-1321.

[18] Allain H, et al. *Clin Ther*. 1993;15:549-558.

[19] Semlitsch H, et al. *Pharmacopsychiatry*. 1995;28(4):134-142.

[20] Holgers K, et al *Audiology*. 1994;33(2):85-92.

[21] Nazzaro P, et al. *Minerva Med*. 1973;79:4198.

[22] Herrschaft H. *Pharm Unserer Zeit*. 1992;21(6):266-275.

[23] Itil T, et al. *Psychopharmacol Bull*. 1995;31(1):147-158.

[24] Reisecker F. *Wien Med Wochenschr*. 1996;146(21-22):546-548.

[25] Kanowski S, et al. *Pharmacopsychiatry.* 1996;29(2):47-56.

[26] Haase J, et al. *Z Gerontol Geriatr.* 1996;29(4):302-309.

[27] LeBars P, et al. *JAMA.* 1997;278(16):1327-1332.

[28] DeSmet P, et al. Ginkgo Biloba. Berlin: Springer-Verlag 1997;51-66.

[29] Schneider B. *Arzneimittelforschung.* 1992;42(4):428-436.

[30] Haramaki N, et al. *Free Radic Biol Med.* 1994;16(6):789-794.

[31] Shen J, et al. *Biochem Mol Biol Int* .1995;35(1):125-134.

[32] Belougne E, et al. *Thromb Res.* 1996;82(5):453-458.

[33] Koltringer P, et al. *Fortschr Med.* 1993;111:170.

[34] Bauer U. *Arzneimittelforschung.* 1984;34:716.

[35] Drabaek H, et al. *Ugeskr Laeger.* 1996;158(27):3928-3931.

[36] Ernst E. *Fortschr Med.* 1996;114(8):85-87.

[37] Smith P, et al. *J Ethnopharmacol.* 1996;50(3):131-139.

[38] Emerit I, et al. *Radiat Res.* 1995;144(2):198-205.

[39] Kenzelmann R, et al. *Arzneimittelforschung.* 1993;43:978.

[40] Tamborini A, et al. *Ref Fr Gynecol Obstet.* 1993;88:447-457.

[41] Droy-Lefaix M, et al. *Int J Tissue React.* 1995;17(3):93-100.

[42] Atzori C, et al. *Antimicrob Agents Chemother.* 1993;37:1492.

[43] Agar A, et al. *Int J Neurosci.* 1994;76(3-4):259-266.

[44] Punkt K, et al. *ACTA Histochem.* 1997;99(3):291-299.

[45] Bartolo M. *Minerva Med.* 1973;79:4192.

[46] Li W, et al. *Chung Kuo Chung Hsi I Chieh Ho Tsa Chih.* 1995;15(10):593-595.

[47] Kobayashi N, et al. *Yakugaku Zasshi.* 1993;113(10):718-724.

[48] Paick J, et al. *J Urol.* 1996;156(5):1876-1880.

[49] Yagi M, et al. *Yakugaku Zasshi.* 1993;113:596.

[50] Long R, et al. *Hua Hsi I Ko Ta Hsueh Hsueh Pao.* 1992;23:429.

[51] Rowin J, et al. *Neurology.* 1996;46(6):1775-1776.

❧❧❧ PATIENT INFORMATION ❧❧❧

Uses: Ginseng is popular for a variety of uses, including adaptogenic, antine-oplastic, immunomodulatory, cardiovascular, CNS, endocrine, and ergogenic effects, but these uses have not been confirmed by clinical trials.

Interactions: Possible interactions with warfarin, loop diuretics, and phenelzine have been reported.

Side Effects: The most commonly reported side effects with ginseng are nervousness and excitation. However, there have been reports of diffuse mammary nodularity and vaginal bleeding. A hypoglycemic effect has also been reported; use with caution in those who must control their blood glucose levels.

Dosing: Ginseng root is standardized on content of ginsenosides, which should be greater than 1.5%. Extracts typically contain from 4% to 7% ginsenosides. Note that the profile of particular ginsenosides differs between American and Asian ginseng; however, the total ginsenoside content is similar. In numerous clinical trials, dosage of crude root has been from 0.5 to 3 g/day and dosage of extracts generally from 100 to 400 mg.[1-4]

BOTANY: Ginseng commonly refers to *Panax quinquefolius* L. or *Panax ginseng* C.A. Meyer, two members of the family Araliaceae. The ginsengs were classified as members of the genus Aralia in older texts.

Scientific name	Synonyms	Common name	Distribution
P. ginseng C.A. Meyer	*P. pseudoginseng* Wallich; *P. schinseng* Nees	Asian, Chinese, Korean, or Oriental ginseng;[1,5] red ginseng (steamed)	NE China, Korea, Eastern Siberia
P. japonicus var *bipinnatifidus*[5]			China
P. japonicus C.A. Meyer[5]	*P. pseudoginseng* (Will.) subsp. *japonicus*	Japanese ginseng[1,5] Chikusetsu ginseng,[6] or zhu je ginseng [4]	India, Southern China, Japan
P. japonicus var. *major*[5]			China
P. notoginseng (Burkhill) Hoo & Tseng;[5] ([Buck] F.H.Chen)	*P. pseudoginseng* Wallich var. *notoginseng*	Western ginseng; Five-fingers; Sang;[5] San-chi;[1,8] Tien-chan[1] or tienqi[7] ginseng	Asia
P. pseudoginseng subsp. himalaicus		Himalayan ginseng	Nepal
P. pseudoginseng var. *major*		Zhuzishen	China
P. quinquefolius L.		American or Canadian ginseng[1,9]	Eastern and Central USA and Canada
P. vietnamensis Ha et Grushv.		Vietnamese ginseng[1,8]	Vietnam

In the eastern and central United States and Canada,[6] ginseng is found in rich, cool woods; a significant crop is also grown commercially. The short plant grows from 3 to 7 compound leaves that drop in the fall. It bears a cluster of red or yellowish fruits from June to July. The shape of the root can vary between species and has been used to distinguish types of ginseng. Medicinally, it is the root that is considered most valuable in providing the pharmacologically active ginsenosides. Ginsenoside content varies with the age of the root, season of harvest, and preservation method. While at least 4 ginsenosides are detectable in most young roots, this number more than doubles after 6 years of growth. High quality ginseng is generally collected in the fall after 5 to 6 years of growth.[6]

HISTORY: Ginseng is perhaps the most widely recognized plant used in traditional medicine and now plays a major role in the herbal health care market. For more than 2000 years, various forms have been used in medicine. The name *Panax* derives from the Greek word for "all healing" and its properties have been no less touted. Ginseng root's man-shaped figure (shen-seng means "man-root") led proponents of the "Doctrine of Signatures" to believe that the root could strengthen any part of the body. Through the ages, the root has been used in the treatment of asthenia, atherosclerosis, blood and bleeding disorders, colitis, and to relieve the symptoms of aging, cancer, and senility.

Evidence that the root possesses a general strengthening effect, raises mental and physical capacity, and exerts a protectant effect against experimental diabetes, neurosis, radiation sickness, and some cancers has been reported. Today, its popularity is because of the proposed "adaptogenic effect" (stress-protective) of the saponin content.

PHARMACOLOGY:

Adaptogenic effects: From the earliest times, it has been claimed that ginseng exerts a strengthening effect while also raising physical and mental capacity for work. These properties have been defined as an "adaptogenic effect" or a nonspecific increase in resistance to the noxious effects of physical, chemical, or biological stress.[10] Animal studies have shown that ginseng extracts can prolong swimming time, prevent stress-induced ulcers, stimulate the proliferation of hepatic ribosomes, increase natural killer cell activity, and may enhance the production of interferons.[11] Huong, et al (1998), described antistress effects in rats of a saponin in Vietnamese ginseng (MR2); evidence from this study suggested that modulation of opioid, GABA, corticotropin-releasing factor, or interactions thereof were responsible for the effects of MR2.[8] However, a study in mice found no adaptogenic effects.[12]

CNS effects: R_{b1} and R_{g1} appear to play a major role in CNS stimulatory and inhibitory effects and may modulate neurotransmitters. Cholinergic activity implicated in mediating learning and memory processes has been shown to be affected by certain ginsenosides.

In humans, two randomized double-blind, placebo-controlled studies (n = 32 and n = 127) using *P. ginseng* (200 to 400 mg/day for 8 to 12 weeks) were reported to have shown improvements in cognitive functioning, specifically mental arithmetic and abstraction.[1] However, another evaluation of one of these same studies claimed the improvements were not significant.[6] A third study of 50 elderly patients (65 to 80 years of age) comparing *P. ginseng* (dose not reported) to a neurotrophic amino acid/vitamin B_{12} combination reported significant improvements for the ginseng group over baseline however, these results were inferior compared with those of the neurotrophic combination group.[6]

Endocrine effects: Randomized, placebo-controlled human trials have confirmed the hypoglycemic effects of ginseng reported in earlier animal studies.[2,13,14] One study noted statistically significant ($P < 0.01$) improvements in fasting blood glucose and reductions in $HbA1_c$ in subjects with type 2 diabetes mellitus treated 8 weeks with 100 and 200 mg ginseng, respectively (manufacturer listed but species not noted). However, all patients studied also lost weight, which may be touted as equivocal overall results. Two studies have shown that 3 g ground root of *P. quinquefolius* exerts a glucose-lowering effect only postprandially or when stimulated by glucose ingestion.[13,14] Evidence appears to support modulation of insulin sensitization and secretion based on the fact that the cholinergic, dopaminergic, adrenergic, and NO actions found with ginsenosides also have been noted to affect glucose metabolism in animal.[13,14]

Ergogenic effects: Strong evidence supporting the efficacy of ginseng in improving physical performance seems to be lacking. Physical performance in young, active volunteers was found unimproved in 4 studies; however, other studies reported a decrease in heart rate and an increase in maximal oxygen uptake.[1] One comprehensive literature search evaluated data from human studies on *P. ginseng* preparations. Properly controlled studies using higher doses (standardized to 2 g/day of dried root), administered for at least 8 weeks and in larger subject numbers, more often exhibited statistically significant improvements in physical or psychomotor performance. Benefit was most likely to be seen in untrained subjects or those over 40 years of age.[7]

INTERACTIONS: A possible interaction with warfarin has been noted in a case report of a 47-year-old man stabilized on warfarin for 5 years. Four weeks prior to taking ginseng, as *Ginsana* (a commercial product) 3 times daily, his international normalized ratio (INR) was 3.1 and had ranged from 3 to 4 over the previous 9 months; 2 weeks after starting *Ginsana*, his INR decreased to 1.5, but returned to 3.3 within 2 weeks after discontinuing the ginseng. Changes in drug regimens,

dietary consumption of vitamin K, or other nutritional supplements were ruled out as a possible cause of his subtherapeutic INR. No thrombotic episodes occurred during *Ginsana* administration; however, risk of thrombosis prevented rechallenge to confirm this interaction. The mechanism of this interaction is unknown; whether this is a drug interaction or assay interference has yet to be determined.[15]

Refractoriness to the loop diuretic furosemide has been reported in a 63-year-old man approximately 10 days after he started taking 10 to 12 ginseng tablets daily.[16] The patient was hospitalized for edema and hypertension. While in the hospital, he did not receive any nutritional products and responded to IV furosemide. He was discharged from the hospital on oral furosemide. Following discharge, the patient started taking his nutritional supplements and once again developed worsening edema and hypertension.

Two case reports describe hyperstimulation symptoms (eg, insomnia, headache, tremulousness, irritability, and visual hallucinations) when ginseng was taken concomitantly with phenelzine.[17]

For other potential interactions, refer to the "Potential Herb-Drug Interactions" appendix.

TOXICOLOGY: It is estimated that more than 6 million people ingest ginseng regularly in the United States. There have been few reports of severe reactions.

Several reports have implicated ginseng as having an estrogen-like effect in women.[18] One case of diffuse mammary nodularity has been reported,[19] as well as a case of vaginal bleeding in a 72-year-old woman.[20]

Neonatal death has been reported; avoid use during pregnancy and lactation.

The most commonly reported side effects of ginseng are nervousness and excitation, which usually diminish after the first few days of use or with dosage reduction. It has been suggested that methylxanthine constituents of ginseng root (eg, caffeine, theophylline) may contribute to these physiological effects.[6] Inability to concentrate has also been reported following long-term use.[21]

The hypoglycemic effect of the whole root and individual panaxosides has been reported by many investigators. Although no cases of serious reactions in diabetic patients have been reported, people who must control their blood glucose levels should take ginseng with caution.

Ginseng also should not be used by those with high blood pressure.

[1] Vogler B, Pittler MH, Ernst E. *Eur J Clin Pharmacol*. 1999;55:567-575.

[2] Sotaniemi EA, Haapakoski E, Rautio A. *Diabetes Care*. 1995;18:1373-1375.

[3] Ziemba AW, Chmura J, Kaciuba-Uscilko H, Nazar K, Wisnik P, Gawronski W. *Int J Sport Nutr*. 1999;9:371-377.

[4] D'Angelo L, Grimaldi R, Caravaggi M, et al. *J Ethnopharmacol*. 1986;16:15-22.

[5] Newall C, Anderson L, Phillipson J. *Herbal medicines, a guide for health-care professionals*. London: The Pharmaceutical Press, 1996:145-50.

[6] Bahrke M, et al. *Sports Med* 2000;29(2):113-33.

[7] Bucci LR. *Am J Clin Nutr* 2000;72(suppl):624S-636S.

[8] Huong N, et al. *Methods Find Exp Clin Pharmacol* 1998;20(1):65-76.

[9] Wong A, et al. *Arch Gen Psychiatry* 1998;55:1033-44.

[10] Brekhman II, Dardymov IV. *Lloydia* 1969;32:46.

[11] Singh V, et al. *Planta Med* 1984;50:462.

[12] Lewis W, et al. *J Ethnopharm* 1983;8:209.

[13] Vuksan V, et al. *Arch Intern Med* 2000;160:1009-13.

[14] Vuksan V, et al. *Diabetes Care* 2000;23(9):1221-26.

[15] Janetzky K, et al. *Am J Health Syst Pharm* 1997;54:692-3.

[16] Becker B, et al. *JAMA* 1996;276:606.

[17] Klepser T, et al. *Am J Health Syst Pharm* 1999;56:125-38.

[18] Punnonen R, et al. *BMJ* 1980;281:1110.

[19] Palmer B, et al. G*BMJ* 1978;1:1284.

[20] Greenspan E. *JAMA* 1983;249:2018.

[21] Hammond T, et al. *Med J Aust* 1981;1:492.

Glucosamine

SCIENTIFIC NAME(S): 2-Amino-2-deoxyglucose

COMMON NAME(S): Chitosamine

❧❧❧❧ PATIENT INFORMATION ❧❧❧❧

Uses: Glucosamine is being investigated extensively as an antiarthritic in osteoarthritis.

Side effects: Well tolerated. No serious side effects have been associated directly with glucosamine. The potential of glucosamine to alter blood glucose levels warrants caution of use in diabetic patients. The majority of side effects have been mild, including gastric discomfort (eg, heartburn, diarrhea, nausea, vomiting) and itching.

BIOLOGY: Glucosamine is found in mucopolysaccharides, mucoproteins, and chitin. Chitin is found in yeasts, fungi, arthropods, and various marine invertebrates as a major component of the exoskeleton. It also occurs in other lower animals and members of the plant kingdom.[1]

PHARMACOLOGY: Chitin has been described as a vulnerary or wound-healing polymer,[2] while glucosamine has been referred to as a pharmaceutical aid, chondroprotective, antireactive,[3] and antiarthritic.[1] In osteoarthritis (the most common form of arthritis), there is a progressive degeneration of cartilage glycosaminoglycans (GAG). The idea of using glucosamine orally is to provide a "building block" for its regeneration. Glucosamine is the rate-limiting step in GAG biosynthesis. It is biochemically formed from the glycolytic intermediate fructose-6-phosphate by way of amination of glutamine as the donor, ultimately yielding glucosamine-6-phosphate. This is subsequently converted or acetylated to galactosamine before being incorporated into growing GAG. This will stimulate the production of cartilage components and bring about improvement of the articular conditions, thus leading to joint repair.[3,4] Glucosamine also has been reported to protect the articular cartilage from the damages exerted by some nonsteroidal anti-inflammatory drugs (NSAIDs).[5]

Several double-blind studies indicate that glucosamine sulfate may be better than some NSAIDs and placebos in relieving pain and inflammation caused by osteoarthritis.[4,6-9] The relative efficacy of ibuprofen and glucosamine sulfate was compared in the management of osteoarthritis of the knee.[10,11,12] This included 3 studies, 2 at 4 weeks and 1 at 8 weeks, that showed glucosamine (1.5 g/day orally) was more effective in reducing pain when compared with ibuprofen. Oral glucosamine sulfate therapy vs placebo in osteoarthritis was studied (80 patients, 1.5 g/day orally) and researchers found decreased symptoms and improved autonomous motility with glucosamine.[13] These investigators also employed electron microscopy studies on cartilage and found that patients who received placebo showed a typical picture of established osteoarthrosis while those given glucosamine showed a picture similar to healthy cartilage. They concluded that glucosamine tends to rebuild damaged cartilage, thus restoring articular function in most chronic arthrosic patients.[13]

The majority of these early studies were completed outside of North America. Two other studies, one in Canada and one in the United States, did not show any significant difference when glucosamine was compared with placebo in reducing pain in knee osteoarthritis.[14,15]

A Cochrane Systematic Review identified 16 randomized, controlled trials that demonstrated efficacy and safety of glucosamine in osteoarthritis. The formulation of glucosamine used was questioned as most trials used a formulation available in Europe.[16]

A meta-analysis compared 6 glucosamine trials that also concluded that glucosamine has a moderate effect on osteoarthritis. The formulation of glucosamine used was also questioned, along with the short duration of the trials, and potential publication bias.[17,18]

Glucosamine also can be found in combination with chondroitin sulfate with or without manganese. Two randomized, placebo-controlled trials have demonstrated these combinations' ability to relieve symptoms of knee osteoarthritis.[19,20]

A 3-year randomized, double-blind, placebo-controlled trial involving 139 patients over 50 years of age with primary, mild to moderate knee osteoarthritis compared 1500 mg/day of glucosamine to placebo. Symptom improvement was reported, as well as mild adverse events. There was no significant joint-space narrowing in patients who received glucosamine, demonstrating slowing of progression of osteoarthritis. This study excluded obese patients (in whom osteoarthritis is prevalent) and was conducted in Europe where glucosamine is a standardized prescription product. Extrapolation to products available in the United States cannot be made.[21,22]

Deficiencies of studies include short duration (4 to 8 weeks), exclusion of the severe forms of osteoarthritis, sponsorship by the glucosamine manufacturer, use of different formulations of glucosamine and different dosages, use of analgesics in some trials, and use of different outcome assessments of arthritis pain and mobility (ie, Lequesne Index and Western Ontario and McMaster Universities [WOMAC] questionnaire). Different patient populations were studied in various countries, making generalization to individual patients difficult.[9,11,14-16,18,21,23]

Controversy about glucosamine arose with the publication in 1997 of *The Arthritis Cure*. Subsequent response by *The Medical Letter on Drugs and Therapeutics* stated, "glucosamine appears to be safe and might be effective."[24]

A randomized, double-blind, placebo-controlled clinical efficacy study called the Glucosamine/Chondroitin Arthritis Intervention Trial (GAIT) is recruiting patients (as of June 10, 2002) with osteoarthritis of the knee in the United States to determine effect on joint space and to definitively determine the efficacy and safety of glucosamine and chondroitin (alone and in combination) with a 2-year follow-up period. Additional information along with inclusion and exclusion criteria can be found at the clinical trials Web site, http://www.clinicaltrials.gov.[25]

TOXICOLOGY: No direct toxic effects of glucosamine could be found in the scientific literature; however, 1 report describes potential bronchopulmonary complications of antirheumatic drugs including glucosamine.[26]

The majority of side effects have been mild, including gastric discomfort (eg, heartburn, diarrhea, nausea, vomiting) and itching.[9,11,12,19] Occult blood in feces has been reported in patients taking glucosamine.[10]

Concern that glucosamine may increase blood glucose levels in patients with diabetes is the result of several animal and human studies.[27-29] Variability in results was reported because of different glucosamine doses used, from a significant 17% reduction to a marginal effect.[27,30] A study in 10 healthy patients found that an infusion of glucosamine sulfate reduced glucose tolerance.[31] The exact mechanism of the effect of glucosamine on glucose levels has not been elucidated.[32] Until a definitive conclusion has been made, patients with diabetes and osteoarthritis are advised to inform their health care provider prior to starting glucosamine.[33,34]

[1] Budavari S, ed. *The Merck Index*; 11th edition, Merck & Co., Inc., N.J. 1989;4353.

[2] Budavari S, ed. *The Merck Index*; 11th edition, Merck & Co., Inc., N.J. 1989;2049.

[3] Setnikar I. *Int J Tiss Reac*. 1992;14:253-261.

[4] Anonymous. *Am J Natl Med*. 1994;1:10-14.

[5] Rovati LC. *Int J Tiss Reac*. 1992;14:243-251.

[6] Reichelt A, Forster KK, Fischer M, Rovati LC, Setnikar I. *Arzneim-Forsch/Drug Res*. 1994;44:75-80.

[7] Vajaradul Y. *Clin Ther*. 1981;3:336-343.

[8] Pujalte JM, Llavore EP, Ylescupidez FR. *Curr Med Res Opin*. 1980;7:110-114.

[9] Noack W, Fischer M, Forster KK, Rovati LC, Setnikar I. *Osteoarthritis Cartilage*. 1994;2:51-59.

[10] Vaz AL. *Current Med Res Op*. 1982;8:145-149.

[11] Muller-Fassbender H, Bach GL, Haase W, Rovati LC, Setnikar I. *Osteoarthritis Cartilage*. 1994;2:61-69.

[12] Qiu GX, Gao SN, Giacovelli G, Rovati L, Setnikar I. *Arzneim-Forsch/Drug Res*. 1998;48:469-474.

[13] Drovanti A, Bignamini AA, Rovati AL. *Clin Ther*. 1980;3:260-272.

[14] Houpt JB, McMillan R, Wein C, Paget-Dellio SD. *J Rheumatol*. 1999;26:2423-2430.

[15] Rindone JP, Hiller D, Collacott E, Nordhaugen N, Arriola G. *West J Med*. 2000;172:91-94.

[16] Towheed TE, Anastassiades TP, Shea B, Houpt J, Welch V, Hochberg MC. Glucosamine therapy for treating osteoarthritis (Cochrane Review). In: The Cochrane Library, Issue 1, 2002. Oxford: Update Software.

[17] McAlindon TE, LaValley MP, Gulin JP, Felson DT. *JAMA*. 2000;283:1469-1475.

[18] Towheed TE, Anastassiades TP. *JAMA*. 2000;283:1483-1484.

[19] Leffler CT, Philippi AF, Leffler SG, Mosure JC, Kim PD. *Mil Med*. 1999;164:85-91.

[20] Das A Jr, Hammad TA. *Osteoart Cart*. 2000;8:343-350.

[21] Reginster JY, Deroisy R, Rovati LC, et al. *Lancet*. 2001;357:251-256.

[22] McAlindon T. *Lancet*. 2001;357:247-248.

[23] Anonymous. *Bandolier*. 1997;4:1-3.

[24] Anonymous. *Med Let*. 1997;39:91-92.

[25] National Institutes of Health. Glucosamine/chondroitin arthritis intervention trial (GAIT). Sponsors: National Center for Complementary and Alternative Medicine, National Institute of Arthritis and Musculoskeletal and Skin Diseases, and Department of Veterans Affairs Co-operative Studies Program. U.S. National Library of Medicine 2002.

[26] Larget-Piet B, Martigny J, Villiaumey J. *Therapie*. 1986;41:269-277.

[27] Baron AD, Zhu JS, Zhu JH, Weldon H, Maianu L, Garvey WT. *J Clin Invest*. 1995;96:2792-2801.

[28] Virkamaki A, Yki-Jarvinen H. *Diabetes*. 1999;48:1101-1107.

[29] Patti ME, Virkamaki A, Loandaker EJ, Kahn CR, Yki-Jarvinen H. *Diabetes*. 1999;48:1562-1571.

[30] Miles PDG, Higo K, Romeo, OM, Lee MK, Rafaat K, Olefsky JM. *Diabetes*. 1998;47:395-400.

[31] Monauni T, Zenti MG, Cretti A, et al. *Diabetes*. 2000;49:926-935.

[32] Nelson BA, Robinson KA, Buse MG. *Diabetes*. 2000;49:981-991.

[33] Adams ME. *Lancet*. 1999;354:353-354.

[34] Russell AI, McCarty MF. *Lancet*. 1999;354:1641.

SCIENTIFIC NAME(S): *Hydrastis canadensis* L. Family: Ranunculaceae

COMMON NAME(S): Goldenseal, yellowroot, orangeroot, eyebalm, eyeroot, goldenroot, ground raspberry, Indian turmeric, yellow puccoon, jaundice root, sceau d'or

---

❧❧❧ PATIENT INFORMATION ❧❧❧

Uses: Goldenseal may be of use in topical infections and is used as an eyewash. Goldenseal has been included in cold and flu preparations for its anticatarrhal effects but little evidence supports this use and its effects are debatable.

Side Effects: Goldenseal is contraindicated in pregnancy and hypertension; adverse effects with normal doses are rare.

Dosing: Goldenseal has not been the subject of any formal clinical trials for external antiseptic or antiherpes properties. Extracts standardized to 5% hydrastine are available; however, the berberine content may be more important for goldenseal's medicinal uses. Doses of 100 mg hydrastine and 2 g crude root have been proposed.[1]

BOTANY: Goldenseal is a perennial herb found in the rich woods of the Ohio River valley and other locations in the northeastern US. The single, green-white flower, which has no petals, appears in the spring on a hairy stem above a basal leaf and 2 palmate, wrinkled leaves. The flower develops into a red seeded berry. The plant grows from horizontal, bright yellow rhizomes, which have a twisted, knotty appearance.

HISTORY: Goldenseal root was used medicinally by American Indians of the Cherokee, Catawba, Iroquois, and Kickapoo tribes as an insect repellent, a diuretic, a stimulant, and a wash for sore or inflamed eyes.[2] It was used to treat arrow wounds and ulcers,[3] as well as to produce a yellow dye. Early settlers learned of these uses from the Indians and the root found its way into most 19th century pharmacopeias. The Eclectic medical movement was particularly enthusiastic in its adoption of goldenseal for gonorrhea and urinary tract infections. The widespread harvesting of *Hydrastis* in the 19th century, coupled with loss of habitat, resulted in depletion of wild populations. In 1997, *Hydrastis* was listed under Appendix II of the Convention on International Trade in Endangered Species of Wild Fauna and Flora (CITES), which controls exports of the root to other countries. The final listing included roots or live plants but excluded finished products. As an alternative to wild harvesting, goldenseal was cultivated in the Skagit Valley of Washington state and is being promoted as a cash crop in New York, North Carolina,[4] and Canada. Because of its high price, goldenseal, like other expensive herbs, has often been adulterated. Common adulterants include species of *Coptis* and *Xanthorrhiza*,[5] both of which also contain large amounts of the yellow alkaloid berberine. The popular notion that goldenseal can be used to affect the outcome of urinalysis for illicit drugs evolved from the novel *Stringtown on the Pike* by pharmacist John Uri Lloyd, in which goldenseal bitters are mistaken for strychnine in a simple alkaloid test by an expert witness in a murder trial.[6] Goldenseal can be variously ingested prior to testing or added to the urine sample after collection. It is one of several adulterants commonly detected in urinalysis samples.[7]

PHARMACOLOGY: The isoquinoline alkaloids hydrastine, berberine, and canadine are present in goldenseal and viewed as the principle bioactive components.[8] While berberine is widely distributed in plants, hydrastine is characteristic of goldenseal root and is considered to be the most important bioactive alkaloid. There is extensive pharmacologic literature on hydrastine and berberine. The alkaloids are poorly absorbed when taken orally, so studies of parenterally administered goldenseal alkaloids must be interpreted with care. Goldenseal alkaloids have modest antimicrobial activity, which may be relevant when applied topically. Berberine, canadine, and canadaline had disinfectant activity against 6 strains of bacteria, while hydrastine was inactive.[9] Berberine sulfate was bactericidal against *Vibrio cholerae* but bacteriostatic to *Staphylococcus aureus*.[10] Berberine sulfate has been shown to block adherence of *Streptococcus pyogenes* to epithelial cells, which may be a reasonable mode of action for topical antimicrobial use.[11] Berberine has been iden-

tified as the active component of *Hydrastis* in an antitubercular assay,[12] while hydrastine and other isolated compounds had no activity. Berberine has been reported to inhibit uptake of glucose by cancer cells.[13] Berberine showed weak activity in an antioxidant model.[14] While hydrastine is closely related to the convulsant isoquinoline alkaloid bicuculline, hydrastine had no activity in a GABA-receptor binding assay at high concentrations.[15]

TOXICOLOGY: Very high doses of goldenseal may rarely induce nausea, anxiety, depression, seizures, or paralysis. Hydrastine was once used as a uterine hemostatic,[7] but was found inferior to ergot in the treatment of postpartum hemorrhage. Goldenseal is generally contraindicated for use in pregnancy. Because of hypertensive actions of the alkaloids, it is also contraindicated in cardiovascular patients.

[1] Claus E, ed. *Pharmacognosy.* 3rd ed. Philadelphia, PA: Lea & Febiger; 1956.

[2] Hobbs C. *Pharmacy in History.* 1990;32:79.

[3] Bolyard J. *Medicinal Plants and Home Remedies of Appalachia.* Springfield, IL: Charles C. Thomas,1981.

[4] Davis J. *Advances in goldenseal cultivation.* North Carolina Cooperative Extension Service, Horticultural Information Leaflet No. 131, 1996.

[5] Blaque G, et al. *Bull Sci Phar.* 1926;33:375.

[6] Foster S. Goldenseal. Hydrastis canadensis. *Botanical Series,* No. 309, 2nd ed. Austin, TX: American Botanical Council, 1996.

[7] Mikkelsen S, et al. *Clin Chem.* 1988;34:2333-2336.

[8] Genest K. *Can J Pharm Sci.* 1969;4:41-45.

[9] Scazzocchio F, et al. *Fitoterapia.* 1998;64:58.

[10] Amin A, et al. *Can J Microbiol.* 1969;15:1067-1076.

[11] Sun D, et al. *Antimicrobial Agents Chemother.* 1988;32:1370-1374.

[12] Gentry E, et al. *J Nat Prod.* 1998;61:1187-1193.

[13] Creasey W. *Biochem Pharmacol.* 1979;28:1081-1084.

[14] Misík V, et al. *Planta Med.* 1995;61:372-373.

[15] Kardos J, et al.*Biochem Pharmacol.* 1984;33:3537-3545.

Gotu Kola

SCIENTIFIC NAME(S): *Centella asiatica* (L.) Urb. Also: *Hydrocotyle asiatica* Family: Umbelliferae (Apiaceae).

COMMON NAME(S): Gotu kola, hydrocotyle, Indian pennywort, talepetrako

---

❧❧❧ PATIENT INFORMATION ❧❧❧

Uses: Traditionally used as treatment for a variety of ills and as an aphrodisiac, gotu kola has demonstrated some efficacy in treating wounds and varicose veins. Evidence suggests it has antifertility, hypotensive, and sedative effects.

Side Effects: Gotu kola causes contact dermatitis in some individuals.

Dosing: Doses of gotu kola in crude form range from 1.5 to 4 g/day. Various extracts standardized to asiaticoside content also are available and have been studied in clinical trials in venous insufficiency and wound healing at extract doses of 30 to 90 mg/day. Wound-healing studies have involved topical application of an ointment containing the extract.[1]

BOTANY: *Centella asiatica* is a slender, creeping plant that grows in swampy areas of India, Sri Lanka, Madagascar, South Africa, and the tropics.

HISTORY: Gotu kola has been widely used to treat a variety of illnesses, particularly in traditional Eastern medicine. Sri Lankans noticed that elephants, renowned for their longevity, munched on the leaves of the plant. Thus the leaves became known as a promoter of long life, with a suggested "dosage" of a few leaves each day. Among the ailments purported to be cured or controlled by gotu kola are mental problems, high blood pressure, abscesses, rheumatism, fever, ulcers, leprosy, skin eruptions, nervous disorders, and jaundice. Gotu kola has been touted as an aphrodisiac. Gotu kola should not be confused with the dried seed of *Cola nitida* (Vent.), the plant used in cola beverages. *Cola nitida* contains caffeine and is a stimulant, while gotu kola has no caffeine and has sedative properties.[2]

PHARMACOLOGY:

Wound healing: Gotu kola extracts have promoted wound healing.[3] Cell culture experiments have shown that the total triterpenoid fraction of the extracts, at a concentration of 25 mcg/mL, does not affect cell proliferation, total cell protein synthesis, or the biosynthesis of proteoglycans in human skin fibroblasts. However, the fraction increases the collagen content of cell layer fibronectin, which may explain the wound healing action.[4] The glycoside madecassoside has anti-inflammatory properties, while asiaticoside appears to stimulate wound healing.

Titrated extract of gotu kola (TECA) 100 mg/kg has been used as a scarring agent to stimulate wound healing in patients with chronic lesions (eg, cutaneous ulcers, surgical wounds, fistulas, gynecologic lesions). A clinical study evaluated TECA for treating bladder lesions in 102 patients with bilharzial infections. Injections of TECA 2%, usually administered intramuscular for 1 to 3 months, produced cure or improvement in 75% of the cases, as determined from symptoms and urinary and cystoscopic findings. Healing occurred with little scar formation, thus avoiding much of the loss of bladder capacity resulting from bilharzial infections.[5]

Gotu kola has also shown promise in treatment of psoriasis. When creams containing oil and water extracts of the leaves were administered each morning to 7 psoriatic patients, 5 showed complete clearance of lesions within 3 to 7 weeks. One patient showed clearance of most lesions, and one showed improvement without clearance. One patient experienced a mild recurrence 4 months after treatment. Although this study was not controlled, a placebo effect was considered unlikely. The creams were nontoxic and cosmetically acceptable, making them suitable for long-term use.[2]

Antihypertensive Effects: The efficacy of a commercial gotu kola product in the treatment of venous hypertension has been evaluated, using a combined microcirculatory model.[6] The researchers conducted a single-blind, placebo-controlled randomized study of the effects of the total triterpenoid fraction in 89 patients with venous hypertension microangiopathy. The effects were found to be significantly different from placebo in hypotensive activity on all the microcirculatory parameters investigated. No side effects were noted.

Varicose Veins: The effects of gotu kola extract on mucopolysaccharide metabolism were noted in subjects with varicose veins.[7] The total triterpenic fraction of the plant (60 mg/day for 3 months) elevated the basal levels of uronic acids and of lysosomal enzymes, indicating an increased mucopolysaccharide turnover in varicose vein patients. These results confirm the regulatory properties of *C. asiatica* extract on the metabolism in the connective tissue of the vascular wall.

Miscellaneous Effects: A preliminary study showed TECA to produce histologic improvement in 5 of 12 patients with chronic hepatic disorders.[8]

One study of 94 patients with venous insufficiency of the lower limbs indicated that TECA produced clinical improvement in this condition. Improvement occurred in the subjective measures of the sensation of heaviness and pain in the legs, edema, and overall patient assessment of efficacy, and in the objective measure of vein distensibility. The researchers concluded that TECA stimulated collagen synthesis in the vein wall, thus increasing vein tonicity and reducing the capacity of the vein to distend. In contrast, patients receiving placebo exhibited an increase in vein distensibility.[9]

The pharmacokinetics of the total triterpenic fraction of gotu kola have been studied, after single and multiple administrations to healthy volunteers.[10] Using a high performance liquid chromatography procedure for detection of asiatic acid, researchers found that after 2 chronic treatment doses, the peak plasma concentration, area under the concentration-time curve, and half-life were higher than those observed after the corresponding single-dose administration.

Relatively large doses of extract have been found to be sedative in small animals; this property is attributed to the presence of 2 saponin glycosides, brahmoside and brahminoside.

TOXICOLOGY: Preparations of gotu kola have a reputation for having a relative lack of toxicity. However, contact dermatitis has been reported in some patients using preparations of fresh or dried parts of the plant.[11] This is not surprising in light of the topical irritant qualities of certain components of the plant. In the cited study of bilharzial patients, some who received SC injections rather than IM injections experienced pain at the injection site with blackish discoloration of the SC tissues. These side effects may have been diminished with IM injections.[5]

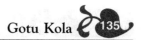
[1] Brinkhaus B, et al. *Centella asiatica. Phytomed.* 2000;7:427-448.

[2] Natarajan S, et al. *Ind J Dermatol.* 1973;18:82.

[3] Poizot A, et al. *C R Acad Sci.* 1978;286:789.

[4] Tenni R, et al. *Ital J Biochem.* 1988;37:69.

[5] Fam A. *Intern Surg.* 1973;58:451.

[6] Becaro G, et al. *Curr Ther Res.* 1989;46:1015.

[7] Arpaia MR, et al. *Int J Clin Pharma Res.* 1990;10:229.

[8] Darnis F, et al. *Sem Hop.* 1979;55:1749.

[9] Pointel JP, et al. *Angiology.* 1987;38(1 Pt 1):46.

[10] Grimaldi R, et al. *J Ethnopharmacol.* 1990;28:235.

[11] Eun HC, et al. *Contact Dermatitis.* 1985;13:310.

SCIENTIFIC NAME(S): *Vitis vinifera* L. and *V. coignetiae* Pulliat. Family: Vitaceae

COMMON NAME(S): Grape seed, muskat, Procyanidolic oligomers (PCO), Proanthocyanidin, Oligomeric procyanidolic complexes (OPC)[1-3]

ᴥ PATIENT INFORMATION ᴥ

Uses: May have antioxidant and cytoprotective effects and provide possible relief from venous insufficiency, although more study is needed.

Side Effects: No toxicity in humans has been reported. It is contraindicated in patients with known hypersensitivity to grape seed. Additional scientific studies are recommended to substantiate the historical claims as well as attain a profile of any potential serious side effects.

Dosing: Extracts of grape seeds containing mostly PCO have been studied in a variety of clinical trials in Europe for antioxidant properties, venous insufficiency, and ophthalmologic complaints at doses of 50 to 300 mg/day.[4]

HISTORY: Both grape seed and pine bark contain PCO. PCO extracts have been marketed in France for decades as treatment for venous and capillary disorders (eg, retinopathies, venous insufficiency, vascular fragility).[1]

Red grape seeds are generally obtained as a by-product of wine production. When ground, these seeds become the source of grape seed oil. Red wine contains PCO, and when used in association with a nonatherogenic diet, may reduce the incidence of cardiovascular disease.[1,3,4]

PHARMACOLOGY: Most trials with grape seed extract are animal studies demonstrating mostly antioxidant, cytoprotective, and vascular effects. The majority of trials in humans study the uses of grape seed extract as an antioxidant and for various venous and capillary disorders.

Microvascular injury: Scavenging by procyanidins from *V. vinifera* seeds of reactive oxygen species involved in the onset and the maintenance of microvascular injury has been studied.[10] It was reported that procyanidins have a remarkable dose-dependent antilipoperoxidant activity. They also inhibit xanthine oxidase activity (the enzyme that triggers the oxy radical cascade). In addition, procyanidins non-competitively inhibit the proteolytic enzymes of collagenase and elastase and the glycosidases of hyaluronidase and beta-glucuronidase. These are involved in the turnover of the main structural components of the extravascular matrix collagen, elastin, and hyaluronic acid.[5]

Antioxidant effects: The antioxidant effects of grape seed proanthocyanidin extract (GSPE is an admixture of proanthocyanidins dimer, trimer, and tetramer: 54%, 13%, and 6.8%) on the generation of nitric oxide in rat primary glial cell cultures have been investigated.[6] The data indicated that GSPE may exert its antioxidant and cytoprotective effect in rat glial cultures by preserving the basal glutathione status during increased nitric oxide generation. Therefore, the authors conclude that GSPE may be utilized under such pathological conditions.[6]

The antioxidant activity of a grape seed extract (300 mg of grape procyanidin extracts in 2 capsules) was investigated in a single-blinded, randomized, placebo-controlled crossover study of 20 young volunteers. Subjects were given 2 capsules or placebo for 5 days. Blood samples were taken at baseline and at the end of the study and then assayed for antioxidant activity as well as vitamin C and E levels. The study was repeated with a second treatment after a washout period of 2 weeks. On day 5, the authors concluded that the extract did not affect serum vitamin C and E levels, but serum total antioxidant activity was statistically significant ($P < 0.01$).[7]

Nutrition: The effects of dietary grape seed tannins on nutritional balance and on some enzymatic activities along the crypt-villus axis of rat small intestine have been studied.[8] This study did not reveal a significant tannin toxicity, except for a reduced dry matter and nitrogen digestibility. However, the tannins directly interfere with mucosal proteins, stimulating the cell renewal.[8] Another study involved a 1-year investigation in rats to determine if age-related insulin resistance could be overcome through the use of natural products (ie, included grape seed extract).[9] Although a combination of agents was used in the study, the authors concluded that the activity of the antioxidant supplements (eg, chromium polynicotinate, grape seed extract, zinc monomethionine) markedly lowered systolic blood pressure in normotensive rats, lowered HbA_{1c}, and reduced lipid peroxidation.[9]

The wine grape seeds can be used as health oils because of their high content of essential fatty acids and tocopherols.[10] A methanol extract of the Oriental medicinal plant *V. coignetiae* exhibited protective effects for liver cells in the in vitro assay method using primary cultured rat hepatocytes. Activity-guided fractionation of this extract produced epsilon-viniferin as an active principle. It also exhibited protection against carbon tetrachloride-induced hepatic injury in mice, shown by serum enzyme

assay and pathological examination. Ampelopsin C and the mixture of vitisin A and cis-vitisin A were found to be strong hepatotoxins.[11] One study concluded that GSPE may offer a cytoprotective role in acetaminophen-induced hepatic DNA damage and apoptotic and necrotic cell death of liver cells.[12]

Capillary disorders: The effect of grape seed extract on capillary resistance disorders was studied in hypertensive and diabetic patients. Overall, results were obtained in an open trial of 28 patients and during a double-blind vs placebo-controlled trial of 25 patients. Patients received 150 mg/day of grape seed extract (ie, *Endotelon*). The drug was well tolerated in both groups and capillary resistance improved significantly ($P < 0.0005$ and $P < 0.005$).[13]

Miscellaneous: Other studies have shown that polyphenolic substances from the seeds and skin of the wine grapes ("Koshu") can strongly inhibit 5'-nucleotidase activities from snake venom and rat liver membrane; have significant therapeutic activity in Ehrlich ascites carcinoma; have inhibitory action against the growth of *Streptococcus mutans*, a carcinogenic bacteria; and inhibit glucan formation from sucrose.[14] The latter 2 actions may indicate that these principles can aid in the prevention of dental caries. Grape seed oil has been shown to be a safe and efficient hand-cleansing agent.[15]

TOXICOLOGY: No human toxicity has been reported for the grape seed, its oil, or its isolated constituents. Scientific evidence for the use of grape seed extract during pregnancy also is unknown. Grape seed is contraindicated in patients with known hypersensitivity.

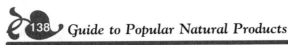

1 Murray M, Pizzorno J. *Encyclopedia of Natural Medicine*. 2nd ed. Rocklin CA: Prima Publishing; 1998.

2 Lininger S, ed. *The Natural Pharmacy*. Rocklin CA: Prima Publishing; 1998.

3 Somerville R, ed. *The Drug and Natural Medicine Advisor: The Complete Guide to Alternative and Conventional Medications*. Alexandria, VA:Time-Life Custom Publishing; 1997.

4 Lagrue G, Olivier-Martin F, Grillot A. *Sem Hop*. 1981;57:1399-1401.

5 Augustin M, Vivas N. *J Wine Res*. 1997;8:159-169.

6 Maffei Facino R, Carini M, Aldini G, Bombardelli E, Morazzoni P, Morelli R. *Arzneimittelforschung*. 1994;44:592-601.

7 Roychowdhury S, Wolf G, Keilhoff G, Bagchi D, Horn T. *Nitric Oxide*. 2001;5:137-149.

8 Nuttall SL, Kendall MJ, Bombardelli E, Morazzoni P. *J Clin Pharm Ther*. 1998;23:385-389.

9 Vallet J, Rouanet JM, Besancon P. *Ann Nutr Metab*. 1994;38:75-84.

10 Preuss HG, Montamarry S, Echard B, Scheckenbach R, Bagchi D. *Mol Cell Biochem*. 2001;223:95-102.

11 El-Mallah MH, Murui T. *Seifen-Oele-Fette-Wachse*. 1993;119:45.

12 Oshima Y, et al. *Experientia*. 1995;51:63.

13 Ray SD, Kumar MA, Bagchi Det. *Arch Biochem Biophys*. 1999;369:42-58.

14 Toukairin T, Uchino K, Iwamoto M, et al. *Chem Pharm Bull*. 1991;39:1480-1483.

15 Krogsrud NE, Larsen Al. *Contact Dermatitis*. 1992;26:208.

SCIENTIFIC NAME(S): *Camellia sinensis* (L.) Kuntze. Family: Theaceae

COMMON NAME(S): Tea, green tea

❧❧❧❧ PATIENT INFORMATION ❧❧❧❧

Uses: Green tea retains many chemicals of the fresh leaf. It is thought to reduce cancer, lower lipid levels, help prevent dental caries, and possess antimicrobial, antimutagenic, and antioxidative effects.

Side Effects: Green tea contains caffeine. The FDA advises those who are or may become pregnant to avoid caffeine. Tea may impair iron metabolism.

Dosing: Green tea has been studied as a component of diet for its cancer preventative and caries preventative properties. A typical tea bag contains 2 g of leaf. Doses of 4 to 5 cups/day (corresponding to ca. 300 mg caffeine) are considered high, depending on the patient's caffeine tolerance. The content of polyphenols increases with extended brewing time. Green tea extracts are available standardized to 25%, 60%, and 80% total polyphenols, compared with a content of 8% to 12% in the leaf. Use of this extract can avoid the inconvenience of drinking large volumes of liquids.[1,2]

BOTANY: *C. sinensis* is a large shrub with evergreen leaves native to eastern Asia. The plant has leathery, dark green leaves and fragrant, white flowers with 6 to 9 petals.[3,4]

HISTORY: The dried, cured leaves of *C. sinensis* have been used to prepare beverages for more than 4000 years.[5] The method of curing determines the nature of the tea. Green tea is prepared from the steamed and dried leaves; by comparison, black tea leaves are withered, rolled, fermented, and then dried.[6] Oolong tea is semifermented and considered to be intermediate in composition between green and black teas.[4,7] The Chinese regarded the drink as a cure for cancer, although the tannin component is believed to be carcinogenic. The polyphenol presence in tea may play a role in lowering heart disease and cancer risk.[5]

PHARMACOLOGY:

Pharmacokinetics: Blood and urine levels of humans have been investigated.[8] Drinking green tea daily may maintain plasma catechin levels that may exert antioxidant activity against lipoproteins in blood circulation.[9] High performance liquid chromatography (HPLC) determination of catechins and polyphenol components have been performed.[9,10,11,12]

Lipid effects: Green tea consumption has been associated with a decrease in total cholesterol levels but not in triglycerides or HDL cholesterol levels.[13] In this survey, at least 9 cups of tea had to be consumed per day for a significant effect.[14] One report did not support the tea's beneficial actions on serum lipid levels.[15]

Dental caries: Green tea exhibits antimicrobial actions against oral bacteria.[16] After 5 minutes of contact with a 0.1% green tea polyphenol solution, *Streptococcus mutans* was completely inhibited. Plaque and gingival index were decreased after a 0.2% solution was used to rinse and brush teeth.[17] Data suggest green tea's fluoride content may increase the cariostatic action, along with the other tea components.[18] After rinsing with green tea extract, the catechin components present in saliva have been determined by HPLC, and were present in the saliva for up to 1 hour.[19] Green tea consumption may also be effective in reducing the cariogenic potential of starch-containing foods by inhibiting salivary amylase, which hydrolyzes food starch to fermentable carbohydrates.[20]

Antimicrobial/Antifungal: Green tea inhibited the growth of diarrhea-causing bacteria *Staphylococcus aureus*, *S. epidermidis*, *Vibrio cholerae* O1, *V. cholerae* non-O1, *V. parahaemolyticus*, *V. mimicus*, *Campylobacter jejuni*, and *Plesiomonas shigelloides*.[21] Green tea extract inhibits a wide range of pathogenic bacteria including methicillin-resistant *S. aureus*. This activity may be caused by the catechin and theaflavin components.[22] In addition, green tea extract had antibacterial actions against 24 bacterial strains in infected root canals.[23]

Antimutagenic: Antimutagenic activity against a variety of organisms has been evaluated from different tea components.[24,25] Flavonol constituents in both green and black teas contributed to antimutagenic potential against dietary carcinogens.[26] The catechin components have been shown to contribute to antimutagenicity as well.[27] The antimutagenic potential of green tea extracts may be caused by a direct interaction between reactive genotoxic species of various promutagens and nucleophilic tea components present in the aqueous extracts.[28]

Antioxidative: Antioxidative activity was studied in 25 tea types, actions due, in part, to catechins present.[29-32] Tea consumed with milk may affect in vivo antioxidation thought to be caused by the complexation of tea polyphenols by milk proteins.[33]

Anticancer: Some reports find that tea possesses anticarcinogenic effects, protecting against cancer risk.[29,34-38] One epidemiologic review explains favorable effects from tea only if high intake

occurs in high-risk populations.[39] Another study finds data unsupportive in the hypothesis that black tea consumption protects against 4 major cancers.[40] One other epidemiological study suggests modest anticancer benefits with several investigations leading to the possibility of decreased risks of digestive tract cancer from tea.[41]

The polyphenol components of green tea may have chemopreventative properties.[42-49] Various catechins exhibit inhibitory actions on tumor cell lines, including breast, colon, lung, and melanoma.[50] A report on the nonpolyphenolic fraction of green tea finds pheophytins to be potent antigenotoxic substances as well.[51]

Tea and curcumin used in combination on certain cell types were noted to have a synergistic effect in chemoprevention.[52,53] There are many proposed mechanisms as to how green tea expresses its anticancer effects.[29,43,44,47,49]

Anticancer, gastrointestinal reports: Green tea may offer protective effects against digestive tract cancers.[54] One study suggests a protective effect against esophageal cancer.[55] Findings of another report concluded that green tea may lower the risk of colon, rectum, and pancreas cancers, as well.[56] Affected stomach cells treated with green tea catechin extract led to growth inhibition and induction of apoptosis, suggesting possible stomach cancer protection.[58] Catechins have also contributed to inhibition of small intestine carcinogenesis.[57] In tube-fed patients positive effects were seen against colon carcinoma.[59] One conflicting study found a direct correlation between drinking 5 or more cups of green tea a day and a diet high in salty foods as a risk factor for pancreatic cancer among Japanese men.[60]

Anticancer, skin: Green tea offers chemopreventative effects against skin cancers of varying stages and is useful against inflammatory responses in cancers caused by known skin tumor promoters such as chemicals or radiation.[61] Green tea and its polyphenol fractions display a protective effect against ultraviolet radiation-induced skin cancer.[62]

Anticancer, various: Green tea's chemopreventative activities against hepatic and pulmonary carcinogenesis have been addressed,[63,64] as well as effects against lung tumorigenesis,[65] smoke-induced mutations,[66] pancreatic carcinogenesis,[67] and leukemia.[68] Green tea can inhibit the carcinogenic effects of female hormones, as well.[69] One report addresses the unconventional use of green tea to treat breast cancer.[70]

Miscellaneous effects: Two well-known components of green tea from a pharmacologic basis are caffeine and tannin. Caffeine is an effective central nervous system stimulant that can induce nervousness, insomnia, tachycardia, elevated blood sugar and cholesterol levels, high levels of stomach acid, and heartburn.[71] These components are also useful for headaches, enhancement of renal excretion of water, weight loss, and as a cardiotonic. Green tea is also used as an astringent, for wounds and skin disorders, and soothing insect bites, itching, and sunburn. Tea is a sweat-inducer, a nerve tonic, and has been used for functional asthenia, eye problems, and as an analgesic.[3,4,6] Green tea has been employed in hepatitis treatment and for protection of the liver.[3,72] Green tea's role in stroke prevention,[73] as a thromboxane inhibitor,[74] and as a hypotensive has been described.[75]

TOXICOLOGY: The FDA has advised that women who are or may become pregnant should avoid caffeine-containing products.[71] Drinking moderate amounts of caffeine has shown inconsistent results, with more recent studies not demonstrating adverse effects on the fetus.[76,77] Caffeine-containing beverages may also alter female hormone levels, including estradiol.[78]

There is evidence that condensed catechin tannin of tea is linked to a high rate of esophageal cancer in regions of heavy tea consumption. This effect may be overcome by adding milk, which binds the tannin, possibly preventing its detrimental effects.[6] Catechins have also been linked to tea-induced asthma.[79] One study reports that catechins may have antiallergic effects, inhibiting type I allergic reactions.[80] Green tea harvesters experienced shortness of breath, stiffness, pain in neck and arms, and other occupation-related problems.[81]

The daily consumption of an average of 250 mL of tea by infants has been shown to impair iron metabolism, resulting in a high incidence of microcytic anemia.[82]

[1] Lecomte A. *Rev Assoc Mond Phytother.* 1985:36-40.

[2] Gruenwald J, ed. *PDR for Herbal Medicines.* 2nd ed. Montvale, NJ: Thomson Medical Economics; 2000: 369-372.

[3] Chevallier A. *Encyclopedia of Medicinal Plants.* New York, NY: DK Publishing, 1996;179.

[4] Bruneton J. *Pharmacognosy, Phytochemistry, Medicinal Plants.* Paris, France: Lavoisier, 1995; 885-887.

[5] Weisburger J. *Cancer Lett.* 1997; 114(1-2):315-317.

[6] Duke JA. *Handbook of Medicinal Herbs.* Boca Raton, FL: CRC Press, 1985.

[7] Graham H. *Prev Med.* 1992; 21(3):334–350.

[8] Yang CS, et al. *Cancer Epidemiol Biomarkers Prev.* 1998;7(4):351-354.

[9] Nakagawa K, et al. *Biosci Biotechnol Biochem.* 1997;61(12):1981-1985.

[10] Unno T, et al. *Biosci Biotechnol Biochem.* 1996;60(12):2066-2068.

[11] Dalluge J, et al. *Rapid Commun Mass Spectrom.* 1997;11(16):1753-1756.

[12] Maiani G, et al. *J Chromatogr B Biomed Sci Appl.* 1997;692(2):311-317.

[13] Watanabe J, et al. *Biosci Biotechnol Biochem.* 1998;62(3):532-534.

[14] Kono S, et al. *Prev Med.* 1992;21(4):526.

[15] Tsubono Y, et al. *Ann Epidemiol.* 1997;7(4):280-284.

[16] Saeki Y, et al. *Bull Tokyo Dent Coll.* 1993;34(1):33-37.

[17] You S. *Chung Hua Kou Hsueh Tsa Chih.* 1993;28(4):197-199.

[18] Yu H, et al. *Fukuoka Igaku Zasshi.* 1992;83(4):174-180.

[19] Tsuchiya H, et al. *J Chromatogr B Biomed Sci Appl.* 1997;703(1-2):253-258.

[20] Zhang J, et al. *Caries Res.* 1998;32(3):233-238.

[21] Toda M, et al. *Nippon Saikingaku Zasshi.* 1989;44(4):669-672.

[22] Yam T, et al. *FEMS Microbiol Lett.* 1997;152(1):169-174.

[23] Horiba N, et al. *J Endod.* 1991;17(3):122-124.

[24] Nagao M, et al. *Mutat Res.* 1979;68(2):101-106.

[25] Yen G, et al. *Mutagenesis.* 1996;11(1):37-41.

[26] Bu-Abbas A, et al. *Mutagenesis.* 1996;11(6):597-603.

[27] Constable A, et al. *Mutagenesis.* 1996:11(2):189-194.

[28] Bu-Abbas A, et al. *Mutagenesis.* 1994;9(4):325-331.

[29] Katiyar S, et al. *J Cell Biochem Suppl.* 1997;(27):59-67.

[30] Cheng T. *J Am Coll Cardiol.* 1998;31(5):1214.

[31] Yamanaka N, et al. *FEBS Lett.* 1997;401(2-3):230-234.

[32] Kumamoto M, et al. *Biosci Biotechnol Biochem.* 1998;62(1):175-77.

[33] Serafini M, et al. *Eur J Clin Nutr.* 1996;50(1):28-32.

[34] Mukhtar H, et al. *Prev Med.* 1992;21(3):351-360.

[35] Yang C, et al. *J Natl Cancer Inst.* 1993;85(13):1038-1049.

[36] Mukhtar H, et al. *Adv Exp Med Biol.* 1994;354:123-124.

[37] Mitscher L, et al. *Med Res Rev.* 1997;17(4):327-365.

[38] Dreosti I, et al. *Crit Rev Food Sci Nutr.* 1997;37(8):761-770.

[39] Kohlmeier L, et al. *Nutr Cancer.* 1997;27(1):1-13.

[40] Goldbohm R, et al. *J Natl Cancer Inst.* 1996;88(2):93-100.

[41] Blot W, et al. *Eur J Cancer Prev.* 1996;5(6):425-438.

[42] Cheng S, et al. *Chin Med Sci J.* 1991;6(4):233-238.

[43] Komori A, et al. *Jpn J Clin Oncol.* 1993;23(3):186-190.

[44] Stoner G, et al. *J Cell Biochem Suppl.* 1995;22:169-180.

[45] Han C. *Cancer Lett.* 1997;114(1-2):153-158.

[46] Yang C, et al. *Environ Health Perspect.* 1997;105(Suppl. 4):971-976.

[47] Chan M, et al. *Biochem Pharmacol.* 1997;54(12):1281-1286.

[48] Ahmad N, et al. *J Natl Cancer Inst.* 1997;89(24):1881-1886.

[49] Tanaka K, et al. *Mutat Res.* 1998;412(1):91-98.

[50] Valcic S, et al. *Anticancer Drugs.* 1996;7(4):461-468.

[51] Okai Y, et al. *Cancer Lett.* 1997;120(1):117-123.

[52] Khafif A, et al. *Carcinogenesis.* 1998;19(3):419-424.

[53] Conney A, et al. *Proc Soc Exp Biol Med.* 1997;216(2):234-245.

[54] Inoue M, et al. *Cancer Causes Control.* 1998;9(2):209-216.

[55] Gao Y, et al. *J Natl Cancer Inst.* 1994;86(11):855-858.

[56] Ji B, et al. *Int J Cancer.* 1997;70(3):255-258.

[57] Hibasami H, et al. *Oncol Rep.* 1998;5(2):527-529.

[58] Ito N, et al. *Teratogenesis Carcinog Mutagen.* 1992;12(2):79.

[59] Hara Y. *J Cell Biochem Suppl.* 1997;27:52-58.

[60] Mizuno S, et al. *Jpn J Clin Oncol.* 1992;22(4):286.

[61] Mukhtar H, et al. *J Invest Dermatol.* 1994;102(1):3-7.

[62] Ley R, et al. *Environ Health Perspect.* 1997;105(Suppl 4):981-984.

[63] Klaunig J, et al. *Prev Med.* 1992;21(4):510-519.

[64] Cao J, et al. *Fundam Appl Toxicol.* 1996;29(2):244-250.

[65] Katiyar S, et al. *Carcinogenesis.* 1993;14(5):849-855.

[66] Lee I, et al. *J Cell Biochem Suppl.* 1997;27:68-75.

[67] Majima T, et al. *Pancreas.* 1998;16(1):13-18.

[68] Asano Y, et al. *Life Sci.* 1997;60(2):135-142.

[69] Gao F, et al. *SCI CHINA B.* 1994;37(4):418-429.

[70] Kaegie E. *CMAJ.* 1998;158(8):1033-1035.

[71] Tyler V. *The New Honest Herbal.* Philadelphia, PA: G.F. Stickley Co., 1987.

[72] Sugiyama K, et al. *Biosci Biotechnol Biochem.* 1998;62(3):609-611.

[73] Sato Y, et al. *Tohoku J Exp Med.* 1989;157(4):337-343.

[74] Ali M, et al. *Prostaglandins Leukot Essent Fatty Acids.* 1990;40(4):281-83.

[75] Taniguchi S, et al. *Yakugaku Zasshi.* 1988;108(1):77-81.

[76] Briggs G, et al. *Drugs in Pregnancy and Lactation,* 3rd ed. Baltimore, MD: Williams and Wilkins, 1990.

[77] Mills J, et al. *JAMA.* 1993;269(5):593.

[78] Nagata C, et al. *Nutr Cancer.* 1998;30(1):21-24.

[79] Shirai T, et al. *Ann Allergy Asthma Immunol.* 1997;79(1):65-69.

[80] Shiozaki T, et al. *Yakugaku Zasshi.* 1997;117(7):448-454.

[81] Mirbod S, et al. *Ind Health.* 1995;33(1):101-117.

[82] Merhav H, et al. *Am J Clin Nutr.* 1985;41:1210.

SCIENTIFIC NAME(S): *Paullinia cupana* Kunth var. *sorbilis* (Mart.) Ducke or *P. sorbilis* (L.) Mart. Family: Sapindaceae

COMMON NAME(S): Guarana, guarana paste or gum, Brazilian cocoa, Zoom

---

⁂ PATIENT INFORMATION ⁂

Uses: Guarana has been used as a natural energizer, cognitive stimulant, flavoring for beverages, and as a component in natural weight loss products; however, it cannot be recommended as a natural energizer or weight loss aid.

Side Effects: Excessive nervousness, insomnia, and other health risks in patients sensitive to caffeine.

Dosing: Guarana paste is used as a stimulant at a dose of 1 g, usually dissolved in water or juice. The caffeine content is between 3.6% and 5.8%.[1]

BOTANY: Guarana is the dried paste made from the crushed seeds of *P. cupana* or *P. sorbilis*, fast-growing woody perennial shrubs native to Brazil and other regions of the Amazon.[2] It bears orange-yellow fruits that contain up to 3 seeds each. The seeds are collected and dry-roasted over fire. The kernels are ground to a paste with cassava and molded into cylindrical sticks, which are then sun-dried. Today, the most common forms of guarana include syrups, extracts, and distillates used as flavorings and a source of caffeine by the soft drink industry. Guarana also is used as an ingredient in herbal weight loss preparations usually in combination with ephedra (ma huang).

HISTORY: Guarana has played an important role in the Amazonian Indians' society. It is often taken during periods of fasting to improve tolerance of dietary restrictions. In certain regions, the extract is believed to be an aphrodisiac and to protect from malaria and dysentery.[3,4] In the 19th century, guarana became popular as a stimulating drink in France,[2] and in 1880 was introduced as an official drug in the US Pharmacopeia, where it remained listed until 1910.[5] Natural diet aids, which rely on daily doses of guarana, have been advertised in the lay press. Guarana is occasionally combined with glucomannan in natural weight loss tablets. The advertisements indicate that the ingredients in guarana have the same chemical makeup as caffeine and cocaine but can be used for weight reduction without any of the side effects of these drugs. This is not entirely correct.

The stems, leaves, and roots of guarana are used to kill fish in Central and South America.

PHARMACOLOGY: Guarana is used by Brazilian Indians in a stimulating beverage used like tea or coffee; it is sometimes mixed with alcohol to prepare a more intoxicating beverage. In 1840, caffeine was identified as guarana's principal constituent, with a level ranging from 3% to greater than 5% by dry weight.[3]

By comparison, coffee beans contain approximately 1% to 2% caffeine and dried tea leaves vary from 1% to 4% caffeine content.[6] The related alkaloids theophylline and theobromine have also been identified in the plant. Guarana is also high in tannins (primarily catechutannic acid and catechol), present in a concentration of 5% to 6% dry weight; these impart an astringent taste to the product. Guarana contains no cocaine.

The appetite suppressant effect is related to the caffeine content. The "zap of energy" that guarana tablets are reported to give is also due to caffeine. This stimulating effect is so widely recognized that guarana is sometimes called "Zoom."

Trace amounts of a saponin known as timbonine, related to compounds reported in timbo fish poisons used by Amazonian Indians, have been reported.[3]

Guarana extracts have been shown to inhibit aggregation of rabbit and human platelets following either parenteral or oral administration, possibly due to inhibition of platelet thromboxane synthesis.[7]

Some researchers claim that part of the revitalizing effects of guarana may be because of its antioxidant action.[8]

Numerous investigational studies have shown the ability of the sympathetic stimulant ephedrine, when coupled with caffeine, to have a synergistic effect on increasing metabolic rates with subsequent increased energy expenditure (thermogenesis), and to have lipolytic effects.[9] These effects have resulted in a statistically significant weight loss in animal and human trials when combined with diet.

There are few human clinical trials concerning the safety and efficacy of guarana. In a small study, 3 groups of normal volunteers ranging from 20 to 35 years of age were given either placebo, 25 mg caffeine, or 1000 mg of guarana containing 2.1% caffeine daily. After 4 days, no reproducible improvement in cognition was noted in any group using neuropsychological testing, assessment of sleep quality, and a State-Trait Anxiety Inventory.[10] In another study, the effects of long-term administration of guarana on the cognition of healthy, elderly volunteers were studied. Guarana did not cause statistically significant memory improvement.[11]

TOXICOLOGY: There are no published reports describing severe toxicity from guarana, but people sensitive to caffeine should use guarana with caution. This includes patients taking herbal weight loss preparations. Guarana use has led to excessive nervousness and insomnia. Use of guarana is contraindicated in pregnancy and lactation.[12]

[1] Claus E, ed. *Pharmacognosy.* 3rd ed. Philadelphia, PA: Lea & Febiger; 1956.

[2] Angelucci E, et al. *Bol Inst Tecnol Aliment.* 1978;56:183-192.

[3] Henman A. *J Ethnopharmacol.* 1982;6(3):311-338.

[4] Lewis W, et al. *Medical Botany: Plants Affecting Man's Health.* New York: Wiley, 1977.

[5] Steinmetz E. Guarana. *Quart J Crude Drug Res.* 1965:749-751.

[6] Der Marderosian A, et al. *Natural Product Medicine: A Scientific Guide to Foods, Drugs, Cosmetics.* Philadelphia, PA: G.F. Stickley Co., 1988.

[7] Bydlowski S, et al. *Braz J Med Biol Res.* 1991;24(4):421-424.

[8] Mattei R, et al. *J Ethnopharmacol.* 1998;60(2):111-116.

[9] Breum L, et al. *Int J Obes Relat Metab Disord.* 1994;18(2):99-103.

[10] Galduroz J, et al. *Rev Paul Med.* 1994;112(3):607-611.

[11] Galduroz J, et al. *Rev Paul Med.* 1996;114(1):1073-78.

[12] Brinker F. *Herb Contraindications and Drug Interactions,* 2nd ed. Sandy, OR: Eclectic Medical Publications, 1998.

SCIENTIFIC NAME(S): *Crataegus oxyacantha* L., *C. laevigata* (Poir.) DC, and *C. monogyna* Jacquin. Family: Rosaceae

COMMON NAME(S): Hawthorn, English hawthorn, haw, maybush, whitethorn[1]

ꙮꙮꙮ PATIENT INFORMATION ꙮꙮꙮ

Uses: Hawthorn has been used to regulate blood pressure and heart rhythm, to treat atherosclerosis and angina pectoris, and as an antispasmodic and sedative.

Drug Interactions: Hawthorn may pharmacodynamically interfere with digoxin or digoxin monitoring. Consult a physician for dosing information.

Side Effects: Hawthorn is reportedly toxic in high doses, which may induce hypotension and sedation.

Dosing: The usual recommended dose of hawthorn leaves and flowers is 4.5 to 6 g/day. Several standardized extracts (*Crataegutt, Faros 300, Cardiplant*) are available that have been used in clinical trials at doses from 160 to 900 mg/day. The content of oligomeric proanthocyanidins or flavonoids is used for standardization of these extracts.[2-6]

BOTANY: Hawthorn is a spiny bush or small tree that grows up to 7.5 m in height. Its deciduous leaves are divided into 3 to 5 lobes. The white, strong-smelling flowers grow in large bunches and bloom from April to June. The spherical bright red fruit contains one nut (*C. monogyna*) or 2 to 3 nuts (*C. oxyacantha*).[1]

HISTORY: The use of hawthorn dates back to Dioscorides, but the plant gained widespread popularity in European and American herbal medicine only toward the end of the 19th century. The flowers, leaves, and fruits have been used in the treatment of either high or low blood pressure, tachycardia, or arrhythmias.[7] The plant is purported to have antispasmodic and sedative effects. Hawthorn has been used in the treatment of atherosclerosis and angina pectoris. Hawthorn preparations remain popular in Europe[8,9] and have gained some acceptance in the US.[10]

PHARMACOLOGY: Hawthorn's role in controlling cardiovascular disease has been extensively reviewed.[11-14] Pharmacokinetic, pharmacodynamic, and metabolic studies on hawthorn have been performed.[15-17]

Because of its strong cardiac activity, hawthorn has been suggested to be of use in congestive heart failure (CHF)[18,19] and cardiac performance.[20] The plant is known to contain cardiotonic amines.[21] The flavonoids contained in the leaves, flowers, bark, and fruits of hawthorn cause an increase in coronary flow and heart rate and a positive inotropic effect. In isolated animal hearts, the inhibition of the enzyme 3′,5′-cyclic adenosine menophosphate phosphodiesterase may be a mechanism by which hawthorn exerts its cardiac actions.[22] Another study evaluated hawthorn in combination with digoxin to treat heart disease.[23] At least one report exists on the plant's potential antiarrhythmic effects.[24]

Hawthorn flavonoid components also possess vasodilatory action.[22,25] Extracts of hawthorn dilate coronary blood vessels, resulting in reduced peripheral resistance and increased coronary circulation.

Hawthorn is known to be beneficial in myocardial ischemia.[26,27] Other studies concerning circulation aspects have been addressed, including peripheral arterial circulation disorder[28] and varicose symptom complex.[29]

Hawthorn has been studied in the prevention and treatment of atherosclerosis. Hawthorn was also found to enhance cholesterol degradation.[30]

A drink containing hawthorn has lipid-lowering effects when studied in rats and humans.[31]

Hawthorn has been studied for its effects on hypertension,[2,32] its oxygen species scavenging activity,[33] anticomplementary activity,[34] and the ability to effectively treat elective mutism, a rare syndrome in which children with normal verbal capabilities refuse to speak for prolonged time periods.[35]

TOXICOLOGY: The acute parenteral LD_{50} of *Crataegus* preparations has been reported to be in the range of 18 to 34 mg/kg, with that of individual constituents ranging from 50 to 2600 mg/kg.[11] Acute oral toxicity has been reported to be in the range of 18.5 to

33.8 mg/kg.[36] In humans, low doses of hawthorn are usually devoid of adverse effects.[11] No serious adverse drug reactions have been reported from hawthorn, and it appears to be safe and effective for CHF.[18] However, higher doses have the potential to induce hypotension and sedation. The health professional and user must be aware of the potential of hawthorn to affect heart rate and blood pressure. Hawthorn may pharmacodynamically interfere with digoxin.[37] This proposed interaction has not been documented clinically. Since digoxin has a narrow therapeutic index, it would be prudent for patients taking digoxin to avoid hawthorn.

Hawthorn extract may increase the intracellular concentrations of cyclic adenosine monophosphate by influencing the activity of the enzyme phosphodiesterase, and it also may influence other mechanisms that activate adenylcyclase.[11] At least one report is available on hypersensitivity reaction to hawthorn,[38] and toxiderma as a result of the fruits of the plant.[39]

[1] Dobelis IN. *Magic and Medicine of Plants.* Pleasantville, NY: Reader's Digest Association, 1986.

[2] Iwamoto M, et al. *Planta Med.* 1981;42:1.

[3] Weikl A, et al. *Fortschr Med.* 1996;114:291-296.

[4] Schmidt U, et al. *Phytomed.* 1994;1:17-24.

[5] O'Conolly M, et al. *Therapiewoche.* 1987;37:3587-3600.

[6] Leuchtgens H. *Fortschr Med.* 1993;111:352-354.

[7] Stepka W, et al. A survey of the genus *Lloydia.* 1973;36:431.

[8] Duke J. *Handbook of Medicinal Herbs.* Boca Raton, FL: CRC Press, 1985.

[9] Tyler V. *The Honest Herbal: A Sensible Guide to the Use of Herbs and Related Remedies.* Binghamton, NY: The Haworth Press, 1993.

[10] Rodale J. *The Hawthorn Berry for the Heart.* Emmaus, PA: Rodale Books, 1971.

[11] Hamon NW. *Canad Pharm J.* 1988(Nov):708, 724.

[12] Petkov V. *Am J Chin Med.* 1979;7(3):197-236.

[13] Kendler B. *Prog Cardiovasc Nurs.* 1997;12(3):3-23.

[14] Miller A. *Altern Med Rev.* 1998;3(6):422-431.

[15] Ammon H, et al.*Planta Med.* 1981;43(4)313-322.

[16] Ammon H, et al. *Planta Med.* 1981;43(3):209-239.

[17] Hammerl H, et al. *Arzneimittelforschung.* 1967;21(7):261-264.

[18] Weittmayr T, et al. *Fortschr Med.* 1996;114(1-2):27-29.

[19] Gildor A. *Circulation.* 1998;98(19):2098.

[20] O'Conolly M, et al. *Fortschr Med.* 1986;104(42):805-808.

[21] Wagner H, et al. *Planta Med.* 1982;45(2):98-101.

[22] Schussler M, et al.*Arzneimittelforschung.* 1995;45(8):842-845.

[23] Wolkerstorfer H. *Munch Med Wochenschr.* 1966;108(8):438-441.

[24] Thompson E, et al. *J Pharm Sci.* 1974;63(12):1936-1937.

[25] Blesken R. *Fortschr Med.* 1992;110(15):290-292.

[26] Piotti L, et al. *Med Klin*. 1965;60(53):2142-2145.

[27] Massoni G. *G Gerontol*. 1968;16(9):979-984.

[28] Di Renzi L, et al. *Boll Soc Ital Cardiol*. 1969;14(4):577-585.

[29] Gehrels P. *Ther Ggw*. 1970;109(8):1163-1166.

[30] Rajendran S, et al. *Atherosclerosis*. 1996;123(1-2):235-241.

[31] Chen J, et al. *World Rev Nutr Diet*. 1995;77:147-154.

[32] Rigo J, et al. *Orv Hetil*. 1968;109(37):2059-2060.

[33] Bahorun T, et al. *Arzneimittelforschung*. 1996;46(11):1086-1089.

[34] Shahat T, et al. *Planta Medica*. 1996;62(1):10-13.

[35] Krohn D, et al. *J Amer Acad Child Adolesc Psychiatry*. 1992;31(4):711-718.

[36] Ammon H, et al. *Planta Med*. 1981;43:105.

[37] Miller L. *Arch Intern Med*. 1998;158(20):2200-2211.

[38] Steinman H, et al. *Contact Dermatitis*. 1984;11(5):321.

[39] Rogov V. *Vestn Dermatol Venerol*. 1984;7:46-47.

Hibiscus

SCIENTIFIC NAME(S): *Hibiscus sabdariffa* L. Family: Malvaceae

COMMON NAME(S): Hibiscus, karkade, red tea, red sorrel, Jamaica sorrel, rosella, soborodo (Zobo drink), Karkadi, roselle, sour tea

---

❧❧❧❧ PATIENT INFORMATION ❧❧❧❧

Uses: The leaves and calyxes have been used as food and the flowers steeped for tea. Hibiscus has been used in folk medicine as a diuretic, mild laxative, and treatment for cardiac and nerve diseases and cancer. Mucilaginous leaves have been used as a topical emollient. Roselle juice is used to quench thirst.

Interactions: Hibiscus beverage has the potential to decrease effectiveness of the antimalarial medication, chloroquine.

Side Effects: The flowers are considered relatively nontoxic.

BOTANY: Hibiscus is native to tropical Africa but today grows throughout many tropical areas. This strong annual herb grows to at least 1.5 m and produces elegant red flowers. The flowers (calyx and bract portions) are collected when slightly immature. The major producing countries are Jamaica and Mexico.[1]

HISTORY: The hibiscus has a long history of use in Africa and neighboring tropical countries. Its fragrant flowers have been used in sachets and perfumes. In areas of northern Nigeria, this plant has been used to treat constipation.[2] Fiber from *H. sabdariffa* has been used to fashion rope as a jute substitute.[3] The fleshy red calyx is used in the preparation of jams, jellies, and cold and warm teas and drinks.[3,4] The leaves have been used like spinach.[3] The plant is used widely in Egypt for the treatment of cardiac and nerve diseases[5] and has been described as a diuretic. In Iran, drinking sour tea for the treatment of hypertension is a popular practice.[6] It has been used in the treatment of cancers.[1] The mucilaginous leaves are used as a topical emollient in Africa.[7] In Western countries, hibiscus flowers often are found as components of herbal tea mixtures. People of Thailand consume roselle juice to quench thirst.[8] Karkade seed products (ie, karkade defatted flour, protein concentrate, protein

isolate) have been studied for their nutritional and functional value.[4]

PHARMACOLOGY: The plant has been used as a mild laxative, an effect that may be in part caused by the acids or saponins described above. Pharmacologic evaluations of hibiscus extracts have produced conflicting results. A 5% solution caused a slight increase in intestinal motility in vitro, while higher concentrations reduced it. Complete inhibition of intestinal motility was observed in vitro with more concentrated water extracts.[9] In a different study, extract prepared from the fresh and fleshy calyx of hibiscus demonstrated a mild cathartic activity in rats at doses of 400 and 800 mg/kg without increases in peristaltic activity.[2]

Assessment of the water and oil absorption capacity, bulk density, and emulsifying activity has estimated that karkade seeds might be harvested for sources of protein and oil to increase cultivation and economic value.[4]

Comparison of consumption of 16 and 24 g/day of roselle juice did not demonstrate a beneficial effect on the prevention of renal stones. Urinary changes seen in the 16 g/day group (ie, increased ion concentration of calcium and oxalate) actually may increase the risk of stone formation. However, the

24 g/day group showed a tendency to decrease ion concentration of calcium and oxalate; thus, a study with higher doses may be valuable to ascertain potential effects in preventing renal stone formation.[8]

The extract reduced uterine motility in vitro and had essentially no effect on respiratory rate.[9] There is no evidence that doses of hibiscus from teas have a sedative effect. When injected IV in dogs, a 10% aqueous extract of the flowers caused a rapid but short-lived dose-dependent decrease in mean blood pressure. A randomized clinical trial evaluated the effect of sour tea available commercially in Iran on essential hypertension on 54 otherwise healthy volunteers. A decrease in systolic and diastolic pressure, when compared with controls, was seen in the sour tea group. After cessation of drinking the sour tea, a rise in both systolic and diastolic pressures occurred. The exact mechanism of how tea prepared from *H. sabdariffa* decreases blood pressure is still unknown.[6] Although no adverse effects were seen in this study, the use of sour tea for treating hypertension requires further study.

Aqueous extracts of hibiscus appear to exert a slight antibacterial effect. Extracts have been found to inhibit the movement of human and canine taenias and a 4% solution killed the worms in approximately 30 minutes in vitro.[9] A 15% aqueous extract prevented the growth of *Mycobacterium tuberculosis* in vitro, and 10 mL doses of a 20% extract prevented growth of the bacillus in infected rabbits.[10] However, these data require confirmation and the antibacte-

rial effect of the plant should not be considered clinically relevant.

Roselle tea extract has shown high inhibition against porcine pancreatic α-amylase (PPA). Proposed uses for this inhibition are for decreased glucose absorption and to inhibit replication of HIV.[11]

PCA has shown potential as a chemopreventive agent against tumor promotion and possesses anti-inflammatory properties. A study in mice demonstrated that topical application of PCA inhibited 12-*O*-tetradecanoylphorbol-13-acetate-induced tumor promotion and edema.[12] PCA also has been found to inhibit the survival of human promyelocytic leukemia HL-60 cells by inducing apoptosis in vitro.[13]

Additionally, hibiscus anthocyanins have shown antioxidant activity in protecting against *tert*-butyl hydroperoxide-induced hepatotoxicity in rats. Application and action in humans has yet to be investigated.[14]

INTERACTIONS: Consumption of the Sudanese beverage, Karkadi (*H. sabdariffa*), concomitantly with the antimalarial agent, chloroquine, produced a statistically significant reduction in the area under the curve of chloroquine, thus potentially reducing its antimalarial efficacy.[15]

TOXICOLOGY: Hibiscus flowers generally are considered to be relatively nontoxic. However, a 30% aqueous extract of the flowers had an LD-50 of 0.4 to 0.6 mL in mice following intraperitoneal injection.[9] Animals injected with this toxic dose were dull and apathetic and died within 24 hours.

[1] Leung AY. *Encyclopedia of Common Natural Ingredients Used in Food, Drugs, and Cosmetics.* New York, NY: J Wiley and Sons; 1980.

[2] Haruna AK. *Phytother Res.* 1997;11:307-308.

[3] Mabberley DJ. *The Plant-Book: A Portable Dictionary of the Higher Plants.* New York, NY: Cambridge University Press; 1987.

4 Abu-Tarboush HM, Ahmed SA, Al Kahtani HA. *Cereal Chem.* 1997;74:352-355.

5 Osman AM, et al. *Phytochemistry.* 1975;14:829.

6 Haji Faraji M, Haji Tarkhani AH. *J Ethnopharmacol.* 1999;65:231-236.

7 Duke JA. *CRC Handbook of Medicinal Herbs.* Boca Raton, FL: CRC Press; 1985.

8 Kirdpon S, Nakorn S, Kirdpon W. *J Med Assoc Thai.* 1994;77:314-321.

9 Sharaf A. *Planta Medica.* 1962;10:48.

10 Sharaf A, Gineidi A. *Planta Med.* 1963;11:109.

11 Hansawasdi C, Kawabata J, Kasai T. *Biosci Biotechnol Biochem.* 2000;64:1041-1043.

12 Tseng TH, Hsu JD, Lo MH, et al. *Cancer Lett.* 1998;126:199-207.

13 Tseng TH, Kao TW, Chu CY, Chou FP, Lin WL, Wang CJ. *Biochem Pharmacol.* 2000;60:307-315.

14 Wang CJ, Wang JM, Lin WL, Chu CY, Chou FP, Tseng TH. *Food Chem Toxicol.* 2000;38:411-416.

15 Mahmoud BM, Ali HM, Homeida MM, Bennett JL. *J Antimicrob Chemother.* 1994;33:1005-1009.

SCIENTIFIC NAME(S): *Humulus lupulus* L. Family: Moraceae or Cannabaceae

COMMON NAME(S): Hops, European hops, common hops, lupulin

⋆⋆⋆⋆ PATIENT INFORMATION ⋆⋆⋆⋆

Uses: Hops have been used as a flavoring, diuretic, sedative, and treatment for intestinal cramping, tuberculosis, cancer, cystitis, menstrual problems, and nervous conditions.

Side Effects: Contact dermatitis has been reported after exposure to hops pollen.

Dosing: Hops has been used as a mild sedative or sleep aid, with the dried strobile given in doses of 1.5 to 2 g. An extract combination with valerian, Ze 91019 (*ReDormin*, Ivel), has been studied at a hops extract dose of 60 mg for insomnia.[1]

BOTANY: Hops are climbing perennial plants with male and female flowers on separate plants. Hops can attain heights of 7.5 m.[2] Commercially, the female cone-like flowering parts are collected and dried. Lupulin is composed of the separated glandular hairs and contains more resins and volatile oil than hops but may also contain more adulterants.

HISTORY: The major use of hops is in beer production, where oxidation of the bitter principle humulene yields the characteristic flavor.[3] Extracts are used as flavors in foods and beverages. Traditionally, hops had been used as a diuretic and in the treatment of intestinal cramping, tuberculosis, cancer, and cystitis.[2] Brewery sludge baths were used medicinally for their rejuvenating effects and for menstrual problems.[4]

As sedation sometimes occurred in hop pickers, the flowers were used as sedatives and were placed in pillows to relieve nervous conditions.[5] Some extracts are used as emollients in skin preparations.

PHARMACOLOGY: The bitter acids (eg, lupulone, humulone) are reported to have antimicrobial activity,[2] with the more hydrophobic compounds being the most active. In addition, the extracts are said to inhibit smooth muscle spasticity. A volatile alcohol, 2-methyl-3-butene-2-ol may account in part for the plant's sedative and hypnotic effects.[5]

Reports have suggested that hops contain compounds that impart estrogenic activity. An early study found a high level of estrogenic activity in the beta-bitter acid fraction of the plant.[4] One poorly designed study, which subsequently became something of a legend, reported that women who participated in hops collection often began menstruating 2 days after starting to reap the hops. However, neither estrogenic nor any other hormonal activity has been observed in a variety of hops extracts tested in several animal models under carefully controlled conditions.[6] Hops are related botanically to marijuana and have been smoked as a mild sedative.[5]

TOXICOLOGY: Extracts can be allergenic, contact dermatitis has been reported after exposure to hops pollen.[2] However, bronchial hyperresponsiveness among hops packagers occurred with an incidence similar to that in the general population.[7]

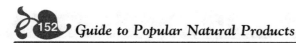

[1] Fussel A, et al. *Eur J Med Res.* 2000;5:385-390.

[2] Leung AY. *Encyclopedia of Common Natural Ingredients Used in Food, Drugs, and Cosmetics.* New York, NY: John Wiley and Sons, 1980.

[3] Lam KC, et al. *J Agric Food Chem.* 1987;35:57.

[4] Zenisek A, et al. *Am Perfumer Arom.* 1960;75:61.

[5] Tyler VE. *The New Honest Herbal.* Philadelphia, PA: G.F. Stickley Co., 1987.

[6] Fenselau C, et al. *Food Cosmet Toxicol.* 1973;11:597.

[7] Meznar B, et al. *Plucne Bolesti.* 1990;42(1-2):27.

SCIENTIFIC NAME(S): *Marrubium vulgare* (Tourn.) L. Family: Labiatae

COMMON NAME(S): Horehound, hoarhound, white horehound

◄◄◄◄ PATIENT INFORMATION ►►►►

Uses: Horehound has been used as a flavoring, expectorant, vasodilator, diaphoretic, diuretic, and treatment for intestinal parasites.

Side Effects: Large doses may induce cardiac irregularities.

Dosing: Horehound is given for digestive complaints as a crude herb at a daily dose of 4.5 and as a pressed juice of the herb at 30 to 60 mL.[1]

BOTANY: Horehound is native to Europe and Asia and has been naturalized to other areas, including the United States.[2] It is a perennial aromatic herb of the mint family. The plant grows to a height of approximately 0.9 m and has oval leaves covered with white, woolly hairs. Horehound bears small, white flowers in dense whorls, which bloom from June to August.

HISTORY: The leaves and flower tops of the horehound have been used in home remedies as a bitter tonic for the common cold. They are now used primarily as flavorings in liqueurs, candies, and cough drops. In addition, extracts of the plant were used for the treatment of intestinal parasites and as a diaphoretic and diuretic. A different genus, the black horehound (*Ballota nigra*), is a fetid perennial native to the Mediterranean area that is sometimes used as an adulterant of white horehound.

PHARMACOLOGY: Horehound is used in cough lozenges and cold preparations. The volatile oil, marrubiin, has been reported to have expectorant and vasodilatory effects. Similarly, marrubiin stimulates secretion by the bronchial mucosa.[3]

TOXICOLOGY: While marrubiin has been reported to have antiarrhythmic properties, it may also induce cardiac irregularities in larger doses.

[1] Blumenthal M, Brinckmann J, Goldberg A, eds. *Herbal Medicine: Expanded Commission E Monographs.* Newton, MA: Integrative Medicine Communications; 2000: 197-200.

[2] Windholz M, ed. *Merck Index,* 10th ed. Rahway, NJ: Merck and Co., 1983.

[3] Tyler VE. *The New Honest Herbal.* Philadelphia: G.F. Stickley, 1987.

SCIENTIFIC NAME(S): *Aesculus* Family: Hippocastanaceae. The most common member of the genus in the US and Europe is *A. hippocastanum* L.

COMMON NAME(S): Chestnut, horse chestnut

❧❧❧ PATIENT INFORMATION ❧❧❧

Uses: Horse chestnuts are potentially useful against edema, inflammation, and venous insufficiency.

Side Effects: All parts of plants in the *Aesculus* family are potentially toxic, especially the seeds. Horse chestnut has been classified by the FDA as an unsafe herb. Horse chestnut components in skin cleansers are potentially carcinogenic.

Dosing: Horse chestnut extracts typically are standardized on content of triterpene glycosides, calculated as the major component, escin. Doses corresponding to 20 to 120 mg of escin have been used for venous insufficiency.[1,2]

BOTANY: Members of the genus *Aesculus* grow as trees and shrubs, often attaining heights of 22.5 m. The fruit is a capsule with a thick, leathery husk that contains from 1 to 6 dark seeds (the nuts). As the husk dries, the nuts are released. The pink and white flowers of the plant grow in clusters. The tree is native to the Balkan woods and western Asia but is now cultivated worldwide.[3]

HISTORY: Because of its widespread prevalence, horse chestnut has been used in traditional medicine and for other commercial applications for centuries. Extracts of the bark have been used as a yellow dye, and the wood has been used for furniture and packing cases. In the western US, the crushed unripe seeds of the California buckeye were scattered into streams to stupefy fish, and leaves were steeped as a tea for congestion. The horse chestnut has been used as a traditional remedy for arthritis and rheumatism.[4] Extracts are available commercially for oral, topical, and parenteral administration for the management of varicose veins and hemorrhoids.[4]

Even though the seeds are toxic, several methods were used to reduce their toxicity. Seeds were buried in swampy, cold ground during the winter to free them of toxic bitter components, then eaten in the spring after boiling.[5] Native Americans roasted the poisonous nuts, peeled, and mashed them, then leached the meal in lime water for several days and used it to make breads.[6]

PHARMACOLOGY: Commerical extracts of horse chestnut have been evaluated in the treatment of several disease states. An extract of the plant (containing 50 mg of triterpene glycosides) decreases venous capillary permeability and appears to have a "tonic" effect on the circulatory system.[7] The bark yields aesculin, which improves vascular resistance and aids in toning vein walls. This is desirable for such ailments as hemorrhoids, varicose veins, leg ulcers, or frostbite.[3] In another report, triterpene and steroid saponins from horse chestnut were effective in treating or preventing venous insufficiency. Enzyme studies show that elastase (enzymes involved in turnover or perivascular substances) inhibition may be a mechanism involved.[8] Aesculin reduces capillary wall permeability by decreasing fluid retention, by increasing the permeability of capillaries, and by allowing reabsorption of excess fluid back into the circulatory system.[3] Anti-inflammatory effects also have been reported.[3,9] One reference reported a dosage of 20 mg/day (max) intravenous administration of aescin to be effective in preventing or treating postoperative edema.[10] In patients with chronic venous insufficiency, extracts have reduced patient complaints, along with objective measures of edema.[11] In a placebo-controlled study, horse chestnut seed extract improved edema in patients suffering from venous edema of chronic deep-vein incompetence.[12] The bark of the horse chestnut possesses anti-inflammatory activity, primarily because of the presence of the steroids stigmasterol, alpha-spinasterol, and beta-sitosterol.[13]

Other pharmacological effects of horse chestnut preparations include the following: treatment of whooping cough from a decoction of the leaves,[3] fever reduction,[3,6] in sunscreens for absorption of skin-damaging UV-B radiation,[14] and antimicrobial actions from recently isolated antifungal proteins.[15]

TOXICOLOGY: The FDA classifies *Aesculus* (horse chestnut) as an unsafe herb;[6] all members of this genus are potentially toxic.[16]

The most significant toxic principle is esculin. Poisoning is characterized by muscle twitching, weakness, incoordination, dilated pupils, vomiting, diarrhea, depression, paralysis, and stupor.[17] The nut is the most toxic part of the plant.[18] Children have been poisoned by drinking tea made from the leaves and twigs and by eating the seeds; deaths have followed such ingestion. Gastric lavage and symptomatic treatment have also been suggested.[17]

A potential association between nasal cancer and long-term exposure to wood dusts, including dust from chestnut trees, has been reported.[19] Aflatoxins have been identified in some commercial skin-cleansing products containing horse chestnut. Because aflatoxins are potent carcinogens that can be absorbed through the skin, it is imperative that strict quality control be applied to topical products containing potentially contaminated horse chestnut material.[20]

Horse chestnut pollen is allergenic and often associated with allergic sensitization, particularly in urban children.[21] A case report describes drug-induced hepatic injury to a 37-year-old man caused by venoplant (horse chestnut extract preparation) given for treatment of bone fracture inflammation.[22]

[1] Pauschinger K. *Phlebology Proctology.* 1987;2:57-61.

[2] Diehm C, et al. *Lancet.* 1996;347:292-294.

[3] Chevallier A. *Encyclopedia of Medicinal Plants.* New York, NY: DK Publishing, 1996;159.

[4] Tyler V, et al. *Pharmacognosy.* Philadelphia, PA: Lea & Febiger, 1988.

[5] Sweet M. *Common Edible & Useful Plants of the West.* Healdsburg, CA: Naturegraph Publishers, 1976.

[6] Duke J. *Handbook of Medicinal Herbs.* Boca Raton, FL: CRC Press, 1985.

[7] Bisler H, et al. *Dtsch Med Wochenschr.* 1986;111(35):1321.

[8] Facino R, et al. *Arch Pharm.* 1995;328(10):720-724.

[9] Tsutsumi S, et al. *Shikwa Gakuho.* 1967;67(11):1324-1328.

[10] Reynolds J, ed. *Martindale: The Extra Pharmacopoeia,* 31st ed. London, England: Royal Pharmaceutical Society, 1996:1670.

[11] Hitzenberger G. *Wien Med Wochenschr.* 1989;139(17):385.

[12] Diehm C, et al. *Vasa.* 1992;21:188.

[13] Senatore F, et al. *Boll Soc Ital Biol Sper.* 1989;65(2):137.

[14] Bisset N. *Herbal Drugs and Phytopharmaceuticals.* Stuttgart, Germany: CRC Press, 1994;268-272.

[15] Osborn R, et al. *Febs Lett.* 1995;368(2):257-262.

[16] Nagy M. *JAMA.* 1973;226(2):213.

[17] Hardin J, et al. *Human Poisoning From Native and Cultivated Plants,* 2nd ed. Durham, NC: Duke University Press, 1974.

[18] Anon. *Vet Hum Toxicol.* 1983;25:80.

[19] Battista G, et al. *Scand J Work Environ Health.* 1983;9(1):25.

[20] el-Dessouki S. *Food Chem Toxicol.* 1992;30:993.

[21] Popp W, et al. *Allergy.* 1992;47:380.

[22] Takegoshi K, et al. *Gastroenterol Jpn.* 1986;21(1):62-65.

Jiaogulan

SCIENTIFIC NAME(S): *Gynostemma pentaphyllum* (Thunb.) Makino. Family: Cucurbitaceae (Squashes)

COMMON NAME(S): Jiaogulan, Penta tea, Amachazuru (Japan), Southern ginseng, Dungkulcha (Korea)

ꜜꜜꜜ PATIENT INFORMATION ꜜꜜꜜ

Uses: Gynostemma is effective in regulating blood pressure, strengthening the immune system, lowering cholesterol, and in increasing stamina and endurance properties. *Gynostemma* has also been found to have hyperlipidemic, lipid peroxidation, adaptogenic, anticancer, cardiovascular and cerebrovascular effects.

Side effects: The side effects of *Gynostemma* include severe nausea and increased bowel movements.

Dosing: The adaptogenic use of jiaogulan is standardized on an extract containing 85% gypenosides, with a daily dose of 60 to 180 mg gypenosides recommended; however, published studies to justify this dose are lacking.

BOTANY: *Gynostemma pentaphyllum* is a climbing, perennial vine native to China, Japan, and parts of southeast Asia. The plant is dioecious, that is, it carries male and female flowers on separate plants. While the plant grows abundantly and is harvested from the wild, it has been brought under cultivation and tissue culture has been achieved.[1-4] Adulteration by *Cayratia japonica* has been noted.[3]

HISTORY: Jiaogulan has been incorporated into traditional Chinese medicine only in the last 20 years. The plant has a history of folk use in the Guizhou province in China. Its properties are said to have been investigated when a Chinese census revealed a large number of elderly people in the province reported using the plant. Investigation as a potential sweetening agent stimulated chemical investigations in Japan. Commercialization and scientific study of the leaves have been promoted by provincial Chinese authorities, and the discovery that several ginseng saponins occur in the leaves has prompted aggressive promotion of the product as a substitute for ginseng. The appearance of jiaogulan in American commerce has been heralded by publication of a popular book.[5]

PHARMACOLOGY: A large series of dammarane triterpene saponins, gypenosides 1-82, have been isolated from the leaves of jiaogulan.[6-13] Several of these saponins are identical to those found in ginseng. Though the plant contains ginseng and ginseng-like saponins, it has not been reported to contain the other types of biologically active compounds, acetylenes, and polysaccharides found in ginseng. Thus, while ginseng pharmacology presents a reasonable starting point for investigation, jiaogulan cannot be considered as pharmacologically identical to ginseng.

Hyperlipidemia: A clinical study of hyperlipoproteinemic subjects also found a decrease in total cholesterol (TC) with increased HDL/TC at a dose of 10 mg given 3 times daily for 30 days.[14] A study of 105 patients confirmed these effects.[15]

Lipid peroxidation: An antioxidant effect of gypenosides was reported in phagocyte, endothelial cell, and liver microsome systems.[16] Further study by the same group[17] explored these effects in vascular endothelial cells injured by hydrogen peroxide.

Adaptogenic: Despite the wide reputation of ginseng as an adaptogen, few studies have been published on the topic.

Cardiovascular and cerebrovascular effects: The hot water extract of *Gynostemma pentaphyllum* was found to activate platelet aggregation. However, the active principle was not elucidated.[18] Gypenosides inhibited platelet aggregation in another study.[19]

Cancer and immunologic effects: An extract of *Gynostemma* inhibited the growth of a rectal adenocarcinoma cell line,[20] while total gypenosides inhibited growth of A549, Calu 1, and 592/9 carcinoma cells more potently (1 to 10 mg/L) than Hela and Colo 205 cells.[21] Cancer patients given jiaogulan granules after chemotherapy showed improved immune function by several endpoints.[22]

TOXICOLOGY: One study found an oral LD50 of 49 g/kg for the crude extract with no organ toxicity at 4 g/kg daily for 90 days.[23] Side effects reported in clinical studies included severe nausea and increased bowel movements.[24]

[1] Zhang ZH, et al. *China J Chinese Materia Medica* 1989;14(6):335-36.

[2] Liu X, et al. *Journal of Chinese Medicinal Materials* 1989;12(6):8-10.

[3] Wu M, et al. *Zhongyaocai* 1987;(4):22-25.

[4] Ding S, et al. *Chinese Pharmaceutical Journal* 1994;29(2):79-83.

[5] Blumert M, et al. *Jiaogulan (Gynostemma pentaphyllum)* China's immortality herb. Badger, CA: Torchlight Publishing, 1999.

[6] Takemoto T, et al. *Yakugaku Zasshi* 1983;103:173.

[7] Takemoto T, et al. *Yakugaku Zasshi* 1983;103(10):1015-23.

[8] Takemoto T, et al. *Yakugaku Zasshi* 1984;104(10):1043-49.

[9] Takemoto T, et al. *Yakugaku Zasshi* 1984;104(11):1155-62.

[10] Takemoto T, et al. *Yakugaku Zasshi* 1986;106(8):664-70.

[11] Yoshikawa K, et al. *Yakugaku Zasshi* 1986;106(9):758-63.

[12] Yoshikawa K, et al. *Yakugaku Zasshi* 1987;107(4):262-67.

[13] Yoshikawa K, et al. *Yakugaku Zasshi* 1987;107(5):361.

[14] Hu X, et al. *Fujian Medical Journal* 1988;10(5):4-6.

[15] Zhou H, et al. *Hunan Med J* 1991;8(5):259-60.

[16] Li L, et al. *Cancer Biother* 1993;8(3):263-72.

[17] Li L, et al. *Phytother Res* 1993;7(4):299-304.

[18] Takagi J, et al. *Chem Pharm Bull* 1985;33(12):5568-71.

[19] Wu J, et al. *Chinese J Pharmacol Toxicol* 1990;4(1):54-57.

[20] Jin M, et al. *Modern Applied Pharmacy* 1992;9(2):49-52.

[21] Liu H, et al. *Journal of Xi'an Medical University* 1994;15(4):346-48.

[22] Wang J, et al. *Zhejiang Journal of Traditional Chinese Medicine* 1989;24(10):449.

[23] Li R, et al. *Journal of New Chinese Medicine* 1988;20(4):51-53.

[24] Chen Z, et al. *Journal of Chinese Medicinal Materials* 1989;12(6):42-44.

SCIENTIFIC NAME(S): *Piper methysticum* Forst. f. Family: Piperaceae

COMMON NAME(S): Kava, kawa, kava-kava, awa, yangona

❧❧❧ PATIENT INFORMATION ❧❧❧

Indications: Kava is used in the treatment of mild-to-moderate anxiety and for sedation, although limited clinical information is available.

Drug Interactions: Other sedatives, alprazolam, levodopa.

Side Effects: Kava is contraindicated in pregnancy and lactation and should not be used in patients with depression. Heavy consumptoms of kava can produce a scaly skin rash similar to pellagra; however, supplementation with niacin did not reverse the condition. Disturbances in visual accomodation have been described. Limit kava use to 3 months to avoid habituation.

Dosing: The dried rhizome of kava usually is taken at daily doses of 1 to 3.4 g/day, standardized to 3.5% kava pyrones, although ceremonial use has involved much higher doses. The many cultivars have been shown to have different kava pyrone profiles and somewhat different pharmacologic effects. There are several concentrated extracts of kava available, with 30%, 55%, and 70% kava pyrone content, respectively. Total daily doseshave ranged from 35 to 230 mg of kava pyrones in studies of anxiety, muscle relaxant, sleep, and menopause.[1-6]

BOTANY: Kava is the dried rhizome and roots of *Piper methysticum*, a large shrub widely cultivated in many Pacific islands ranging from Hawaii and Tahiti to New Guinea.[6] It has large, heart-shaped leaves and is propagated exclusively by root cuttings. It is thought to be derived from the wild species *P. wichmannii* C. DC.[7] Many kava cultivars are recognized, and the comparative chemistry and ethnopharmacology have been studied in detail by Lebot,[8] who grouped 121 named cultivars from 51 islands into 6 chemotypes.

HISTORY: The kava beverage is prepared from the roots of the plant, which were traditionally chewed or pulverized and steeped in water. The cloudy mixture is filtered and served at room temperature. Kava has been an important part of Pacific island ceremonial cultures for many centuries, with elaborate rituals attending its consumption.[9] Traces of kava extract on artifacts from Fiji have been identified by mass spectrometry.[10] Its main use has been as a relaxation inducer in kava ceremony participants, facilitating discussion and interaction.

PHARMACOLOGY: Chewing kava causes numbness in the mouth due to a local anesthetic action of the kava lactones, the primary bioactive constituents of the kava root.[11] In addition, it produces a mild euphoria characterized by feelings of contentment and fluent and lively speech. Higher doses may lead to muscle weakness, especially in the legs, although some observers relate this to sitting for long periods during the kava ceremony rather than to kava itself. Very high doses may induce a deep sleep. Kava lactones, especially kawain, have been shown to have modest anticonvulsant activity in electroshock and metrazol models.[12]

The molecular mechanism of action of kava lactones and kava is not entirely clear. Kava lactones at concentrations from 0.1 to 100 mcM were found to enhance the binding of bicuculline to the GABA receptor by only 20% to

30%.[13] The observation that strychnine-induced convulsions are effectively antagonized by several kava lactones supports a possible effect on the glycine receptor.[14] Inhibition of uptake of noradrenaline but not serotonin by kava lactones at high doses was observed.[15]

Kavain, one of the major kava lactones,[16] had an antithrombotic effect on platelets, dose-dependently blocking platelet aggregation, adenosine triphosphate (ATP) release, and synthesis of prostaglandins at high micromolar concentrations.[17] Despite a reputation as an antimicrobial agent in urinary tract infections, kava extracts showed minimal antifungal, and no antimicrobial or antiviral activity.[18]

Concerns about impaired performance under the influence of kava have motivated several studies in humans. Insignificant changes in cognitive function under kava, with only the extent of body sway showing an increase have been found.[19] Subjects' rating of intoxication under kava was low to moderate, while respiration, heart rate, and blood pressure were unaffected. Kava lowered arousal rating without affecting the stress rating, although the decrease was not statistically significant.[19] Another small study compared kava with oxazepam in their effects on behavior and event-related potentials in a word recognition task. While oxazepam produced pronounced effects on performance, no effects were seen with kava.[20] A study of reaction time by the same authors concluded that kava may increase attention slightly, in contrast to oxazepam, which impaired attention.[21] In EEG studies, kavain showed mild sedation at high doses (600 mg) but not at lower doses (200 mg).[22] Kava had no effect on alertness and long-term memory in a further study.[23] Minor changes in vision and balance were detected with kava in a single subject.[24]

Clinical studies on kava have produced evidence of efficacy in mild-to-moderate anxiety. Several studies have been reviewed in comparison with other CNS-active herbal products.[25] Kavain was compared with oxazepam in a double-blind study and was equally effective and safe.[1] Over 4 weeks, kava extract progressively reduced anxiety compared with placebo with no reported side effects.[2] Menopause-related anxiety was successfully treated with kava extract in an 8-week study, with rapid onset of efficacy.[3] A longer, 25-week, double-blind, placebo-controlled study of 101 patients with anxiety disorders found that Hamilton anxiety (HAMA) scores decreased faster than with placebo.[4] A similar 4-week study using HAMA and Clinical Global Impression (CGI) scores found kava extract effective.[26] All of the preceding studies were conducted in Germany. The first US study of kava in anxiety was recently reported at a conference but has not yet been published. It found similar therapeutic effects of kava extract under double-blind, placebo-controlled conditions.[27]

TOXICOLOGY: Kava's actions are additive with those of alcohol and benzodiazepines, although this well-known interaction is poorly documented in the clinical toxicology literature.[28,29] Heavy consumption of kava produces a scaly skin rash similar to pellagra. However, supplementation with niacin did not reverse the condition.[30] Cessation of kava use causes reduction or disappearance of the dermopathy. Shulgin suggested that the flavokawain pigments were responsible for this toxicity;[31] despite the lack of any scientific proof, these pigments are commonly removed in the production of commercial extracts.[32] Poor nutritional status and other general adverse effects were seen in an Australian aboriginal community where (nontraditional) kava consumption was very heavy.[33] Disturbances in visual accomodation have also been described.[24]

Kava is contraindicated in pregnancy and lactation and should not be used in patients with depression. Do not use while operating heavy machinery. There is a possible interaction between kava and other sedatives and levodopa. Limit kava use to 3 months to avoid habituation.

1 Lehmann E, et al. *Phytomedicine*. 1996;3:113.
2 Kinzler E, et al. *Arzneim-Forsch*. 1991;41:584.
3 Warnecke V. *Fortschr Med*. 1991;109:119.
4 Volz H, et al. *Pharmacopsychiatry*. 1997;30:1.
5 Emser W, et al. *TW Neurologie Psychiatrie*.. 1991;5:636-642.
6 Singh Y. *J Ethnopharmacol*. 1992;37:13.
7 Lebot V, et al. *Biochem Syst Ecol*. 1996;24:775.
8 Lebot V, et al. *Phytochem*. 1996;43:397.
9 Holmes L. The function of kava in modern Samoan culture. In: Efron DH, *Ethnopharmacologic Search for Psychoactive Drugs*. Washington, DC: Public Health Service Pub. No. 1645,1967;107.
10 Hocart C, et al. *Rapid Comm Mass Spectrom* 1993;7:219.
11 Lewin L. *Über Piper methysticum (kawa-kawa)*. Berlin: Medical Society,1886.
12 Furgiuele A, et al. *J Pharm Sci*. 1965;54:247.
13 Boonen G, et al. *Planta Med*. 1998;64:504.
14 Kretzschmar R, et al. *Experientia*. 1970;26:283.
15 Seitz U, et al. *Planta Med*. 1997;63:548.
16 Smith R. *Phytochem*. 1983;22:1055.
17 Gleitz J, et al. *Planta Med*. 1997;63:27.
18 Locher CP, et al. *J Ethnopharmacol*. 1995;49:23.
19 Prescott J, et al. *Drug and Alcohol Review*. 1993;12:49.
20 Münte T, et al. *Neuropsychobiology*. 1993;27:46.
21 Heinze H, et al. *Pharmacopsychiatry*. 1994;27:224.
22 Saletu B, et al. *Human Psychopharmacology*. 1989;4:169.
23 Russell P, et al. *Bulletin of the Psychonomic Society*. 1987;25:236.
24 Garner L, et al. *J Ethnopharmacol*. 1985;13:307.
25 Schulz V, et al. *Phytomedicine*. 1997;4:379.
26 Lindenberg D, et al. *Fortschr Med*. 1990;108:31.
27 Singh N, et al. *Alternative Therapies*. 1998;4:97.
28 Almeida J, et al. *Ann Intern Med*. 1996;125:940.
29 Miller L. *Arch Intern Med*. 1998;158:2200.
30 Ruze P. *Lancet*. 1990;335:1442.
31 Shulgin A. *Bull Narc*. 1973;25:59.
32 Schwabe K-P. *Kava-kava extract, process for the production thereof and use thereof*. 1994;United States Patent No.5296224.
33 Mathews J, et al. *Med J Aust*. 1988;148:548.

SCIENTIFIC NAME(S): N6-furfuryladenine, N-(2-furanylmethyl)-1H-purin-6-amine, 6-furfurylaminopurine

COMMON NAME(S): Kinetin

٭٭٭٭ PATIENT INFORMATION ٭٭٭٭

Uses: Kinetin functions as an essential growth hormone, which can influence cell growth and differentiation. It can delay and offset aging characteristics such as cell growth rate and size. It is claimed to reduce wrinkles and improve skin texture, telangiectasia, and mottled hyperpigmentation though there is little information to support this.

Side effects: There is a very low incidence of side effects when used topically. Commn side effects include erythema, peeling, burning, and stinging.

Dosing: There is no available information on appropriate human doses of this plant growth hormone.

BOTANY: Kinetin, a cytokinin and plant hormone, is a cell division factor found in plant parts and yeast.[1] Kinetin has also been detected in freshly extracted DNA from human cells.[2]

HISTORY: Plant hormones, or cytokinins, were named for their ability to stimulate cell division (cytokinesis).[3] The first known cytokinin was a component of coconut milk. This was used as a standard additive to plant tissue cultures in the lab because of its ability to make plants divide. Cytokinins were eventually isolated from coconut milk, immature organs of corn, and various other sources.[4] Studies dating back to the mid-1950s describe the structure and synthesis of kinetin specifically.[1]

Kinetin has been advertised as an antiaging product for wrinkled skin treatment. *Kinerase* is a cream/lotion containing a 0.1% kinetin concentration.[5]

PHARMACOLOGY: Cytokinins function as essential growth hormones, which can influence cell growth and differentiation in plant and non-plant tissues.[6,7] Kinetin can be formed in vivo, neutralizing harmful properties of hydroxyl radical reaction products. This is a defense mechanism in response to oxidative stress of cells.[8] Degradation of sugar residues in DNA is a major route of this cellular damage.[7] Kinetin-activated, major nucleolar organizer regions in basal, equatorial, and near-apical tissue of onion (leaf base) suggest it to be a regulator.[9] Single-celled yeast, *Saccharomyces cerevisiae*, used as a model, demonstrated spore formation at micromolar concentrations of kinetin.[6] Addition of kinetin in a culture medium of human cells can delay and offset aging characteristics such as growth rate and cell size.[10] The amount of DNA in the nucleii of the fibroblast cells increased in the presence of kinetin from human skin.[11]

The skin care product *Kinerase* claims to be a "nature-identical" plant growth factor, which "delays and improves unwanted changes in appearance and texture of photodamaged skin." It allegedly reduces wrinkles and improves skin texture, telangiectasia, and mottled hyperpigmentation. Results are typically seen in 4 to 6 weeks. Product literature compares *Kinerase* with the prescription cream *Renova* (0.05% tretinoin), finding *Kinerase* to be superior to *Renova* parameters by patient self-assessment at a 24-week period. There was an incidence of side effects using

Kinerase vs *Renova* (eg, erythema, peeling, burning, and stinging).[5]

TOXICOLOGY: Computer literature searches found no information on toxicology of kinetin. The makers of *Kinerase* claim its use is associated with virtually no skin irritation, no thinning of the skin, no restrictions in pregnant or nursing women, no restrictions on duration of use, etc. The product is reportedly hypoallergenic and noncomedogenic and has no known interactions with drugs or other products.[5]

[1] Budavari S, et al, eds. *The Merck Index 11th ed.* Rahway, NJ: Merck & Co., Inc. 1989;5195.

[2] Barciszewski J, et al. *FEBS Letters.* 1996;393(2-3):197-200.

[3] Starr C, et al. *Biology — The Unity and Diversity of Life, 4th ed.* Belmont, CA: Wadsworth Publishing Co. 1987;286.

[4] Arms K, et al. *Biology, 2nd ed.* New York, NY: Saunders Publishing, Co. 1982:786.

[5] http://www.dermcosmetic.com/kinerase.html.

[6] Laten H. *Biochimica et Biophysica Acta.* 1995;1266(1):45-49.

[7] Barciszewski J, et al. *Biochem Biophys Res Commun.* 1997;238(2):317-319.

[8] Barciszewski J, et al. *FEBS Lett.* 1997;414(2):457-460.

[9] Karagiannis C, et al. *Mech Ageing Dev.* 1994;76(2-3):145-155.

[10] Rattan S, et al. *Biochem Biophys Res Commun.* 1994;201(2):665-672.

[11] Kowalska E. *Folia Morphol (Warsz).* 1992;51(2):109-118.

SCIENTIFIC NAME(S): *Pueraria lobata* (Willd) Ohwi. Also known as *P. thunbergiana*. Family: Leguminosae. Other species include the following:[1] *P. mirifica* (Thailand herb known as kwaao khruea, used for hormonal content),[1] *P. tuberosa* DC (also studied for hormonal effects),[2,3] and *P. thomsonii* Benth.[4]

COMMON NAME(S): Japanese arrowroot, kudzu vine[5], ge gen (Chinese)

⚜⚜⚜ PATIENT INFORMATION ⚜⚜⚜

Uses: Kudzu has been used as a ground cover and fodder. It is also used as medicinal herb for treating alcoholism and for muscular aches, heart disease, and related disorders, although there is limited documentation to support these uses.

Side Effects: No known toxic effects; safety undefined.

Dosing: Kudzu root has been studied at a dose of 2.4 g/day in alcoholism.[6]

BOTANY: Kudzu is a fast-growing vine native to the tropics of China and Japan. It has been used as fodder and as a ground cover crop. Because it produces long stems that can attain 20 m in length and extensive roots, it has been used to control soil erosion. The plant was introduced into the US where it has become established and proliferates particularly in the moist southern regions. It is in the southern regions that it grows vigorously and is now considered a pest. The leaves of the plant contain 3 broad oval leaflets with purple flowers and curling tendril spikes.[7]

HISTORY: Although kudzu has been widely recognized as a ground cover and fodder crop in the Western world, the plant has a long history of medicinal use in Asian cultures. As far back as the 6th century BC, Chinese herbalists have used the plant for muscular pain and for the treatment of measles.[7] Kudzu is cited in botanical herbals from Japan, China, and Fiji.[8] The Chinese have also used extracts of the plant to treat alcoholism.[7,9]

PHARMACOLOGY: Kudzu has gained attention because the isoflavones contained in the root have been found to be reversible inhibitors of the enzyme alcohol dehydrogenase. Derivatives of these compounds are also potent inhibitors of aldehyde dehydrogenase. Both of these enzymes are required for the normal metabolic degradation of alcohol and its byproducts.[10]

Traditional Chinese medicine still employs kudzu for treatment of muscular aches and pain, such as neck pain and stiffness and upper back problems.[7] It is also a traditional remedy for gastritis, dysentery, and the flu.[11]

Kudzu's beneficial effects on heart disease and related disorders have been documented. Plant extracts increased cerebral blood flow in arteriosclerosis patients,[7] and decreased oxygen consumption by myocardium and exerted spasmolytic activity.[11] Kudzu has been used in the treatment of hypertension,[12] arrhythmia,[13] ischemia,[14] angina pectoris, and migraines.[11] At least one report is available discussing one kudzu glycoside and its antioxidant acitivity.[15]

Related species *P. mirifica* and *P. tuberosa* have been studied for their contraceptive effects.[7]

TOXICOLOGY: Kudzu has been used as a medicinal herb for centuries without any reported toxic side effects.[10] However, the safety profile of the plant and its extracts has yet to be defined through systematic pharmacologic screens. Acute toxicity of 4 species of *Pueraria* has been comparatively studied.[14]

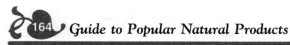

1 http://www.ostc-was.org.

2 Mathur R, et al. *Acta Eur Fertil.* 1984;15(5):393-394.

3 Prakash A, et al. *Acta Eur Fertil.* 1985;16(1):59-65.

4 Yu S, et al. *Chung Kuo Chung Yao Tsa Chih.* 1992;17(9):534-536, 575.

5 Mabberley D. *The Plant-Book.* Cambridge: Cambridge University Press, 1987.

6 Shebek J, et al. *J Altern Complement Med.* 2000;6:45-48.

7 Chevallier A. *Encyclopedia of Medicinal Plants.* New York: DK Publishing, 1996;256.

8 Penso G. *Inventory of Medicinal Plants Used in the Different Countries.* World Health Organization, 1982.

9 Anonymous. *Am J Hosp Pharm.* 1994;51:750.

10 Keung W. *Alcohol Clin Exp Res.* 1993;17:1254.

11 Bruneton J. *Pharmacognosy, Phytochemistry, Medicinal Plants.* Paris: Lavoisier Publishing, 1995;298.

12 Qicheng F. *J Ethnopharmacol* . 1980;2(1):57-63.

13 Lai X, et al. *Chung Kuo Chung Yao Tsa Chih.* 1989;14(5):277, 308-311.

14 Zhou Y, et al. *Chung Kuo Chung Yao Tsa Chih.* 1995;20(10):619-621, 640.

15 Sato T, et al. *Chem Pharm Bull.* 1992;40(3):721-724.

SCIENTIFIC NAME(S): *Citrus limon* (L.), family *Rutaceae*

COMMON NAME(S): Lemon

༂.༂.༂ PATIENT INFORMATION ༂.༂.༂

Uses: Lemon has been used in food preparations and the agricultural industry to gel and stabilize foods. Important for its nutritional value, lemon possesses vitamin C, which is necessary to sustain the body's resistance to infection and heal wounds. Lemon also contains antioxidant, anticancer, hydrophilic, and antimicrobial properties.

Side Effects: Toxicology reports include erosive effects on tooth enamel.

Dosing: No dosage information is available on the medicinal use of lemon or lemon oil.

BOTANY: The lemon tree is an ever-green, growing to over 6 m in height. Its toothed leaves are light green. The citrus fruit (lemon) is small, green to yellow in color, and oval in shape. Unlike other citrus varieties, the lemon tree bears fruit continuously. The plant is cultivated in Mediterranean and sub-tropical climates worldwide.[1,2]

HISTORY: The lemon originated in southeast Asia, probably in India or southern China. Its history is some-times unclear because of the confusion with the similarly appearing "citron," a closely related species. The lemon was thought to have been depicted in Ro-man artwork as early as the first century A.D.[2] Other sources state that the fruit was first grown in Europe in the second century A.D.[1]

In the 1600s, physicians became aware that daily intake of lemon juice would prevent outbreaks of scurvy among sail-ors on long sea voyages. Scurvy is a vitamin deficiency disease character-ized by muscle wasting, inability of wound healing, bruising, and gum de-terioration.[3] English ships were re-quired by law to carry enough lemon or lime juice for each sailor to get 1 ounce daily, earning them the nickname "lim-eys."[3]

More than 50% of the US lemon crop is processed into juice and other drink products. The peel, pulp, and seeds are also used to make oils, pectin, or other products. Lemon juice has long been used as a diuretic, diaphoretic, astrin-gent, tonic, lotion, and gargle.[2]

PHARMACOLOGY: Pharmacologi-cally, the lemon is also important for its nutritional value. Vitamin C is neces-sary to sustain the body's resistance to infection and heal wounds. The potas-sium content in the fruit is useful to offset the potassium loss caused by blood-pressure lowering drugs in some patients.[4] In addition, lemon juice may increase iron absorption as described in a report of 234 women.[5]

Lemons also play a role as antioxidants. German studies in the late 1980s related this effect to the peel.[3] The pectin fiber and lemon oil also possess antioxidant properties.[4]

Lemons have anticancer properties illus-trated in animal and human studies.[4,6] Citrus fruit intake is inversely related to cancer rates, especially stomach cancers. Vitamin C blocks formation of carcino-genic nitrosamines, after consumption of nitrites or nitrates (ie, in smoked food).[4]

The pectin component in lemons, be-cause of the hydrophilic properties, acts to thicken gastric contents, regulating transit. This is useful to treat both vomiting and diarrhea.[7] Pectin also lowers blood cholesterol and aids in prevention of cardiovascular disease.[3,4,7] Bioflavonoids strengthen the inner lining of the blood vessels, including veins and capillaries. This is important for treatment of varicose veins, easy bruising, arteriosclerosis, or bleeding gums.[1]

Lemon's role as an antimicrobial agent has been reported. The volatile oil is said to be both antiseptic and antibacterial.[1] It has inhibited growth of *Aspergillus* mold in 1 report.[8] The juice has been evaluated as a natural biocide to disinfect drinking water.[9] Lemon juice also has sterilized rabies-virus-contaminated areas, to inactivate the virus in patients bitten by affected dogs.[10] The lemon has also been useful for infections, fevers, colds, flu, sore throat, gingivitis, and canker sores. It is also a liver and pancreas tonic.[1]

Skin ailments have also benefitted from lemons. It has been externally used for acne, fungus (ringworm and athlete's foot), sunburn, and warts.[1] One study reports lemon juice in the treatment of keloid, a scarring condition.[11]

Once digested, lemon (despite its acidity) has an alkaline effect in the body, rendering it useful in such conditions as rheumatism, arthritis, and gout, where acidity is a negative contributing factor.[1]

Other actions of lemon preparations include increasing citrate levels inexpensively as therapy in patients with hypocitraturic calcium nephrolithiasis[12] and behavior modification.[13-17]

TOXICOLOGY: The erosive effects of lemon juice on tooth enamel have also been evaluated.[18,19,20,21] One study finds loss of gloss, alteration in enamel color, and irregular dental tissue loss upon morphological analysis.[21]

[1] Chevallier, A. *Encyclopedia of Medicinal Plants*. New York, NY: DK Publishing,1996;81.

[2] Ensminger A, et al. *Foods & Nutrition Encyclopedia*, 2nd edition. Boca Raton, FL: CRC Press Inc., 1994;1299-1302.

[3] Carper, J. *The Food Pharmacy*. New York, NY: Bantam Publishing, 1988;222-223.

[4] Polunin, M. *Healing Foods*. New York, NY: DK Publishing, 1997;64-65.

[5] Ballot D, et al. *Br J Nutr.* 1987;57(3):331-43.

[6] Murray, M. *The Healing Power of Food*. Rocklin, CA: Prima Publishing Co., 1993;143,366.

[7] Bruneton, J. *Pharmacognosy, Phytochemistry, Medicinal Plants*. Paris, France: Lavoisier Publishing, 1995;107-9.

[8] Alderman G, et al. *Z Lebensm Unters Forsch.* 1976;160(4):353-358.

[9] D'Aquino M, et al. *Bull Pan Am Health Organ.* 1994;28(4):324-330.

[10] Larghi O, et al. *Rev Asoc Argent Microbiol.* 1975;7(3):86-90.

[11] Rueter, G. *Zentralbl Chir.* 1973;98(16):604-606.

[12] Seltzer M, et al. *J Urol.* 1996;156(3):907-909.

[13] Eysenck S, et al. *Percept Mot Skills.* 1967;24(3):1047-1053.

[14] Casey J, et al. *Percept Mot Skills.* 1971;33(3):1059-1065.

[15] Sajwaj T, et al. *J Appl Behav Anal.* 1974;7(4):557-563.

[16] Cook J, et al. *Behav Res Ther.* 1978;16(2):131-133.

[17] Hogg, J. *Br J Clin Psychol.* 1982;21(Pt 3):227-228.

[18] Allan, D. *Br Dent J.* 1967;122(7):300-302.

[19] Takaoka S, et al. *Koku Eisei Gakkai Zasshi.* 1971;21(1):6-11.

[20] Pias, M. *Chronicle.* 1972;35(8):217-218.

[21] Grando L, et al. *Caries Res.* 1996;30(5):373-378.

SCIENTIFIC NAME(S): *Melissa officinalis* L. Family Lamiaceae (Mints)

COMMON NAME(S): Lemon balm, balm, melissa, sweet balm

ᴥᴥ PATIENT INFORMATION ᴥᴥ

Uses: Lemon balm has been used for Graves disease, as a sedative, antispasmodic, and a topical agent for cold sores.

Side Effects: No side effects have been reported.

Dosing: Crude lemon balm herb typically is dosed at 1.5 to 4.5 g/day. A standardized preparation of lemon balm extract, *Euvegal forte* (Spitzner Arz.) contains 80 mg lemon balm leaf extract and 160 mg valerian root extract, given 2 or 3 times/day as a sleep aid.[1,2] A 1% extract cream also has been studied as a topical agent for herpes.[3]

BOTANY: Lemon balm is a low perennial herb with ovate- or heart-shaped leaves that have a lemon odor when bruised. The small yellow or white flowers are attractive to bees and other insects. It is indigenous to the Mediterranean region and western Asia, and widely naturalized in Europe, Asia, and North America. The leaves are harvested before flowering and used medicinally.

HISTORY: Lemon balm has been used in herbal medicine since the times of Pliny, Dioscorides, Paracelsus, and Gerard. The name "melissa" corresponds to the Greek word for bee, while "balm" is a contraction of balsam. The plant had culinary and medicinal uses, with the principal historical medicinal uses being carminative, diaphoretic, and antipyretic.

PHARMACOLOGY: Lemon balm's traditional medicinal use was as a sedative and antispasmodic.

Lemon balm has antiviral activity against a variety of viruses, including herpes simplex virus (HSV) and HIV-1. The activity has been attributed to caffeic acid and its di- and trimeric derivatives as well as to tannins.[4,5] A clinical trial of a cream formulation of lemon balm extract demonstrated evidence of activity against HSV cold sores.[6]

Another use of lemon balm has been in Graves' disease, in which the thyroid is abnormally activated by thyroid-stimulating immunoglobulin (TSI). Freeze-dried extracts of lemon balm bound thyrotropin and prevented it and the Graves' TSI from activating its receptor[7-10] although with less potency than the extracts of *Lithospermum officinales*, *Lycopus virginicus*, and *Lycopus europaeus*. In all cases, the activity was traced to caffeic acid oligomers such as rosmarinic acid and lithospermic acid. Auto-oxidation of the caffeic acid derivatives to ortho-quinones was postulated to be important for the biological activity.

Rosmarinic acid has also been found to inhibit the C3 and C5 convertase steps in the complement cascade.[11-13]

Lemon balm is approved in the German Commission E monographs for nervous sleeping disorders and functional gastrointestinal complaints.[14]

TOXICOLOGY: The antithyroid activity of lemon balm extract mentioned above is weak enough that it does not present a serious safety concern in patients without Graves' disease. The topical use for herpes cold sores has not produced any reports of dermal toxicity. Lemon balm extract was not found to be genotoxic in a screen of several medicinal plants.[15]

[1] Dressing H, et al. *Psychpharmakotherapie.* 1996;3:123-130.

[2] Cerny A, et al. *Fitoterapia.* 1999;70:221-228.

[3] Koytchev R, et al. *Phytomed.* 1999;6:225-230.

[4] Kucera LS, et al. *Proc Soc Exp Biol Med.* 1967;124(3):865.

[5] Herrmann EC Jr, et al. *Proc Soc Exp Biol Med.* 1967;124(3):869.

[6] Wöbling RH, et al. *Phytomedicine.* 1994;125.

[7] Auf'mkolk M, et al. *Endocrinology.* 1984;115(2):527.

[8] Auf'mkolk M, et al. *Endocrinology.* 1985;116(5):1687.

[9] Auf'mkolk M, et al. *Endocrinology.* 1985;116(5):1677.

[10] Sourgens H, et al. *Planta Med.* 1982;45:78.

[11] Rampart M, et al. *Biochem Pharmacol.* 1986;35(8):1397.

[12] Engelberger W, et al. *Int J Immunopharmacol.* 1988;10(6):729.

[13] Peake PW, et al. *Int J Immunopharmacol.* 1991;13(7):853.

[14] Barrett, M. *CRN: Reference on Evaluating Botanicals* Washington, D.C.: Council for Responsible Nutrition, 1998.

[15] Ramos Ruiz A, et al. *J Ethnopharmacol.* 1996;52(3):123.

SCIENTIFIC NAME(S): *Aloysia triphylla* (L'Her.) Britt. Formerly described as *A. citriodora* (Cav.) Ort., *Verbena citriodora* Cav., *V. triphylla, Lippia citriodora* (Ort.) HBK Family: Verbenaceae

COMMON NAME(S): Lemon verbena, louisa

◄◄◄◄ PATIENT INFORMATION ◄◄◄◄

Uses: Lemon verbena is used in teas, flavorings, fragrances, antispasmodics, carminatives, sedatives, and stomachics.

Side Effects: Some individuals may experience contact hypersensitivity.

Dosing: Lemon verbena is used as a digestive aid in doses of approximately 5 g/day; however, there are no clinical studies to substantiate the safety or efficacy of this dose.

BOTANY: Lemon verbena is an aromatic plant native to Argentina and Chile.[1] It is a deciduous plant that is commonly cultivated in the tropics and Europe. It is grown commercially in France and North Africa. The plant grows to 3 m and is characterized by fragrant, lemon-scented narrow leaves. It bears small white flowers in terminal panicles.[1]

HISTORY: Lemon verbena has been used medicinally for centuries, having been touted for use as an antispasmodic, antipyretic, carminative, sedative, and stomachic. The leaves and flowering tops are used in teas and as beverage flavors. The plant is grown as an ornamental and its fragrance is used in perfumery. The plant requires shelter during cold periods.[1]

PHARMACOLOGY: The essential oil is said to be acaricidal and bactericidal. An alcoholic leaf extract has been reported to have antibiotic activity in vitro against *Escherichia coli, Mycobacterium tuberculosis*, and *Staphylococcus aureus,* although it had no antimalarial activity. A 2% emulsion of the oil has been reported to kill mites and aphids.[2]

A component of the related plant, *Verbena officinalis,* has been reported by Chinese investigators to have antitussive activity.[3]

TOXICOLOGY: Lemon verbena generally is recognized as safe for human consumption and for use as a flavoring in alcoholic beverages. Contact hypersensitivity has been associated with members of the related *Verbena genus.*

[1] Simon JE, et al. *Herbs: an indexed bibliography, 1971-1980.* Hamden, CT: The Shoe String Press, 1984.

[2] Duke JA. *Handbook of Medicinal Herbs.* Boca Raton, FL: CRC Press, 1985.

[3] Gui CH. *Chung Yao Tung Pao* 1985;10:35.

Lemongrass

SCIENTIFIC NAME(S): *Cymbopogon citratus* (DC.) Stapf. *Andropogon citratus* DC, *A. schoenathus*. *C. flexuosus*, *A. flexuosus*. Family: Poaceae (Gramineae), Grass.

COMMON NAME(S): Lemongrass. *C. citratus*, is known as Guatemala, West Indian, or Madagascar lemongrass. *C. flexuosus*, is known as cochin lemongrass, British Indian lemongrass, East Indian lemongrass, or French Indian verbena.

ꙮꙮꙮ PATIENT INFORMATION ꙮꙮꙮ

Uses: Lemongrass is used as a fragrance and flavoring, and in folk medicine as an antispasmodic, hypotensive, anticonvulsant, analgesic, antiemetic, antitussive, antirheumatic, antiseptic, and treatment for nervous and GI disorders and fevers. Because there is little human evidence to support its effectiveness in an oral dosage, lemongrass may be considered a placebo.

Drug Interactions: Constituent beta-myrcene was found to interfere with cytochrome P450 liver enzymes, suggesting possible toxicities.

Side Effects: Lemongrass is considered to be of low toxicity. Lemongrass should not be used in pregnancy because of uterine and menstrual flow stimulation.

Dosing: No information is available on dosage in the medicinal use of lemongrass oil.

BOTANY: *Cymbopogon* is a tall, aromatic perennial grass that is native to tropical Asia. *C. citratus* is cultivated in the West Indies, Central and South America, and tropical regions. The linear leaves can grow up to 90 cm in height and 5 mm wide. Freshly cut and partially dried leaves are used medicinally and are the source of the essential oil.[1,2]

HISTORY: Lemongrass is one of the most widely used traditional plants in South American folk medicine. It is used as an antispasmodic, analgesic, for the management of nervous and gastrointestinal disorders, to treat fevers, and as an antiemetic. In India, it is commonly used as an antitussive, antirheumatic, and antiseptic. It is usually taken by ingesting an infusion made by pouring boiling water on fresh or dried leaves. Lemongrass is an important part of Southeast Asian cuisine, especially in Thai food and has been used in flavoring. In Chinese medicine, lemongrass is used in the treatment for headaches, stomachaches, abdominal pain, and rheumatic pain.[3]

PHARMACOLOGY: Lemongrass has been widely used in South American traditional medicine. A report of Guatemalan use lists lemongrass as a popular medicinal plant.[4] Brazilian folk medicine uses the plant for nervous conditions or gastrointestinal disturbances.[5] Traditional Indian medicine employs lemongrass for fever, infection, and sedation.[1] Other uses include astringent, fragrance in beauty products, food flavoring, and treatment for skin conditions, muscle pain, infections, fever, colitis, and indigestion.[1,2] However, effectiveness of lemongrass has not been sufficiently evaluated to help substantiate these claims.

The general lack of pharmacologic activity of oral doses of lemongrass has been substantiated in humans. Volunteers who took a single oral dose or 2 weeks of oral intake of the tea showed no changes in any hematologic or urinary tests, or in EEG or ECG tracings. Some subjects showed mild elevations of direct bilirubin and amylase levels, but none were accompanied by any clinical manifestations. The hypnotic effect was further investigated in 50 volunteers who ingested a tea prepared under double-blind conditions for 3 nights, 3 to 5 days apart. The parameters tested (sleep induction time, sleep quality, dream recall, reawakening) did not show any effect of lemongrass compared with placebo. Furthermore, 18 patients with documented anxiety traits showed no differences in their anxiety scores after taking a single 150 mL dose of lemongrass tea under double-blind conditions.[5]

Antimicrobial effects: Several reports demonstrating the antimicrobial effects of lemongrass are available discussing its activity against animal and plant pathogens, gram-positive and gram-negative bacteria, and fungus.[6] Constituents geraniol (alpha-citral) and neral (beta-citral) were found to possess these antibacterial effects in 1 report.[7] The citral content in the oil greatly affected the antibacterial actions as shown in another report testing fresh oil against oils up to 12 years old.[8] Some organisms inhibited by lemongrass oil include *Acinetobacter baumanii*, *Aeromonas veronii*, *Candida albicans*, *Enterococcus faecalis*, *Escherichia coli*, *Klebsiella pneumoniae*, *Pseudomonas aeruginosa*, *Salmonella enterica*, *Serratia marcescens*, *Staphlycoccus aureus*, and *Proteus mirabilis*.[9,10] One mechanism of action explained in a report evaluating lemongrass oil and its antibacterial effects on *E. coli* determined that the oil elicits morphological alterations on the host, including filamentation, inhibition of septum formation, production of bulging, abnormal shaping of cells, as well as cell lysis, all of which deter bacterial growth.[11]

Antifungal effects: Antifungal effects of the oil have been studied as well, and include actions against such dermatophytes as *Trichophyton mentagrophytes*, *T. rubrum*, *Epidermophyton floccosum*, and *Microsporum gypseum*.[12] In a 13-oil study, lemongrass oil was found to be among the most active against human dermatophyte strains, inhibiting 80% of strains, with inhibition zones greater than 10 mm in diameter.[13] Other studies report lemongrass actions against keratinophilic fungi,[14] ringworm fungi,[15,16] and food storage fungi.[17] Lemongrass oil is discussed as being effective as an herbicide[18] and an insecticide[19,20] because of these naturally occurring antimicrobial effects.

Anticarcinogenic effects: There are also numerous reports demonstrating the anticarcinogenic (or antitumor) properties of lemongrass. Edible plants (including lemongrass), in general, are discussed.[21,22] Another report finds the plant extract to possess antimutagenic properties against certain *S. typimurium* strains.[23] A Japanese patent application discusses how constituent geraniol markedly inhibits Epstein-Barr virus.[24] Oil of *C. citrans* possessed high antiradical power, as well as some antioxidant activity.[25]

TOXICOLOGY: Lemongrass is generally recognized as safe (GRAS) in the US.

Topical application of lemongrass has rarely led to an allergic reaction. Two cases of toxic alveolitis have been reported from inhalation of the oil.[2] No laboratory test abnormalities were noted after ingestion of lemongrass tea. Achara, an herbal tea made from dried lemongrass leaves, was found to be atoxic.[26] Aqueous extracts of the plant used as an insecticide led to some mitotic abnormalities in *Allium cepa* root tips grown in these extracts, which may have implications in humans.[27] In addition, constituent beta-myrcene was found in reports to interfere with cytochrome P450 liver enzymes, suggesting possible toxicities.[28-30]

Lemongrass should not be used in pregnancy because of uterine and menstrual flow stimulation.[31]

[1] Lawless, J. *The Illustrated Encyclopedia of Essential Oils*. Element Books, Inc. Rockport, MA 1995;132.

[2] Blumenthal, M, ed. *The Complete German Commission E Monographs*. American Botanical Council, Austin TX; 1998;341-42.

[3] Leung A. *Encyclopedia of Common Natural Ingredients Used in Food, Drugs, and Cosmetics*. New York, NY: J Wiley and Sons, 1980.

[4] Giron L, et al. *J Ethnopharmacol*. 1991;34(2-3):173-187.

[5] Leite J, et al. *J Ethnopharmacol*. 1986;17(1):75-83.

[6] Baratta M, et al. *Flavour Fragrance J*. 1998;13(4):235-244.

[7] Onawunmi G, et al. *J Ethnopharmacol*. 1984;12(3):279-286.

[8] Syed M, et al. *Pak J Sci Ind Res*. 1995;38(3/4):146-148.

[9] Hammer K, et al. *J Appl Microbiol*. 1999;86(6):985-990.

[10] Chalcat J, et al. *J Essent Oil Res*. 1997;9(1):67-75.

[11] Ogunlana E, et al. *Microbios*. 1987;50(202):43-59.

[12] Wannissorn B, et al. *Phytother Res*. 1996;10(7):551-554.

[13] Lima E, et al. *Mycoses*. 1993;36(9-10):333-336.

[14] Qureshi S, et al. *Hindustan Antibiot Bull*. 1997;39(1-4):56-60.

[15] Yadav P, et al. *Indian J Pharm Sci*. 1994;56(6):227-230.

[16] Kishore N, et al. *Mycoses*. 1993;36(5-6):211-215.

[17] Mishra A, et al. *Appl Environ Microbiol*. 1994;60(4):1101-1105.

[18] Dudai N, et al. *J Chem Ecol*. 1999;25(5):1079-1089.

[19] Ahmad F, et al. *Insect Sci Its Appl*. 1995;16(3/4):391-393.

[20] Gilbert B, et al. *An Acad Bras Cienc*. 1999;71(2):265-271.

[21] Murakami A, et al. *Fragrance J*. 1994;22(7):71-79.

[22] Murakami A, et al. *Mem Sch Biol-Oriented Sci Technol*. Kinki Univ. 1997;1-23.

[23] Vinitketkumnuen U, et al. *Mutat Res*. 1994;341(1):71-75.

[24] Nagamine K et al. *Jpn Kokai Tokkyo Koho.*. 1994 (4pp). App number: JP 93-71649 19930330.

[25] Menut C, et al. *J Essent Oil Res*. 2000;12(2):207-212.

[26] Orisakwe O, et al. *Asia Pac J Pharmacol*. 1998;13(2 and 3):79-82.

[27] Williams G, et al. *Cytobios*. 1996;87(350):161-168.

[28] Kauderer B, et al. *Environ Mol Mutagen*. 1991;18(1):28-34.

[29] De-Oliveira A, et al. *Toxicol Lett*. 1997;92(1):39-46.

[30] De-Oliveira A, et al. *Toxicology*. 1997;124(2):135-140.

[31] McGuffin M, et al. *American Herbal Products Association's Botanical Safety Handbook*. Boca Raton, FL: CRC Press; 1997.

SCIENTIFIC NAME(S): *Lentinula edodes* (Berk.) Pegler, syn. with *Tricholomopsis edodes* Sing., *Lentinus edodes* (Berk.) Singer

COMMON NAME(S): Shiitake, snake butter, pasania fungus, forest mushroom, hua gu

---

⋙⋙ PATIENT INFORMATION ⋘⋘

Uses: Lentinan is proving to be a valuable component in cancer and infection treatments. It has also demonstrated cholesterol-lowering and immune-regulatory properties.

Side Effects: Lentinan is derived from the Shiitake mushroom, which is edible and is not generally associated with side effects. Reports of lentinan side effects are rare.

Dosing: The isolated polysaccharide lentinan from shiitake culture has been used IV at doses of 2 to 10 mg on a weekly schedule as adjunctive therapy in HIV as well as cancer, primarily in Japan.[1]

BOTANY: Lentinan is a polysaccharide derived from the vegetative parts of the edible Japanese shiitake mushroom. It is the cell wall constituent extracted from the fruiting bodies or mycelium of *L. edodes*.[2] The light, amber fungi are found on fallen broadleaf trees, such as chestnut, beech, or mulberry. They have decurrent, even, or ragged gills, a stem, and are covered with delicate, white flocking.[3] Shiitake mushrooms are commonly sold in food markets in the Orient and are now widely available in the United States, Canada, and Europe.

HISTORY: Lentinan is a complex polysaccharide that possesses immuno-stimulating antitumor properties. Lentinan was isolated from edible shiitake mushrooms that have been used in traditional Asian cooking and herbal medicine. Shiitake has been renowned in Japan and China as a food and medicine for thousands of years and is now commonplace throughout the world. Extracts of these mushrooms are being incorporated into over-the-counter dietary supplements designed to improve the status of the immune system.

PHARMACOLOGY: The antitumor activity of lentinan has been recognized for almost 30 years. Because a number of naturally occurring polysaccharides had previously been found to have antitumor activity, lentinan (a water-soluble beta-1,3 glucan polysaccharide) was considered for detailed evaluation. In addition to antitumor activity, lentinan also possesses immune-regulatory effects, anti-viral activity, antimicrobial properties, and cholesterol-lowering effects. The following is a brief outline of key aspects of lentinan pharmacology.

Antitumor activity: Therapeutic effects of lentinan in cancers of the gastrointestinal tract have been noted. Lentinan used as an agent for postoperative adjuvant therapy was investigated in patients with stages II to IV gastrointestinal cancer. Stage IV patients had higher lymphocyte counts than control patients, suggesting lentinan's immunopotentiating efficacy in advanced gastrointestinal cancer.[4] Another study reports lifespan prolongation in stomach cancer patients, using lentinan combination therapy.[5] Other successful chemotherapies using lentinan include: cisplatin (CDDP) and fluorouracil (5-FU),[6] mitomycin and 5-FU,[7] cisplatin with radiation,[8] and interleukin-2.[9] Another study involving gastric cancer describes how lentinan caused marked development of reticular fibers related to antitumor effect and enhanced interstitial response.[10] Intracavitary injection of lentinan is useful for malignant effusions in gastric carcinoma patients.[11] Resistance to lentinan chemoimmunotherapy is also reported.[12]

Lentinan's effects on other cancers have also been reported. In prostatic cancer, lentinan 2 mg weekly in combination with *Tegafur* was evaluated. A 5-year average survival rate of treated patients was 43% compared with 29% in the control group.[13] Another report referred to the safety and efficacy of lentinan post-treatment with surgical therapy in 33 breast cancer patients.[14] Lentinan has also been evaluated in cervical cancer patients.[15-17]

Survival rates using lentinan therapies have increased. One study reports 129 days vs 49 days in malignant ascites and pleural effusion patients given lentinan 4 mg/week for 4 weeks.[18] A 4-year follow-up survey of stomach cancer patients reports increased survival at 1, 2, and 3 years, with few reported side effects.[5]

Immune system effects: Although not directly cytotoxic, beta-1,3 glucan has been shown to enhance natural immunity. When administered intraperitoneal to mice with implanted tumors, lentinan effectively increased the activity of cytotoxic peritoneal exudate cells.[19] Direct action of lentinan on tumor cells in mice by scanning electron microscopy has been reported. Lentinan contributes to antitumor immunity enhancement, but not to direct killing activity against tumor cells.[20] Evidence suggests that lentinan preferentially acts on T-cells and may enhance T-helper cell function. Furthermore, lentinan augments natural killer cell activity and activates macrophages.[21] Lentinan also triggers production of interleukin–1 by a direct

action on macrophages or indirectly by augmenting colony-stimulating factor.[22] Many other studies are available where lentinan is found to improve immune function by stimulating T-cell/killer cell/monocyte production,[4,9,11,23-28] increasing natural cell-mediated cytotoxicity,[29] stimulating production of acute-phase transport proteins,[30] affecting lymphocyte and enzyme concentrations,[31] and activating complement.[32]

Anti-viral activity: Lentinan has antiviral activity and has been found to protect against encephalitis caused by the intranasally infected vesicular stomatitis virus in mice.[33] Lentinan enhances zidovudine's effects when used in combination against HIV for in vitro studies.[34]

Antimicrobial properties: Rabbits with induced septic insult without lentinan treatment were reported to have low platelet counts, and elevated bilirubin and creatinine. In lentinan-treated septic animals, platelet counts did not decrease, and elevation of plasma bilirubin and creatinine levels were less prominent. Findings suggest a modified septic process by administration of lentinan.[35] Host resistance against microbial infection by lentinan is reviewed in another report.[36]

Cholesterol-lowering effects: The compound lentinacin has been shown to reduce cholesterol levels in rats by 25% after 7 days of oral administration in a dose as low as 0.005% of feed intake.[37] Other compounds isolated from Shiitake have also been shown to lower blood cholesterol and lipids as well.[38]

TOXICOLOGY: The shiitake mushroom is edible and has not been associated with toxicity. In animals, lentinan shows little toxicity. In a phase I study conducted in 50 patients with advanced cancer, minor side effects were observed in 3 patients; in a study of 185 patients, 17 experienced minor adverse reactions.[7] Few toxic effects are mentioned in 2 reports of lentinan use.[39,40]

[1] Gordon M, et al. *J Med.* 1998;29:305-330.

[2] Chihara G, et al. *Cancer Res.* 1970;30:2776.

[3] Hobbs C. *Medicinal Mushrooms* Santa Cruz, CA: Botanica Press, 1995;125.

[4] Tanabe H, et al. *Nippon Gan Chiryo Gakki Shi.* 1990;25(80):1657-1667.

[5] Tagachi T. *Cancer Detect Prev.* 1987;1(Suppl):333-349.

[6] Mio H, et al. *Gan To Kagaku Ryoho.* 1994;21(4):531-534.

[7] Jeannin JF, et al. *Int J Immunopharm.* 1988;10:855.

[8] Egawa S, et al. *Nippon Hinyokika Gakki Zasshi.* 1989;8(2):249-255.

[9] Suzuki M, et al. *Int J Immunopharm.* 1990;12(6):613-623.

[10] Ogawa K, et al. *Gan To Kagaku Ryoho.* 1994;21(13):2101-2104.

[11] Hazama S, et al. *Gan To Kagaku Ryoho.* 1995;22(11):1595-1597.

[12] Hamuro J, et al. *Br J Cancer.* 1996;73(4):465-471.

[13] Tari K, et al. *Hinyokika Kiyo-Acta Urologica Japonica.* 1994;40(2):199-123.

[14] Kosaka A, et al. *Gan To Kagaku Ryoho.* 1987;14(2):516-522.

[15] Shimizu H, et al. *Nippon Sanka Fujinka Gakkai Zasshi.* 1988;40(12):1899-1900

[16] Shimizu Y, et al. *Nippon Sanka Fujinka Gakkai Zasshi.* 1988;40(10):1557-1558.

[17] Shimizu Y, et al. *Nippon Sanka Fujinka Gakkai Zasshi.* 1990;42(1):37-44.

[18] Oka M, et al. *Biotherapy.* 1992;5(2):107-112.

[19] Hamuro J et al, *Immunology.* 1980;39:551.

[20] Kurokawa T, et al. *Nippon Gan Chiryo Gakki Shi.* 1990;25(12):2822-2827.

[21] Reed FC, et al. *Int J Immunopharm.* 1982;4:264.

[22] Hamuro J, et al. *Int J Immunopharm.* 1982;4:267.

[23] Hanaue H, et al. *Nippon Gan Chiryo Gakki Shi.* 1989;24(8):1566-1571.

[24] Hanaue H, et al. *Clin Ther.* 1989;11(5):614-622.

[25] Tani M, et al. *Anticancer Res.* 1993;13(5C):1773-1776.

[26] Tani M, et al. *Eur J Clin Pharmacol.* 1992;42(6):623-627.

[27] Arinaga S, et al. *Int J Immunopharm.* 1992;14(4):535-539.

[28] Arinaga S, et al. *Int J Immunopharm.* 1992;14(1):43-47.

[29] Peter G, et al. *Immunopharm Immunotox.* 1988;10(2):157–163.

[30] Suga T, et al. *Int J Immunopharm.* 1986;8(7):691-699.

[31] Feher J, et al. *Immunopharm Immunotox.* 1989;11(1):55-62.

[32] Takeshita K, et al. *Nippon Geka Gakkai Zasshi.* 1991;92(1):5-11.

[33] Chang KSS, *Int J Immunopharm.* 1982;4:267.

[34] Tochikura T, et al. *Jpn J Cancer Res.* 1987;78(6):583-589.

[35] Tsujinaka T, et al. *Eur Surg Res.* 1990;22(6):340-346.

[36] Kaneko Y, et al. *Adv Exp Med Biol.* 1992;319:201-215.

[37] Chibata I et al, *Experientia.* 1969;25:1237.

[38] Hobbs C. *Medicinal Mushrooms,* Santa Cruz, CA: Botanica Press, 1995;p. 133-134.

[39] Chihara G, et al. *Cancer Detect Prev.* 1987;1:423-443.

[40] Chihara G. *Dev Biol Stand.* 1992;77:191-197.

Licorice

SCIENTIFIC NAME(S): *Glycyrrhiza glabra* L, *G. uralensis* Fisch. ex DC, *G. pallidiflora* Maxim Family: Leguminosae

COMMON NAME(S): Licorice, Spanish licorice, Russian licorice

⁂ PATIENT INFORMATION ⁂

Uses: Used historically for gastrointestinal complaints, licorice is used today as a flavoring and in shampoos.

Side Effects: Large amounts of licorice taken daily for a long time can cause a range of side effects from lethargy to quadriplegia (body paralysis). Do not over-consume licorice.

Dosing: Licorice root has been used in daily doses from 2 to 15 g for ulcer and gastritis, as well as for coughs; higher doses given for extended periods of time run a risk of hyperkalemia. Deglycyrrhizinated licorice extracts are available. Doses of glycyrrhizin of 200 to 600 mg/day are acceptable.[1-3]

BOTANY: *Glycyrrhiza glabra* is a 1.2 to 1.5 m shrub that grows in subtropical climates with rich soil. The name "glycyrrhiza" is derived from Greek words meaning "sweet roots." The roots are harvested to produce licorice. Most commercial licorice is extracted from varieties of *G. glabra*. The most common variety, *G. glabra* var. *typica* (Spanish licorice), has blue flowers, and *G. glabra* var. *glandulifera* (Russian licorice) has violet blossoms. Turkey, Greece, and Asia Minor supply most commercial licorice.

HISTORY: Therapeutic use of licorice dates back to the Roman Empire. Hippocrates and Theophratus extolled its uses, and Pliny the Elder (A.D. 23) recommended it as an expectorant and carminative. Licorice also figures prominently in Chinese herbal medicine as a "drug of first class" — an agent that exerts godly influence on the body and lengthens life. Licorice is used in modern medicinals chiefly as a flavoring agent that masks bitter agents, such as quinine, and in cough and cold preparations for its expectorant activity. [4]

PHARMACOLOGY: As a result of licorice's extensive folk history for gastric irritation, it has undergone extensive research for use as an anti-

ulcerogenic agent. While the specific mechanism of action is unknown, carbenoxolone, a semisynthetic succinic acid ester of 18β glycyrrhetic acid, a compound combined in licorice, acts to enhance mucous secretions, increase the lifespan of gastric epithelial cells, inhibit back diffusion of hydrogen ions induced by bile, and possibly inhibit peptic activity.

Controlled trials show carbenoxolone is less effective than cimetidine in treating gastric and duodenal disease. In one study, 78% of patients receiving cimetidine demonstrated ulcer improvement by gastroscopy compared with 52% of those receiving carbenoxolone. Additionally, carbenoxolone patients experienced more side effects including edema, hypertension, and hypokalemia. These side effects are more pronounced in elderly patients and those with underlying renal, hepatic, or cardiovascular disease. A proposed mechanism of action for these side effects involves carbenoxolone's action on the renin-aldosterone-angiotensin axis. Spironolactone relieves the side effects but also attenuates the therapeutic effects.

Another licorice product tested as an anti-ulcer agent is deglycyrrhizinated licorice (DGL), which consists of licorice that has had virtually all of its glycyrrhizin removed. Several studies have evaluated the efficacy of DGL, but all have been inconclusive. These agents have not shown consistent results nor the serious side effects exhibited by carbenoxolone.

Another use for glycyrrhizins is suppression of scalp sebum secretion. A 10% glycyrrhizin shampoo prevented sebum secretion for 1 week compared with citric acid shampoo, which delayed oil accumulation by 1 day.

Alcohol extracts of *G. glabra* have in vitro antibacterial activity and weak in vivo antiviral activity.

Prepared Chinese licorice, *Zhigancao*, was found to have antiarrhythmic effects, such as prolonging P-R and Q-T intervals.[5]

TOXICOLOGY: The toxic manifestations of excess licorice ingestion are well documented. One case documented the ingestion of 30 to 40 g of licorice/day for 9 months as a diet food. The subject became increasingly lethargic with flaccid weakness and dulled reflexes. She also suffered from hypokalemia and myoglobinuria. Treatment with potassium supplements re-

versed her symptoms. Excessive licorice intake can result in sodium and fluid retention, hypertension, and inhibition of the renin-angiotensin system.[6]

After consuming large amounts of licorice, human intoxication with aldosterone-like effects was found.[7]

A 70-year-old patient with hypertension and hypokalemia caused by chronic licorice intoxication in excess of approximately 80 candies (each having 0.3 glycyrrhizic acid) a day for 4 to 5 years, discontinued use 1 week before hospital admission. After discontinuing licorice and monitoring a treatment plan including licorice, the activity of 11-β-hydroxysteroid dehydrogenase was suppressed when the patient had been without licorice, but the 11-β-hydroxysteroid dehydrogenase increased as the levels of urinary glycyrrhetic acid decreased.[8]

Other documented complications include paraparesis, hypertensive encephalopathy, and one case of quadriplegia. Products that contain licorice as a flavoring, such as chewing tobacco, have also been implicated in cases of toxicity. Hypersensitivity reactions to glycyrrhiza-containing products have also been noted.

[1] Kassir ZA. *Ir J Med.* 1985;78:153-156.
[2] Morgan AG, et al. *Gut.* 1982;23:545-551.
[3] Morgan AG, et al. *Gut.* 1985;26:599-602.
[4] Shibata S. *Int J Pharmacog.* 1994;32(1):75-89.
[5] Chen RX, et al. *Chung Kuo Chung Yao Tsa Chih.* 1991;16(10):617-619.

[6] Sigurjonsdottir HA, et al. *J Human Hyperten.* 1995;9(5):345-348.
[7] Bielenberg J. *Pharmazeutische Zeitung.* 1989;134(12):9-12.
[8] Farese RV, et al. *N Engl J Med.* 1991;325(10):1223-1227.

Lycopene

SCIENTIFIC NAME(S): Ψ, Ψ-carotene

COMMON NAME(S): Lycopene

৯৯৯৯ PATIENT INFORMATION ৯৯৯৯

Uses: Lycopene has antioxidant activity and may be used in cancer prevention.

Side Effects: No literature on toxicity was found.

Dosing: Lycopene administered as a pure compound has been studied in clinical trials at doses of 13 to 75 mg/day.[1-5]

BOTANY: Lycopene is a carotenoid, occurring in ripe fruit, especially tomatoes.[6] Other sources include watermelon, grapefruit, and guava.[7]

HISTORY: The tomato (*Lycopersicon esculentum*) continues to be a popular and highly consumed crop in the US, second in production to potatoes.[8] Epidemiological evidence finds the constituent lycopene to be associated with a reduced risk of certain diseases and cancers.[9]

PHARMACOLOGY: Factors affecting uptake and absorption of carotenoids have been reported.[10] Pharmacokinetic parameters of lycopene have been evaluated in humans.[11-19]

Cooking releases desirable antioxidants from tomatoes. Absorption of lycopene, which is lipid soluble, is improved in the presence of oil or fat.[20] Lycopene's protective mechanisms include antioxidant activity, induction of cell-cell communication, and growth control.[16,21]

Lycopene's antioxidant actions are well documented. Its presence as a supplement in liquid form reduces lipid peroxidation in one report. It may ameliorate the oxidative stress of cigarette smoke.[22] Another study reports that certain concentrations of lycopene (and other antioxidants) may protect against cognitive impairment.[23] In 19 subjects, lycopene supplementation decreased serum lipid peroxidation and low-density lipoprotein (LDL) oxidation, suggesting a decreased risk for coronary heart disease (CHD).[24] Lycopene demonstrated a protective effect against MI in the European Community Multicenter Study on Antioxidants (EURAMIC), confirming its beneficial effects on the heart.[25] Carotenoid mixtures display synergistic activity against oxidative damage, most pronounced with the presence of both lycopene and lutein.[26] This combination was also found to have potent anticarcinogenic activity.[27]

Oxidative stress is recognized as a major contributor to increased cancer risk. Lycopene's ideal absorption from tomato products act as antioxidants and may also play important roles in cancer prevention.[28] It achieves high concentrations in testes, adrenal glands, and prostate. The intake of lycopene and decreased cancer risk association have been observed in prostate, pancreas, and stomach cancers.[29,30,31,32] Tocopherol exhibited synergistic inhibitory effects against 2 human prostate carcinoma cell proliferation lines.[33] Lycopene may also play a protective role in the early stages of cervical carcinogenesis as seen in a study.[34] Plasma levels of lycopene and other carotenoids were lower in women with cervical intraepithelial neoplasia and cervical cancer, suggesting protection with higher lycopene concentrations.[11]

Reports are available on the international symposium on lycopene and tomato products in disease prevention.[35,36] Reviews describing lycopene and disease prevention can also be referenced.[37-40]

TOXICOLOGY: No literature on lycopene toxicity was found.

[1] Paetau I, et al. *Am J Clin Nutr.* 1998;68:1187-1195.

[2] Paetau I, et al. *Am J Clin Nutr.* 1999;70:490-494.

[3] Kucuk O, et al. *Cancer Epidemiol Biomarkers Prev.* 2001;55:627-635.

[4] Corridan BM, et al. *Eur J Clin Nutr.* 2001;55:627-635.

[5] Wright AJ, et al. *J Lab Clin Med.* 1999;134:592-598.

[6] Budavari S, et al. eds. *The Merck Index*, 11th ed. Rahway: Merck and Co. 1989.

[7] Murray M. *Encyclopedia of Nutritional Supplements* . Rocklin, CA: Prima Publishing. 1996;27-29.

[8] Beecher G. *Proc Soc Exp Biol Med.* 1998;218(2):98-100.

[9] Nguyen M, et al. *Proc Soc Exp Biol Med.* 1998;218(2):101-105.

[10] Williams A, et al. *Proc Soc Exp Biol Med.* 1998;218(2):106-108.

[11] Palan P, et al. *Clin Cancer Res.* 1996;2(1):181-185.

[12] Johnson E, et al. *J Nutr.* 1997;127(9):1833-1837.

[13] O'Neill M, et al. *Br J Nutr.* 1998;79(2):149-59.

[14] Talwar D, et al. *Clin Chim Acta.* 1998;270(2):85-100.

[15] Johnson E. *Proc Soc Exp Biol Med.* 1998;218(2):115-120.

[16] Sies H, et al. *Proc Soc Exp Biol Med.* 1998;218(2):121-124.

[17] Boucher B. *Br J Nutr.* 1998;80(1):115.

[18] Mayne S, et al. *Am J Clin Nutr.* 1998;68(3):642-647.

[19] Yeum K, et al. *J Am Coll Nutr.* 1998;17(5):442-447.

[20] Weisburger J. *Proc Soc Exp Biol Med.* 1998;218(2):140-143.

[21] Stahl W, et al. *Arch Biochem Biophys.* 1996;336(1):1-9.

[22] Steinberg F, et al. *Am J Clin Nutr.* 1998;68(2):319-327.

[23] Schmidt R, et al. *J Am Geriatr Soc.* 1998;46(11):1407-1410.

[24] Agarwal S, et al. *Lipids.* 1998;33(10):981-984.

[25] Kohlmeier I, et al. *Am J Epidemiol.* 1997;146(8):618-626.

[26] Stahl W, et al. *FEBS Lett.* 1998;427(2):305-308.

[27] Nishino H. *J Cell Biochem Suppl.* 1997;27:86-91.

[28] Rao A, et al. *Nutr Cancer.* 1998;31(3):199-203.

[29] Gerster H. *J Am Coll Nutr.* 1997;16(2):109-126.

[30] Giovannucci E, et al. *J Natl Cancer Inst.* 1995 Dec 6;87(23):1767-1776.

[31] Clinton S, et al. *Cancer Epidemiol Biomarkers Prev.* 1996;5(10):823-833.

[32] Giovannucci E, et al. *Proc Soc Exp Biol Med.* 1998;218(2):129-139

[33] Pastori M, et al. *Biochem Biophys Res Commun.* 1998;250(3):582-85.

[34] Kantesky P, et al. *Nutr Cancer.* 1998;31(1):31-40.

[35] Hoffmann I, et al. *Cancer Epidemiol Biomarkers Prev.* 1997;6(8):643-645.

[36] Weisburger J. *Proc Soc Exp Biol Med.* 1998;218(2):93-94.

[37] Clinton S. *Nutr Rev.* 1998;56(2 pt 1):35-51.

[38] Krinsky N. *Proc Soc Exp Biol Med.* 1998;218(2):95-97.

[39] Singh D, et al. *Oncology.* 1998;12(11):1643-53,1657-58,1659-1660.

[40] Michaud I. *ASHP Midyear Clinical Meeting.* 1998 Dec;33:PI-95.

SCIENTIFIC NAME(S): *Ephedra sinica* Stapf., *E. intermedia* Schrenk et C.A. Meyer, or *E. equisetina* Bge. Family: Ephedraceae (ephedra)

COMMON NAME(S): Ephedra, ma huang, yellow horse, yellow astringent. Ephedra is the major component of supplements such as *Herbal Ecstasy*, *DietMax*, *Metabolife 356*, *Solaray*, *Xenadrine*, *Metabolean*, *Energel*, *Stacker 2*, *Black Beauty*, and *Yellow Jacket*. Note that many manufacturers have recently reformulated their products to remove Ephedra because of legal liability questions.

⋙ PATIENT INFORMATION ⋘

Uses: Ma huang may be effective for bronchodilation in asthma and is used in combination with caffeine for weight loss and to increase athletic performance. However, its use is not recommended.

Interactions: Ma huang should not be taken within 14 days of monoamine oxidase (MAO) inhibitor use.

Side Effects: Ephedra use has been linked to cardiovascular adverse effects, including hypertension, stroke, and MI. Patients with hyperthyroidism, benign prostatic hyperplasia, glaucoma, diabetes mellitus, and seizures and women who are pregnant should exercise particular caution.

Dosing: Current guidelines suggest limiting dosage of ephedrine to less than 90 mg/day. Medical supervision may be the most appropriate mode for safe administration of ma huang.

BOTANY: Ephedra species are low shrubby plants with small leaves on jointed, ribbed, green stems. They are dioecious (male and female flowers are usually found on separate plants). The 3 species that are sources of the drug are native to China, where the aboveground parts are collected in the fall and dried for drug use. The ephedras are gymnosperms and are most closely related to the conifers, although many aspects of their botany are different.[1,2] The root of *E. sinica* or *E. intermedia* is known as ma huang gen and is considered to be a distinct drug, used for its antisudorific properties. A chapter on ephedra has been published in the *Flora of China* project.[3]

HISTORY: Ma huang is one of the earliest and best known drugs of Chinese traditional medicine, mentioned in the *Shen Nong Ben Cao Jing*, one of the foundation books of Chinese medicine, about 100 AD. It was and still is used to induce perspiration and to treat the symptoms of bronchial asthma, colds, and influenza.

PHARMACOLOGY: Ephedrine is the main active principle of ephedra and has sympathomimetic activity, which accounts for its clinical use for bronchial asthma and low blood pressure. It is active when given orally, parenterally, or ophthalmically. It also is regarded as a CNS stimulant but is much weaker than amphetamine.

Experiments in animals have examined various activities of ephedrine and ephedra herb. Antitussive effects were found against sulfur dioxide-induced cough in mice, especially in combination with amygdalin.[4] Rats were trained to discriminate ephedrine stimulation from saline; this stimulus was generalized to amphetamine, cocaine, and caffeine, but the stimulant properties were not entirely identical. In this system, ephedrine was about one tenth as potent as amphetamine.[5] Ephedrine, its congeners, and crude ephedra herb have been shown to have activity in anti-inflammatory models in mice.[6,7] Passive cutaneous anaphylaxis in rats was blocked by oral administration of ephedrine; this effect was not caused by a direct effect on histamine release from mast cells.[8] A component of ephedra herb thought to be an anionic carbohydrate blocked the activation of classical and alternative complement pathways.[9] The growth of influenza virus was inhibited in tissue culture by an extract of ephedra herb, and tannins were identified as the likely active constituents.[10]

The 3 subtypes of beta-adrenergic receptor have different pharmacology; ephedrine and congeners are known to activate all 3 subtypes. The activation of the beta-3 subtype has been shown to be responsible for at least part of the thermogenesis observed on administration of ephedrine; blockade of the type 1 and 2 receptors with selective inhibitors still allows about half of the increase in energy expenditure in human subjects while entirely blocking the increase in heart rate and plasma glucose caused by ephedrine.[11] The pharmacokinetics of ephedra in humans have been studied, with ephedrine in crude herb requiring twice as long to reach the peak plasma concentration as pure ephedrine dosage forms.[12] Similarly, the combination of a single dose of ephedra and caffeine has been studied; ephedrine and pseudoephedrine had similar peak concentrations at 140 to 150 minutes, while caffeine blood levels peaked at 90 minutes. Heart rate was increased a maximum of 15 bpm over baseline. Overall results were similar to the individual compounds in pure form.[13]

While asthma treatment is one of the classical clinical uses for pure ephedrine, dietary supplement use and promotion of ephedra herb is concentrated on weight loss and increasing athletic performance.

Weight loss: For weight loss, a combination of ma huang with a caffeine-containing supplement such as guarana or cola nut is most frequently used. The origin of this combination can be traced to the empirical observation of a Danish physician that obese asthma patients treated with a combination of ephedrine, caffeine, and phenobarbital lost weight.[14] This so-called "Elsinore pill" became popular in Denmark for weight loss. Because of skin rashes attributed to phenobarbital, this component of the combination was removed without affecting weight loss.

Subsequent clinical trials have documented weight loss over various time periods using combinations of ephedrine and caffeine or ephedrine alone but found no statistically significant effect. A double-blind study for 3 months with ephedrine and limited diet, but no caffeine, found no effect for 75 and 150 mg/day ephedrine.[15] In a different trial, treatment with ephedrine for 3 months was shown to lead to higher oxygen consumption and thermogenesis and to reduced body weight.[16] An increase of 3.6% in energy expenditure was observed in patients given 50 mg ephedrine 3 times/day for 1 day, but no increase in mechanical work was observed.[17]

The effect of an ephedrine- and caffeine-containing supplement on peak oxygen consumption was studied in 10 obese females. The combination increased oxygen consumption.[18] Thirty-two obese adolescents given ephedrine and caffeine lost weight and body fat in a double-blind, placebo-controlled pilot study.[19] Another study of ma huang and guarana in 67 adults resulted in fat and weight loss over an 8-week period, although side effects in the treatment arm caused a substantial number of dropouts.[20] The same group conducted a larger 6-month trial in which herbal ephedra and caffeine promoted body weight and body fat reduction and improved blood lipids without adverse effects.[21]

Reviews have concluded that ephedrine and caffeine combinations, whether in pure form or in herbal supplements, can stimulate weight loss through enhanced thermogenesis.[14,22] A survey estimated the use of such products in 5 US states in 1998; ephedra was used by 1% of the total population.[23] Estimates of ephedra sales range as high as 2 to 3 billion doses per year, primarily for weight loss.[24]

Athletic performance: Supplements containing ephedra also have been promoted for increasing athletic performance.[25] While insignificant effects on performance have been noted for ephedra alone, combinations of ephedra and caffeine have been found to increase endurance in running and cycling experiments.[26,27] Ephedrine alkaloids are banned in amateur sports; thus, use of ephedra or other supplements containing ephedra alkaloids are grounds for disqualification.

Other: Polysaccharides named ephedrans A-E have been identified from *Ephedra distachya* herb and have hypoglycemic activity in mice.[28] The roots of Ephedra have yielded a variety of hypotensive compounds, including the flavonoid ephedrannin A,[29] feruloylhistamine,[30] and the spermine alkaloids ephedradines A-D.[31] These latter compounds have not been found in the aboveground parts of ephedra.

INTERACTIONS: The potential for drug-ephedra interactions has been profiled, noting that MAO inhibitors should be avoided within 14 days of ephedra use.[32]

TOXICOLOGY: There is wide agreement that ephedrine and related ephedra alkaloids have a relatively narrow therapeutic index. The major area of concern is their effect on the cardiovascular system because ephedrine increases heart rate and elevates blood pressure. The pharmacokinetics and cardiovascular effects of ma huang were examined in normotensive adults. While ephedrine was well-absorbed after oral ephedra dosage, only 6 of 12 subjects experienced an increase in heart rate, while effects on blood pressure were inconsistent.[12] In another experiment with 8 normotensive subjects, the combination of 200 mg caffeine and 20 mg ephedrine found in ephedra increased systolic blood pressure a maximum of 14 mm Hg 90 minutes after a single dose, while heart rate peaked 6 hours after dosage at 15 bpm over baseline.[13] In obese women, a combination of ephedrine with caffeine had insignificant cardiovascular adverse effects at rest and during exercise.[33] A larger placebo-controlled trial found no adverse cardiovascular effects over 14 days in obese adults.[34]

While these clinical studies have found modest effects under controlled conditions, case reports and spontaneous adverse effect reports (AERs) to the FDA have been interpreted as harbingers of a more serious problem. One hundred forty AERs related to ephedra reported between 1997 and 1999. One third of the AERs were considered definitely or probably related to ephedra and another third possibly related. Of these 87 AERs, half reported cardiovascular symptoms, primarily hypertension, while tachycardia, stroke, and seizures were less frequent. Ten deaths and 13 events resulting in permanent disability were recorded.[35] Responses to this study pointed out that such AERs did not prove causation.[36,37] A review of AERs on ephedra from 1995 through 1997 found 37 serious cases including 16 strokes, 10 MIs, and 11 sudden deaths.[38] Again, these findings were controversial.[39,40] A detailed case report of stroke associated with ephedra use has been published.[41]

Other toxicological data on ephedra are less extensive. While ephedra extracts are cytotoxic to cultivated cells, the cytotoxicity is not primarily due to ephedrine.[42] N-nitrosamines of ephedrine and pseudoephedrine have been formed under physiological conditions. N-nitrosoephedrine has been shown to be a carcinogen.[43,44] Acute hepatotoxicity has been associated with use of ma huang; however, the authors of the case report admitted that contamination with other hepatotoxic herbs was the most likely explanation.[45] Numerous reports of toxicity in dogs accidentally ingesting ephedra/caffeine supplements have been collated.[46] The psychoactive aspects of ephedrine alkaloids in the context of drug abuse have been reviewed.[47]

Due in part to the fact that ephedra AERs constituted the largest single category of adverse events and that a number of them were fatal or severe, the FDA proposed rules limiting dosage and establishing warning labels for ephedra products in June 1997.[24] However, in July 1999, the US General Accounting Office issued a report challenging the FDA's basis for the proposed rules, and the FDA subsequently withdrew part of the proposal.[24] In 2000, the dietary supplement industry provided a comprehensive analysis of safety and appropriate dosing issues concluding that a daily dosage corresponding to 90 mg ephedrine was safe.[48] A government-commissioned study of ephedra by the RAND Corporation was begun in June 2002.[49] A chronology of the ephedra controversy from the FDA viewpoint is contained in Senate testimony.[50] A jury awarded more than $4 million to families of stroke and heart attack patients who had used *Metabolife 356*.[51] An industry group, the Ephedra Education Council, maintains an archive of many relevant documents.[52] Consumers and health professionals should exercise appropriate caution until definitive legislative or regulatory action resolves the status of ephedra.

[1] Chaw SM, Parkinson CL, Cheng Y, Vincent TM, Palmer JD. *Proc Natl Acad Sci U S A.* 2000;97:4086-4091.

[2] Bowe LM, Coat G, dePamphilis CW. *Proc Natl Acad Sci U S A.* 2000;97:4092-4097.

[3] Fu L, Yu Y, Riedl H. *Flora of China.* St. Louis, MO and Beijing, China: Missouri Botanical Garden Press and Science Press; 2000:97.

[4] Miyagoshi M, Amagaya S, Ogihara Y. *Planta Med.* 1986:275-278.

[5] Young R, Glennon RA. *Pharmacol Biochem Behav.* 1998;60:771-775.

[6] Kasahara Y, Hikino H, Tsurufuji S, Watanabe M, Ohuchi K. Oriental medicines. Part 75. *Planta Med.* 1985:325-331.

[7] Hikino H, Konno C, Takata H, Tamada M. *Chem Pharm Bull.* 1980;28:2900-2904.

[8] Shibata H, Nabe T, Yamamura H, Kohno S. *Inflamm Res.* 2000;49:398-403.

[9] Ling M, Piddlesden SJ, Morgan BP. *Clin Exp Immunol.* 1995;102:582-588.

[10] Mantani N, Andoh T, Kawamata H, Terasawa K, Ochiai H. *Antiviral Res.* 1999;44:193-200.

[11] Liu YL, Toubro S, Astrup A, Stock MJ. *Int J Obes Relat Metab Disord.* 1995;19:678-685.

[12] White LM, Gardner SF, Gurley BJ, Marx MA, Wang PL, Estes M. *J Clin Pharmacol.* 1997;37:116-122.

[13] Haller CA, Jacob P III, Benowitz NL. *Clin Pharmacol Ther.* 2002;71:421-432.

[14] Greenway FL. *Obes Rev.* 2001;2:199-211.

[15] Pasquali R, Baraldi G, Cesari MP, et al. *Int J Obes Relat Metab Disord.* 1985;9:93-98.

[16] Astrup A, Lundsgaard C, Madsen J, Christensen NJ. *Am J Clin Nutr.* 1985;42:83-94.

[17] Shannon JR, Gottesdiener K, Jordan J, et al. *Clin Sci.* 1999;96:483-491.

[18] Greenway FL, Raum WJ, DeLany JP. *J Altern Complement Med.* 2000;6:553-555.

[19] Molnár D, Torok H, Erhardt E, Jeges S. *Int J Obes Relat Metab Disord.* 2000;24:1573-1578.

[20] Boozer CN, Nasser JA, Heymsfield SB, Wang V, Chen G, Solomon JL. *Int J Obes Relat Metab Disord.* 2001;25:316-324.

21 Boozer CN, Daly PA, Homel P, et al. *Int J Obes Relat Metab Disord.* 2002;26:593-604.

22 Dulloo AG. *Int J Obes Relat Metab Disord.* 2002;26:590-592.

23 Blanck HM, Khan LK, Serdula MK. *JAMA.* 2001;286:930-935.

24 General Accounting Office. Dietary supplements: uncertainties in analyses underlying FDA's proposed rule on ephedrine alkaloids. 1999;GAO/HEHS/GGD-99-90.

25 Bucci LR. *Am J Clin Nutr.* 2000;72:624S-636S.

26 Bell DG, Jacobs I, Ellerington K. *Med Sci Sports Exerc.* 2001;33:1399-1403.

27 Bell DG, McClellan TM, Sabiston CM. *Med Sci Sports Exerc.* 2002;34:344-349.

28 Konno C, Mizuno T, Hikino H. *Planta Med.* 1985:162-163.

29 Hikino H, Takahashi M, Konno C. *Tetrahedron Lett.* 1982;23:673-676.

30 Hikino H, Kiso Y, Ogata M, et al. *Planta Med.* 1984;50:478-480.

31 Hikino H, Ogata K, Konno C, Sato S. *Planta Med.* 1983;48:290-293.

32 Scott GN, Elmer GW. *Am J Health Syst Pharm.* 2002;59:339-347.

33 Waluga M, Janusz M, Karpel E, Hartleb M, Nowak A. *Clin Physiol.* 1998;18:69-76.

34 Kalman D, Incledon T, Gaunaurd I, Schwartz H, Krieger D. *Int J Obes Relat Metab Disord.* 2002;26:1363-1366.

35 Haller CA, Benowitz NL. *N Engl J Med.* 2000;343:1833-1838.

36 Fleming GA. *N Engl J Med.* 2000;343:1886-1887.

37 Hutchins GM. *N Engl J Med.* 2001;344:1095-1097.

38 Samenuk D, Link MS, Homoud MK, et al. *Mayo Clin Proc.* 2002;77:12-16.

39 Lindsay BD. *Mayo Clin Proc.* 2002;77:7-9.

40 Hutchins GM. *Mayo Clin Proc.* 2002;77:733-735.

41 Kaberi-Otarod J, Conetta R, Kundo KK, Farkash A. *Clin Pharmacol Ther.* 2002;72:343-346.

42 Lee MK, Cheng BW, Che CT, Hsieh DP. *Toxicol Sci.* 2000;56:424-430.

43 Alwan SM, Al-Hindawi MK, Abdul-Rahman SK, Al-Sarraj S. *Cancer Lett.* 1986;31:221-226.

44 Tricker AR, Wacker CD, Preussmann R. *Cancer Lett.* 1987;35:199-206.

45 Nadir A, Agrawal S, King PD, Marshall JB. *Am J Gastroenterol.* 1996;91:1436-1438.

46 Ooms TG, Khan SA, Means C. *J Am Vet Med Assoc.* 2001;218:225-229.

47 Kalix P. *J Ethnopharmacol.* 1991;32:201-208.

48 http://www.crnusa.org/cantoxreportindex.html

49 http://www.hhs.gov/news/press/2002pres/20020614.html

50 http://www.senate.gov/~gov_affairs/100802crawford.htm

51 http://verdictsearch.com/news/docs/1204nws-attack.jsp

52 http://www.ephedrafacts.com/backgroundreport.html

Maca

SCIENTIFIC NAME(S): *Lepidium meyenii* Walp. Family: Brassicaceae (Mustards)

COMMON NAME(S): Peruvian ginseng, Maino, Ayuk willku, Ayak chichira

---

❧❧❧ PATIENT INFORMATION ❧❧❧

Uses: Maca has been used as an aphrodisiac, fertility aid, and to relieve stress although there is little scientific information to support these uses.

Side Effects: There is little information on maca's long-term effects. Its long-time use as a food product suggests low potential for toxicity.

Dosing: Maca root is used at 3 to 5 g/day or as 900 mg of root extract; however, there are no published clinical trials to justify these doses.

BOTANY: Maca is cultivated in a narrow, high-altitude zone of the Andes Mountains in Peru. The plant's frost tolerance allows it to grow at altitudes of 3500 to 4450 meters above sea level in the puna and suni ecosystems, where only alpine grasses and bitter potatoes can survive.[1] It and several related wild species are also found in the Bolivian Andes.[2] The plant grows from a stout, pear-shaped taproot and has a matlike, creeping system of stems. While traditionally cultivated as a vegetable crop, use for its medicinal properties has become more prominent in Peru. Maca is related to the common garden cress, *Lepidium sativum* L.

HISTORY: Maca was domesticated at least 2000 years ago and has been used commonly as a food by Peruvian peasants who live in high altitudes. It was considered to be a "famine food," but recent analyses have shown that the root is high in nutritional value, containing essential amino acids and important fatty acids.[3] The root can be dried and powdered, after which it is stored for several years without serious deterioration. Dried roots are cooked in water to make a sweet, aromatic porridge known as "mazamorra." According to Peruvian folk belief, maca enhances female fertility in both humans and livestock, countering the reduction in fertility seen in high altitudes.[4] However, maca is believed to have an anti-aphrodisiac effect on males.[5]

PHARMACOLOGY: Unreferenced data published on a commercial Web site (www.macaperu.com) claims activity of maca in rat adaptogen models that use swimming time and oxygen consumption as endpoints.

Aphrodisiac and antistress properties have also been claimed. The pharmacology of other *Lepidium* species is documented as the following: *L. capitatum* had anti-implantation activity in rats.[6,7] The ethanolic extract of the seeds of *L. sativum* was found to increase collagen deposition in a rat model of fracture healing.[8] *L. latifolium* was found to have diuretic action in rats.[9]

TOXICOLOGY: The presence of substantial amounts of a cardiac glycoside in the related species, *L. apetalum*,[10] is cause for concern. Cardioactive substances have also been detected in *L. sativum*.[11] However, the fact that dried maca roots have been consumed for many years would argue against a risk for cardiotoxicity. *L. virginicum* was inactive in a screen for genotoxicity.[12]

---

[1] Quiros C, et al. *Econ Bot.* 1996;50(2):216.
[2] Toledo J, et al. *Ann Bot.* 1998;82(4):523.
[3] Dini A, et al. *Food Chem.* 1994;49(4):347.

[4] Eckes L. *Gegenbaurs Morphol Jahrb.* 1976;122(5):761-770.

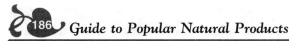

[5] Johns T. *With Bitter Herbs They Shall Eat It. Chemical Ecology and the Origins of Human Diet and Medicine*. Tucson: University of Arizona Press, 1990;119-121.

[6] Singh M, et al. *Planta Med*. 1984;50(2):154-157.

[7] Prakash O, et al. *Acta Eur Fertil*. 1985;16(6):441-448.

[8] Ahsan S, et al. *Int J Crude Drug Res*. 1989;27(4):235.

[9] Navarro E, et al. *J Ethnopharmacol*. 1994;41(1-2):65-69.

[10] Hyun J, et al. *Planta Med*. 1995;61(3):294-295.

[11] Vohora S, et al. *Indian J Physiol Pharmacol*. 1977;21(2):118-120.

[12] Ramos Ruiz A, et al. *J Ethnopharmacol*. 1996;52(3):123-127.

SCIENTIFIC NAME(S): *Grifola frondosa* (Dickson ex Fr.) S.F. Gray (Polyporaceae)

COMMON NAME(S): Maitake, "king of mushrooms," dancing mushroom, "monkey's bench," shelf fungi

---

❧❧❧❧ PATIENT INFORMATION ❧❧❧❧

Uses: Maitake has been used for cancer, diabetes, high blood pressure, cholesterol, and obesity.

Side Effects: Most studies report no side effects.

Dosing: Maitake usually is taken in doses of 3 to 7 g/day; however, there are no clinical studies to substantiate the efficacy or safety of this dose.

BOTANY: The maitake mushroom is from northeastern Japan. It grows in clusters at the foot of oak trees and can reach 50 cm in base diameter. One bunch can weigh up to 45 kg. Maitake has no cap but has a rippling, flowery appearance, resembling "dancing butterflies" (hence, one of its common names "dancing mushroom").[1]

HISTORY: In China and Japan, maitake mushrooms have been consumed for 3000 years. Years ago in Japan, the maitake had monetary value and was worth its weight in silver. This mushroom was offered to Shogun, the national leader, by local lords. In the late 1980s, Japanese scientists identified the maitake to be more potent than lentinan, shiitake, suehirotake, and kawaratake mushrooms, all used in traditional Asian medicine for immune function enhancement.

PHARMACOLOGY: Immunostimulant activity is characteristic of many of the medicinal mushrooms, including shiitake, enokitake, or kawaratake. Maitake exerts its effects by activation of natural killer cells, cytotoxic T-cells, interleukin-1, and superoxide anions, all of which aid in anticancer activity.[2] It has also been determined that the large molecular weight of the polysaccharide molecule and branched structure are necessary for its antitumor effect or immunological enhancement.[3-5]

There is a small number of clinical trials investigating maitake's effects in cancer therapy. Additional controlled studies are needed. In a 165-patient study, quality of life indicators improved, including cancer symptoms (eg, nausea, hair loss) and pain reduction.[6] Cancers that were improved by maitake in clinical cases include liver, lung, breast, brain, and prostate.[1]

Maitake may control blood glucose levels by possible reduction of insulin resistance and enhancement of insulin sensitivity.[1]

Studies are available concerning maitake's antiobesity activity.[7] In an observatory trial, 30 patients lost between 7 and 26 pounds from administration of 20 to 500 mg tablets of maitake powder per day for 2 months.[8]

TOXICOLOGY: Little or no information regarding maitake toxicity is available. Most studies report no side effects.[1] Because potential toxicity exists from mistaken mushroom identity, use caution when obtaining this particular natural product.

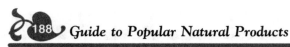

[1] Lieberman S, et al. *Maitake King of Mushrooms*. New Canaan, CT: Keats Publishing, Inc. 1997;7-48.

[2] Adachi K, et al. *Chem Pharm Bull*. 1987;35(1):262-270.

[3] Adachi K, et al. *Chem Pharm Bull*. 1989;37(7):1838-1843.

[4] Adachi K, et al. *Chem Pharm Bull*. 1990;38(2):477-481.

[5] Ohno N, et al. *Biol Pharm Bull*. 1995;18(1):126-133.

[6] Nanba H. *Townsend Letter for Doctors and Patients*. 1996;84-85.

[7] Ohtsuru M. *Anshin*. 1992 Jul:188-200.

[8] Yokota M. *Anshin*. 1992 Jul:202-204.

SCIENTIFIC NAME(S): *Pistacia lentiscus* L. Fam. Anacardiaceae

COMMON NAME(S): Mastic, mastick (tree), mastix, mastich, lentisk

---

❧❧❧ PATIENT INFORMATION ❧❧❧

Uses: Mastic has been used as a flavoring and a breath sweetener. It has also been studied for the treatment of ulcers. Mastic may also have antibacterial, antihypertensive, antioxidant, and cytoprotective effects.

Side Effects: Allergic reactions have occurred.

Dosing: Mastic resin has been studied as a treatment for ulcers at a daily dose of 1 g.[1]

BOTANY: Mastic is collected from an evergreen, dioecious shrub, which can grow to ≈ 3 m in height. It is native to the Mediterranean region, primarily in the Greek Island of Chios. Its leaves are green, leather-like, and oval. The small flowers grow in clusters and are reddish to green. The fruit is an orange-red drupe that ripens to black.

Mastic is "tapped" from the tree from June to August by making numerous, longitudinal gouges in the bark. An oleoresin exudes and hardens into an oval tear shape, about the size of a pea (3 mm). The transparent, yellow-green resin is collected every 15 days. If chewed, it becomes "plastic," with a balsamic/turpentine-like odor and taste. A related species is *P. vera*, the pistachio nut.[2-7]

HISTORY: Mastic resin was used in ancient Egypt as incense and to embalm the dead.[4,8] It has also been used as a preservative and a breath sweetener.[8] Mastic resin is still used as a flavoring in some Greek alcoholic beverages (eg, "retsina" wine) and in chewing gum from the island of Chios.

PHARMACOLOGY: The pharmacology and use of mastic is diverse. Mastic's role in improving benign gastric ulcers is discussed.[9] A double-blind clinical trial in 38 patients with duodenal ulcers given 1 g mastic daily (vs placebo) proved to exhibit ulcer healing effects.[1] A letter in the *New England Journal of Medicine* discusses these studies, as well as others, concluding that 1 g of mastic daily for 2 weeks can cure peptic ulcer rapidly. Its antibacterial actions against *Helicobacter pylori* may explain, in part, these beneficial effects.[10]

Mastic's antibacterial effects have been shown in other reports as well. It has actions against gram-positive and gram-negative bacteria strains,[11] some organisms include *Sarcina lutea*, *Staphylococcus aureus*, and *Escherichia coli*.[12] Mastic also possesses significant antifungal actions. The growth of the fungi *Candida albicans*, *C. parapsilosis*, *Torulopsis glabrata*, and *Trichophyton* sp. have all been inhibited by mastic.[12,13]

Various reports are available discussing miscellaneous uses and effects of mastic, including use as a drug-release vehicle,[14] improvement of adhesive strength in surgical tapes,[15,16,17] and aromatherapy.[8] Mastic has also been reported to be useful in the area of dentistry as a tooth cement and in reducing plaque.[3,18] It can also be used as a flavoring agent, perfume additive,[6] chewed as a gum, or used to retouch photographic negatives.[3] Mastic is also reported to possess some hypotensive effects,[19,20] as well as antioxidant actions because of tocopherol content.[21,22,23] Mastic as an insecticide has proven to be effective.[24]

Other uses include the following: To improve circulation, for muscle aches, bronchial problems,[4,6] as skin care for cuts, and as an insect repellant.[6]

TOXICOLOGY: Most toxicity regarding mastic or source *P. lentiscus* involves allergic reactions. The plant pollen is a major source for allergic reactions.[25-27] The first report of immunological reactions to pollen extracts of *Pistacia* genus occurred in 1987.[25] A monographic review on mastic discussing chemistry, pharmacology, and toxicity is available.[28] Children ingesting mastic may develop diarrhea.[29]

[1] Al Habbal M, et al. *Clin Exp Pharmacol Physiol.* 1984;11(5):541-544.

[2] Youngken H. *Textbook of Pharmacognosy.* 6th ed. Philadelphia, PA: The Blakiston Company, 1950:535-536.

[3] Budavari S, et al, eds. *The Merck Index.* 11th ed. Rahway, NJ: Merck & Co., Inc., 1989:92.

[4] Chevallier A. *The Encyclopedia of Medicinal Plants.* New York, NY: DK Publishing, 1996:249.

[5] Evans W. *Trease and Evans' Pharmacognosy.* 14th ed. Philadelphia, PA: WB Saunders Company Ltd, 1996:290-291.

[6] Lawless J. *The Illustrated Encyclopedia of Essential Oils.* Rockport, MA: Element Books, 1995:203.

[7] www.britannica.com

[8] www.herbnet.com/magazine/mag0003_p04.htm

[9] Huwez F, et al. *Gastroenterol Jpn.* 1986;21(3):273-274.

[10] Huwez F, et al. *N Engl J Med.* 1998;339(26):1946.

[11] Tassou C, et al. *Int Biodeterior Biodegrad.* 1995;36(3/4):411-420.

[12] Iauk L, et al. *J Chemother.* 1996;8(3):207-209.

[13] Ali-Shtayeh M, et al. *Mycoses.* 1999;42(11-12):665-672.

[14] Georgarakis M, et al. *Pharmazie.* 1987;42(7):455-6.

[15] Mikhail G, et al. *J Dermatol Surg Oncol.* 1986;12(9):904-905, 908.

[16] Mikhail G, et al. *J Burn Care Rehabil.* 1989;10(3):216-219.

[17] Lesesne C. *J Dermatol Surg Oncol.* 1992;18(11):990.

[18] www.forthnet.gr/mastic/masticoil.htm

[19] Sanz M, et al. *Pharmazie.* 1992;47(6):466-467.

[20] Sanz M, et al. *Pharmazie.* 1993;48(2):152-153.

[21] Abdel-Rahman A, et al. *J Am Oil Chem Soc.* 1975;52(10):423.

[22] Abdel-Rahman, A. *Grasas Aceites (Seville).* 1976;27(3):175-177.

[23] Cerrati C, et al. *Sostanze Grasse.* 1992;69(6):317-320.

[24] Pascual-Villalobos M, et al. *Ind Crops Prod.* 1998;8(3):183-94.

[25] Keynan N, et al. *Clin Allergy.* 1987;17(3):243-249.

[26] Cvitanovic S, et al. *J Investig Allergol Clin Immunol.* 1994;4(2):96-100.

[27] Keynan N, et al. *Allergy.* 1997;52(3):323-330.

[28] Ford R, et al. *Food Chem Toxicol.* 1992;30(Suppl):71S-72S.

[29] Fernandez A, et al. *J Essent Oil Res.* 2000;12(1):19.

SCIENTIFIC NAME(S): *Filipendula ulmaria* L. Maxim., *Spiraea ulmaria* L. Family: Rosaceae

COMMON NAME(S): Meadowsweet, queen of the meadow, dropwort, bridewort, lady of the meadow

---

❧❧❧ PATIENT INFORMATION ❧❧❧

Uses: Due to its salicylic acid content, meadowsweet has been used for colds and respiratory problems, acid indigestion or peptic ulcers, joint problems, skin diseases, and diarrhea.

Drug Interactions: Aspirin.

Side Effects: Few toxic events have been reported. Do not use in patients with salicylate or sulfite sensitivity, and use caution in asthmatics.

Dosing: Doses of 2.5 to 3.5 g/day of flower and 4 to 5 g of herb are considered conventional; however, no clinical trials support the safety or efficacy of these dosages.[1]

BOTANY: Meadowsweet is a herbaceous perennial shrub growing up to 2 m tall. The plant is native to Europe but also grows in North America, preferring damp, moist soil. The erect stem is red-marbled and hollow. The toothed leaves are dark green in color. Meadowsweet's aromatic, ornamental wildflowers are creamy, yellow-white, and contain 5 petals. The flowers are 5 mm in length and have an aroma reminiscent of wintergreen oil. The dried herb consists of flower petals and some unopened buds, which are the parts used as the drug.[2-9]

HISTORY: In 1682, meadowsweet was mentioned in a Dutch herbal. Holland called the plant "*Filipendula*," while in the rest of Europe, it was known as "*Spiraea*." Queen Elizabeth I adorned her apartments with meadowsweet. The flowers were used to flavor alcoholic beverages in England and Scandinavian countries.[9] In the Middle Ages, meadowsweet was known as "meadwort" because it was used to flavor "mead," an alcoholic drink made by fermenting honey and fruit juices.[6]

In 1838, salicylic acid was isolated from the plant. In the 1890s, salicylic acid was first synthesized to make aspirin.[6] "Aspirin" is derived from "spirin," based on meadowsweet's scientific name, "*Spiraea*."[9]

The plant was used in folk medicine for cancer, tumors, rheumatism, and as a diuretic.[5,8] Today, it is used as a digestive remedy, as supportive therapy for colds, for analgesia, and other indications.

PHARMACOLOGY: Meadowsweet is used for supportive therapy in colds, probably because of its analgesic, anti-inflammatory, and antipyretic actions.[2,3,7,9] The roots have been used to treat respiratory problems such as hoarseness, cough, and wheezing.[5]

The plant is also useful as a digestive remedy for acid indigestion or peptic ulcers. It protects the inner lining of the stomach while providing the anti-inflammatory benefits of salicylates.[6]

Because joint problems may be related to increased acid, the ability of meadowsweet to reduce acidity is also beneficial in treating joint problems.[6] It has also been mentioned that meadowsweet improves the condition of connective tissue of joints.[9] In folk medicine, meadowsweet was used for rheumatism of muscles and joints, and for arthritis.[2]

A heparin-plant protein complex contained in meadowsweet was found to have anticoagulant and fibrinolytic properties.[10] Meadowsweet flowers and seeds demonstrated an increased level of anticoagulant activity in vitro and in vivo in another report.[11] In vitro complement inhibition from the plant's flowers has been studied.[12]

Bacteriostatic activity from meadowsweet flower extracts include actions against *Staphylococcus aureus*, *S. epidermidis*, *Escherichia coli*, *Proteus vulgaris*, and *Pseudomonas aeruginosa*.[4] The salicylic acid in the plant is a known disinfectant used to treat ailments such as skin diseases.[5] Meadowsweet is also a urinary antiseptic, the mechanism of action being its close relation to phenol.[9]

The tannins in the plant possess astringent properties. Root preparations have been used in the treatment of diarrhea.[4,5]

Meadowsweet has been used as a sedative and to soothe nerves.[5]

TOXICOLOGY: The German Commission E Monographs lists no known side effects, contraindications (except those with salicylate sensitivity), or drug interactions with use of meadowsweet.[3] The FDA has classified the plant as an "herb of undefined safety."[5]

Use caution because of the toxicity profile of salicylates. Methyl salicylate can be absorbed through the skin, resulting in fatalities, especially in children.[4,5]

Bronchospasm has also been documented from use of the plant; therefore, use caution in asthmatics. Uteroactivity has also been observed from meadowsweet, warranting avoidance during pregnancy and lactation.[4]

[1] Blumenthal M, Brinckmann J, Goldberg A, eds. *Herbal Medicine: Expanded Commission E Monographs*. Newton, MA: Integrative Medicine Communications; 2000: 253-256.

[2] Bisset N. *Herbal Drugs and Phytopharmceuticals*. Stuttgart, Germany: CRC Press, 1994;480-482.

[3] Blumenthal M, ed. *The Complete German Commission E Monographs*. Boston, MA: American Botanical Council, 1998;169.

[4] Newall C, et al. *Herbal Medicines*. London, England: Pharmaceutical Press, 1996;191-192.

[5] Duke J. CRC *Handbook of Medicinal Herbs*. Boca Raton, FL: CRC Press Inc., 1989;196-197.

[6] Chevallier A. *Encyclopedia of Medicinal Plants*. New York, NY: DK Publishing, 1996;96.

[7] Schulz V, et al. *Rational Phytotherapy*. Berlin Heidelberg, Germany: Springer-Verlag, 1998;143-144.

[8] Bruneton J. *Pharmacognosy, Phytochemistry, Medicinal Plants*. Paris, France: Lavoisier, 1995;221-222, 316-18.

[9] Zeylstra H. *Br J Phytother*. 1998;5(1):8-12.

[10] Kudriashov B, et al. *Izv Akad Nauk SSSR [Biol]*. 1991;6:939-943.

[11] Liapina L, et al. *Izv Akad Nauk Ser Biol*. 1993;(4):625.

[12] Halkes S, et al. *Pharm Pharmacol Lett*. 1997;7(2-3):79.

SCIENTIFIC NAME(S): *Melatonin, MEL*

COMMON NAME(S): Melatonin, MEL

✯✯✯✯ PATIENT INFORMATION ✯✯✯✯

Uses: Melatonin is used to regulate sleep, protect against cancer, and provide a variety of other benefits.

Side Effects: Possible adverse effects include headache and depression.

Dosing: Jet lag: Eastbound travel — Take a preflight early evening treatment of melatonin followed by treatment at bedtime for 4 days after arrival. Westbound travel — Take melatonin for 4 days at bedtime when in the new time zone. *Difficulty falling asleep:* Take 5 mg of melatonin 3 to 4 hours before an imposed sleep period (over a 4-week period). *Difficulty maintaining sleep:* Take a high dose, repeated low doses, or a controlled-release formulation. *Children (6 months to 14 years of age) with sleep disorders:* 2 to 5 mg melatonin has been used.

HISTORY: Melatonin (MEL) is a hormone of the pineal gland that is also produced by extrapineal tissues.[1,2]

Melatonin secretion is inhibited by environmental light and stimulated by darkness, with secretion starting at 9 pm and peaking between 2 and 4 am. Nocturnal secretion of melatonin is highest in children and decreases with age.[3,4] Studies in the past decade have widely expanded melatonin use for easing insomnia, combatting jet lag, preventing pregnancy, protecting cells from free-radical damage, boosting the immune system, preventing cancer, and extending life.[5]

Although melatonin is not approved by the FDA as a drug product, it has been classified as an orphan drug since November 1993 (Sponsor: Dr. Robert Sack, Oregon Health Sciences University)[4] for the treatment of circadian rhythm sleep disorders in blind people with no light perception. It is commercially available as a nutritional supplement either as a synthetic product or derived from animal pineal tissue. Use of the nonsynthetic product is discouraged because of an increased risk of contamination or viral transmission.

PHARMACOLOGY: The FDA does not control melatonin and warns that users are taking it "without any assurance that it is safe or that it will have any beneficial effect."

Blind entrainment: The sleep-wake cycle in humans without light-dark cues is approximately 25 hours, shifting the sleep cycle by 1 hour each day. Blind people with little or no perception of light often develop *free-running* circadian rhythms more than 24 hours and subsequently develop sleep disturbances characterized by chronic fatigue and involuntary napping during the day. In case reports and small controlled studies, oral melatonin (dosage range: 0.5 to 10 mg) has been used to entrain free-running activity rhythms in the blind by advancing and stabilizing the phase of endogenous melatonin secretion.[4,6,7] Although success has varied, the importance of melatonin administration time is recognized. For example, the administration of melatonin (5 or 10 mg for 2 to 4 weeks at bedtime) to an 18-year-old blind man with chronic sleep disturbances produced slightly improved sleep onset but did not reduce daytime fatigue or hypersomnolence.[4,7] However, the administration of melatonin (5 mg for 3 weeks) at 2 to 3 hours prior to habitual bedtime decreased sleep onset (approximately 1.4 hours), slightly increased sleep duration (34 minutes), and improved sleep quality and daytime alertness. The authors suggest that there is a phase response curve (PRC) for the exogenous administration of melatonin; the maximum phase-advancing effects occur when melatonin is administered approximately 6 hours prior to onset of endogenous melatonin secretion.[4,8] The average cumulative phase advancement (CPA) of melatonin rhythms after 3 weeks of treatment with 5 and 0.5 mg/day was 8.41 and 7 hours, respectively.[4,6]

Jet lag: Melatonin's ability to modulate circadian rhythms has prompted several studies on its use in preventing jet lag.[4,9-11] Although the effects have been variable, most patients have reported general improvement in daytime fatigue, disturbed sleep cycles, mood, and recovery times. These studies are limited by the small number of participants and a focus on subjective ratings of effects with little or no evidence of actual changes in circadian shift (ie, changes in oral temperature or cortisol levels). As with entrainment studies in the blind, it appears that timing of administration and the development of optimal regimens require further study. Several melatonin regimens have been examined (5 to 10 mg/day) for various durations. In one study, 52 aircraft personnel were randomized to placebo, early, or late melatonin groups. The early group started melatonin (5 mg/day) 3 days before departure until 5 days after arrival.[4,10] The late group received melatonin upon arrival and for 4 additional days. When compared to placebo, the late melatonin group reported significantly less jet lag, fewer overall sleep disturbances, and faster recovery of energy and alertness. However, the early group (receiving melatonin for 8 days) reported jet lag symptoms similar to the placebo group and a worsened overall recovery. Additional data from uncontrolled studies suggest that benefits were also experienced by international travelers when melatonin was given on the day or night of departure and for 2 to 3 nights after arrival.[4,9,11] (Note: Because driving skills may be affected, one may experience drowsiness within 30 minutes after taking melatonin and then for approximately 1 hour.)

Insomnia: Although melatonin has been shown to shift melatonin secretion and circadian rhythm patterns, its direct hypnotic effect has not been clearly established. Decreased circulating melatonin serum levels have been demonstrated in insomniacs of all ages and in the healthy elderly.[3,4] In small studies of healthy volunteers or chronic insomniacs, large melatonin doses (75 to 100 mg) administered at night (9 pm to 10 pm) produced serum melatonin levels exceeding normal nocturnal ranges and hypnotic effects.[4,12,13] Midday administration of large doses increased serum melatonin levels beyond normal nocturnal ranges, increased subjective fatigue, and decreased cognitive function and vigor.[4,14] Administration of smaller doses (0.3 to 5 mg) has produced inconsistent hypnotic results, possibly due to the inclusion of different sleep disorders, drug formulations, and administration times.[4,15-20] The time to reach peak hypnotic effect was significantly longer when melatonin (5 mg) was administered at 12 noon vs 9 pm (3.66 vs 1 hour).[4,21] Delayed latency with daytime administration may be related to the already low circulating melatonin levels during the day. Low doses (0.3 or 1 mg) administered to healthy volunteers at 6 pm, 8 pm, or 9 pm decreased onset latency and latency to Stage 2 sleep but did not suppress rapid eye movement (REM) sleep nor induce hangover effects.

In patients with difficulty falling asleep, low melatonin doses should be sufficient in promoting sleep onset. However, in patients with difficulty maintaining sleep, low melatonin doses may not produce sufficient blood concentrations to maintain slumber. A 2 mg oral melatonin dose produced peak levels approximately 10 times higher than physiological levels, but it remained elevated for only 3 to 4 hours.[4,22] To maintain effective serum concentrations of melatonin throughout the night, a high dose, repeated low doses, or a controlled-release formulation may be needed. When compared to placebo in a trial of 12 elderly chronic insomniacs, melatonin significantly increased sleep efficiency (75% vs 83%) and decreased wake time after sleep onset (73 vs 49 minutes).[4,19] There were no significant differences between the groups for total sleep time (365 vs 360 minutes) or sleep onset (33 vs 19 minutes). Sleep onset and sleep maintenance were improved in elderly insomniacs after 1 week of immediate (1 mg) and sustained-release (2 mg) melatonin preparations. Sleep onset improved further when the sustained-release form was continued for 2 months.[4,20]

Cancer protection: Melatonin has demonstrated inhibitory effects on tumor growth in animal models and in vitro cancerous breast cell lines.[3] Proposed oncoprotective mechanisms of melatonin include stimulatory effects on circulating natural killer cells and potent antioxidant activity. Preliminary studies have examined the use of melatonin in patients with solid tumors unresponsive to standard therapies, melanoma, and as adjunctive amplifier therapy with interleukin in various metastatic tumors (ie, endocrine, colorectal).[4,21-25] European studies on *B-Oval* (containing melatonin) are ongoing, but it appears to slow the growth rate of human tumor cells. A nightly supplement (10 mg melatonin) has improved 1-year survival rates with metastatic lung cancer patients.[3] Well-controlled trials are needed before the role of melatonin as an oncostatic agent can be confirmed.

Oral contraceptive: Because melatonin plays a role in the endocrine-reproductive system and reduces circulating LH, its use as a contraceptive has been studied.[4,26] Melatonin, in various dosage combinations with a synthetic progestin, in 32 women for 4 months produced anovulatory effects.

TOXICOLOGY: Most studies note the absence of adverse events with melatonin. Minor side effects with doses less than 8 mg have included heavy head, headache, and transient depression.[4,10,11] In psychiatric patients, melatonin has aggravated depressive symptoms.[3,4,27] Toxicological studies have shown that an LD-50 could not be obtained even at extremely high doses. Researchers gave human volunteers 6 g melatonin each night for a month and found no major problems, except for stomach discomfort or residual sleepiness.[5]

[1] Windholz M, et al. *Merck Index*, 11th ed. Rahway, NJ: Merck and Co., 1989.

[2] Bowman WC, et al. *Textbook of Pharmacology*, 2nd ed. St. Louis, MO: Blackwell Scientific Publications, 1980.

[3] Webb SM, et al. *Clin Endocrinol*. 1995;42(3):221.

[4] Generali JA. *Drug Newsletter*. 1996;15(1):3.

[5] Cowley G. *Newsweek*. 1995 Aug 7:46.

[6] Sack RL, et al. *J Biol Rhythms*. 1991;6(3):249.

[7] Tzichinsky O, et al. *J Pineal Res*. 1992;12:105.

[8] Lewy AJ, et al. *Chronobiol Int*. 1992;9(5):380.

[9] Lino A, et al. *Biol Psychiatry*. 1993;34:587.

[10] Petrie K, et al. *Biol Psychiatry*. 1993;33:526.

[11] Claustrat B, et al. *Biol Psychiatry*. 1992;32:705.

[12] Waldhauser F, et al. *Psychopharmacol.* 1990;100:222.

[13] MacFarlane JG, et al. *Biol Psychiatry*. 1991;30:371.

[14] Dollins AB, et al. *Psychopharmacol.* 1993;112:490.

[15] James SP, et al. *Neuropsychopharmacol.* 1989;3:19.

[16] Tzichinsky O, et al. *Sleep*. 1994;17(7):638.

[17] Aldhous M, et al. *Br J Clin Pharmacol.* 1985;19:517.

[18] Nave R, et al. *Eur J Pharmacol*. 1995;275:213.

[19] Zhdanova IV, et al. *Clin Pharmacol & Ther.* 1995;57:552.

[20] Garfinkel D, et al. *Lancet*. 1995;346:541.

[21] Haimov I, et al. *Sleep*. 1995;18(7):598.

[22] Jan JE, et al. *Dev Med and Child Neurol.* 1994;36:97.

[23] Lissoni P, et al. *Oncology*. 1991;48:448.

[24] Zumoff B. *Obstet Gynecol Clin North Am.* 1994;21(4):751.

[25] Lissoni P, et al. *Oncology*. 1995;52:163.

[26] Lissoni P, et al. *Oncology*. 1995;52:360.

[27] Barni S, et al. *Oncology*. 1995;52:243.

SCIENTIFIC NAME(S): *Methylsulfonylmethane, DMSO2*

COMMON NAME(S): MSM

◖◖◖◖ PATIENT INFORMATION ◗◗◗◗

Uses: MSM is said to alleviate gastrointestinal upset, musculoskeletal pain, arthritis, and allergies; to boost the immune system; and to possess antimicrobial effects although there are no known studies in humans to document these uses.

Side effects: No important toxicities were noted in animal reports.

Dosing: MSM commonly is given first at a loading dose of 2 to 5 g/day, then as a maintenance dose of 50 to 200 mg/day for arthritis and other joint conditions.

SOURCE: MSM is a natural chemical in green plants such as *Equisetum arvense*, certain algae, fruits, vegetables, and grains. It is also found in animals (eg, the adrenal cortex of cattle, human and bovine milk, and urine). MSM is naturally occurring in fresh foods; however, it is destroyed with even moderate food processing, such as heat or dehydration.[1]

HISTORY: Literature searches on MSM provide mostly animal studies. MSM has been used as a food supplement.

PHARMACOLOGY: MSM has been said to alleviate gastrointestinal upset, musculoskeletal pain, arthritis, allergies, and to boost the immune system. It is also said to possess antimicrobial effects against such organisms as *Giardia lamblia*, *Trichomonas vaginalis*, and certain fungal infections. The suggested mechanism is that MSM may bind to surface receptor sites, preventing interface between parasite and host.

Tumor onset in colon cancer-induced rats was markedly delayed in animals receiving MSM supplementation vs controls, suggesting a chemopreventative effect.[3] Four percent MSM had a similar delaying effect on rat mammary breast cancer.[4]

MSM showed no effect in preventing diabetes when tested in spontaneously diabetic mice compared with DMSO or dimethylsulfide (DMS).[5]

A 10-day course of MSM also has been evaluated in 13 horses with COPD, and no changes occurred in parameters such as lung sounds, respiratory rate, heart rate, temperature, nasal discharge, or arterial blood gas.[6]

TOXICOLOGY: No important toxicities were noted in animal reports.[3,4]

[1] Richmond V. *Life Sci.* 1986;39(3):263-268.

[2] Bertken R. *Arthritis Rheum.* 1983;26(5):693-694.

[3] O'Dwyer P, et al. *Cancer.* 1988;62(5):944-948.

[4] McCabe D, et al. *Archives of Surgery.* 1986;121(12):1455-1459.

[5] Klandorf H, et al. *Diabetes.* 1989;38(2):194-197.

[6] Traub-Dargatz J, et al. *Am J Vet Res.* 1992;53(10):1908-1916.

Milk Thistle

SCIENTIFIC NAME(S): *Silybum marianum* (L.) Gaertn. Family: Compositae referred to in older texts as *Carduus marianus*. Recently changed to *Carduus marianum*.

COMMON NAME(S): Holy thistle, lady's thistle, marian thistle, Mary thistle, Milk thistle, St. Mary thistle, silybum

---

❧❧❧ PATIENT INFORMATION ❧❧❧

Uses: Treatment or protection against liver damage, as in cirrhosis, Amanita mushroom poisoning, and hepatitis.

Side Effects: Few adverse effects have been seen other than brief gastrointestinal (GI) disturbances and mild allergic reactions; possible urticaria in one patient.

Dosing: Crude milk thistle seed has been administered at 12 to 15 g/day in clinical trials for hepatitis and other liver conditions. Milk thistle also is widely available in several extracts, standardized to 70% to 80% silymarin. These include IdB1016 (*Silipide*, Indena), which is a silybin phosphatidylcholine complex, *Legalon* (Madaus), and *Silimarol*. Doses of these extracts range from 200 to 800 mg/day.[1-3]

BOTANY: This plant is indigenous to Kashmir, but is found in North America from Canada to Mexico. Milk thistle grows from approximately 1.5 to 3 m and has large prickly leaves. When broken, the leaves and stems exude a milky sap. The reddish purple flowers are ridged with sharp spines. The drug consists of the shiny mottled black or grey-toned seeds (fruit). These make up the "thistle" portion, along with its silvery pappus, which readily falls off.[4]

HISTORY: Milk thistle was once grown in Europe as a vegetable. The despined leaves were used in salads; the stalks and root parts were also consumed, even the flower portion was eaten "artichoke-style." The roasted seeds were used as a coffee substitute. Various preparations of milk thistle have been used medicinally for more than 2000 years. Its use as a liver protectant can be traced back to Greek references. Pliny the Elder, a first century Roman writer, (A.D. 23 to 79) noted that the plant's juice was excellent for "carrying off bile."[5] Culpeper (England's premier herbalist) noted milk thistle to be of use in removing obstructions of liver and spleen, and to be good against jaundice. The Eclectics (19th to 20th century) used milk thistle for varicose veins, menstrual difficulty, and congestion in liver, spleen, and kidneys.[6]

In homeopathy, a tincture of the seeds has been used to treat liver disorders, jaundice, gall stones, peritonitis, hemorrhage, bronchitis, and varicose veins.[7]

PHARMACOLOGY: Milk thistle's primary use is as a hepatoprotectant and antioxidant. The properties of silymarin (the extract from milk thistle seeds) are due mainly to its flavonolignan content.[8] Medicinal value may also be attributed in part to the presence of trace metals in the plant.[9]

Hepatoprotection: Silymarin protects liver cells against many hepatotoxins in humans and animals. Some Amanitas (eg, *A. phalloides*, the death cup fungus) contain two toxins: Phalloidin, which destroys the hepatocyte cell membrane; and alpha-amanatin, which reaches the cell nucleus and inhibits polymerase-b activity, thereby blocking protein synthesis. Silymarin is capable of negating both of these effects by blocking the toxin's binding sites, increasing the regenerative capacity of liver cells, and blocking enterohepatic circulation of the toxin.[6] In one study, 60 patients with severe Amanita poisoning were treated with infusions of 20 mg/kg of silybin (one of sylimarin's 3 flavono-lignans) with good results. Although the death rate following this type of mushroom poisoning can exceed 50%, none of the patients treated in this series died.[10] In a clinical trial of 205 patients with Amanita toxicity, 46 patients died; however, all 16 patients who received silybin survived.[11] Administration of silybin within 48 hours of ingestion at a dose of 20 to 50 mg/kg/day was an effective prophylactic measure against severe liver damage.[12] A multicenter trial performed in European hospitals between 1979 and 1982 was conducted using silybin in supportive treatment of 220 Amanita poisoning cases. A 12.8% mortality rate was reported.[13] The death rate using other modern supportive measures such as activated charcoal can be 40%.[36] Silymarin alone or in combination with penicillin reduced death rates from ingestion of death cup fungus to 10%.[14]

In addition to mushroom toxin protection, silymarin also offers liver protection against tetracycline-induced lesions in rats,[15] d-galactosamine-induced toxicity,[16] thallium-induced liver damage,[17] and erythromycin estolate, amitriptyline, nortriptyline, and tert-butylhydroperoxide hepatotoxin exposure of neonatal hepatocyte cell cultures.[18] In a later Italian double-blind, placebo-controlled report, silymarin was elevated in 60 women on long-term phenothiazine or butyrophenone therapy. Results suggested that silymarin treatment can reduce lipoperoxidative hepatic damage caused by chronic use of these psychotropic drugs.[1]

Cirrhosis: Use of milk thistle is inadvisable in decompensated cirrhosis.[19]

In two 1-month, double-blind studies performed on an average of 50 patients with alcoholic cirrhosis treated with silymarin, elevated liver enzyme levels (AST, ALT) and serum bilirubin levels were normalized. It also reduced high levels of gamma-glutamyl transferase, increased lectin-induced lymphoblast transformation and produced other changes not seen in the placebo group.[20-22] A 41-month double-blind study performed in 170 patients with alcoholic cirrhosis indicated silymarin to be effective in treatment as well.[23] Silymarin ameliorated indices of cytolysis in a study also using ursodeoxycholic acid in active cirrhosis patients.[24] However, in a controlled trial of study of 72 patients using 280 mg/day of silymarin, no change in in evolution or mortality of alcoholic liver disease as compared with placebo was found.[25]

Hepatitis: In patients with acute viral hepatitis, silymarin shortened treatment time and showed improvement in serum levels of bilirubin, AST, and ALT.[26,27] Biochemical values returned to normal sooner in silymarin-treated patients.[28] Histological improvement was seen in patients with chronic hepatitis vs placebo in another controlled trial.[29]

In a 116-patient double-blind study of silymarin vs placebo, silymarin 420 mg/day given to histologically proven alcoholic hepatitis patients was shown not to be clinically useful in treating this disease.[30] A later report suggests stable remission in a 6- to 12-month Russian study evaluating treatment of chronic persistent hepatitis.[19] In 20 chronic active hepatitis patients given 240 mg silybin twice daily vs placebo, improved liver function tests related to hepatocellular necrosis were reported.[2]

Blood and immunomodulation: Silymarin's immunomodulatory activity in liver disease patients may also be involved in its hepatoprotective action.[31]

Silybin can increase activity of super-oxide dismutase and glutathione peroxidase, which may also explain its protective effects against free radicals.[32] Silymarin had an anti-inflammatory effect on human blood platelets.[33] Silybin may have antiallergic activity. Its effect on histamine release from human basophils was reversed and may be due to membrane-stabilizing activity.[34] Silybin inhibition of human T-lymphocyte activation is also reported.[35]

Lipid and biliary effects: Administration of silymarin 420 mg/day for 3 months to 14 type II hyperlipidemic patients resulted in slightly decreased total cholesterol and HDL-cholesterol levels.[36] Silybin-induced reduction of biliary cholesterol may be due in part to decreased liver cholesterol synthesis.[37]

Biliary excretion of silybin was evaluated by high performance liquid chromatography (HPLC). Bioavailability of silybin is greater after silipide (a lipophilic silybin-phosphatidylcholine complex) administration than after silymarin administration; therefore, increased delivery of silipide to the liver results.[38] Use of silymarin prevents disturbance of bile secretion, thereby increasing bile secretion, cholate excretion, and bilirubin excretion.[19]

Various other effects: Silybin and silymarin have also been evaluated (including case reports) in diabetes patients for possible value in prophylaxis of diabetic complications[39] and in combination therapy to treat aged skin.[40] Traditional uses of milk thistle include stimulation of milk production in nursing mothers and antidepressant therapy.[8] Other uses include steroid secretory modulation[41] and as therapy of acute promyelocytic leukemia.[42]

Extracts, tablets, or capsules (35 to 70 mg) standardized to 70% silymarin are available as commercial preparations in average daily doses of 200 to 400 mg.[43]

TOXICOLOGY: Human studies of silymarin have shown few adverse effects.[8] Tolerability of silymarin is good; only brief disturbances of GI function and mild allergic reactions have been observed, but rarely enough to discontinue treatment.[19] Mild laxative effects in isolated cases have been reported.[44] A case of urticaria with a foreign commercial milk thistle preparation has been noted.[45]

[1] Palasciano G, et al. *Curr Ther Res.* 1994;55(5):537-45.

[2] Buzzelli G, et al. *Int J Clin Pharmacol Ther Toxicol.* 1993;31(9):456-60.

[3] Mulrow C, et al. Milk thistle: effects on liver disease and cirrhosis and clinical adverse effects. 2000; Agency for Healthcare Research and Quality, Pub. No. 01-E0251.

[4] Bisset N. *Herbal Drugs and Phytopharmaceuticals.* London, England: CRC Press, 1994;121-23.

[5] Foster S. *Botanical Series No. 305.* Austin, TX: American Botanical Council, 1991;3-7.

[6] Hobbs C. *Milk Thistle: The Liver Herb,* 2nd ed., Capitola, CA: Botanica Press, 1992;1-32.

[7] Schauenberg P, et al. *Guide to Medicinal Plants.* New Canaan, CT: Keats Publishing, 1974.

[8] Awang D. *Can Pharm J.* 1993 Oct:403-4.

[9] Parmar V, et al. *Int J Pharmacognosy.* 1993;31(4):324-26.

[10] Vogel G, Proceeding of the International Bioflavonoid Symposium, Munich 1981.

[11] Floersheim GL, et al. *Schweiz med Wochenschr.* 1982;112:1164.

[12] Hruby, et al. *Hum Toxicol.* 1983;2:183.

[13] Hruby K. *Forum.* 1984;6:23-26.

[14] Hruby K. *Intensivmed.* 1987;24:269-74.

[15] Skakun N, et al. *Antibiot Meditsin Biotekh.* 1986;31(10):781-84.

[16] Tyutyulkova N, et al. *Methods Find Exp Clin Pharmacol.* 1981;3:71.

[17] Mourelle M, et al. *J Appl Toxicol.* 1988;8(5):351-54.

[18] Davila J, et al *Toxicology.* 1989;57(3):267-86.

[19] Rumyantseva Z. *Vrach Delo.* 1991;(5):15-19.

[20] Lang I, et al. *Acta Med Hung*. 1988;45(3-4):287-95.

[21] Lang I, et al. *Tokai J Exp Clin Med*. 1990;15(2-3):123–27.

[22] Lang I, et al. *Ital J Gastroenterol*. 1990;22(5):283-87.

[23] Ferneci P, et al. *J Hepatol*. 1989;9(1):105-13.

[24] Lirussi F, et al. *Acta Physiol Hung*. 1992;80(1-4):363-67.

[25] Bunout D, et al. *Rev Med Chil*. 1992;120(12):1370-75.

[26] Magliulo E, et al. *Med Klin*. 1978;73:1060-65.

[27] Cavalieri S. *Gazz Med Ital*. 1974;133:628.

[28] Wilhelm H, et al. *Wien Med Wochenschr*. 1973;123:302.

[29] Kriesewetter E, et al. *Leber Magen Darm*. 1977;7:318-23.

[30] Trinchet J, et al. *Gastroenterol Clin Biol*. 1989;13(2):120-4.

[31] Deak G, et al. *Orv Hetil*. 1990;131(24):1291-92, 1295-96.

[32] Altorjay I, et al. *Acta Physiol Hung*. 1992;80(1-4):375-80.

[33] Max B. *Trends Pharmacol Sci*. 1986 Nov;7:435-37.

[34] Miadonna A, et al. *Br J Clin Pharmacol*. 1987;24(6):747-52.

[35] Meroni P, et al. *Int J Tissue React*. 1988;10(3):177-81.

[36] Somogyi A, et al. *Acta Med Hung*. 1989;46(4):289-95.

[37] Nassuato G, et al. *J Hepatol*. 1991;12(3):290-95.

[38] Schandalik R, et al. *Arzneimittel-Forschung*. 1992;42(7):964-68.

[39] Zhang J, et al. *Chung-Kuo Chung Hsi I Chieh Ho Tsa Chih*. 1993;13(12):725-26, 708.

[40] Esteve M, et al. *Parfuemerie und Kosmetik*. 1991 Dec;72:920, 822, 824, 826, 828-29.

[41] Racz K, et al. *J Endocrinol*. 1990;124(2):341-45.

[42] Invernizzi R, et al. *Haematologica*. 1993;78(5):340-41.

[43] Leung A, et al. *Encyclopedia of Common Natural Ingredients Used in Food, Drugs and Cosmetics*. New York, NY: John Wiley and Sons, Inc., 1996;366-68.

[44] Brown D. *Drug Store News for the Pharmacist*. 1994 Nov;4:58, 60.

[45] Mironets V, et al. *Vrach Delo*. 1990;(7):86-87.

Mistletoe

SCIENTIFIC NAME(S): *Viscum album* L. (European mistletoe) and *Phoradendron flavescens* (Pursh.) Nuttal, *P. serotinum* (Raf.) M.C. Johnston or *P. tomentosum* (DC) Engler (American mistletoes), Family Loranthaceae/Viscaceae

COMMON NAME(S): Mistletoe, bird lime, all heal, devil's fuge, golden bough, mistel (German)

❧❧❧ PATIENT INFORMATION ❧❧❧

Uses: Mistletoe has been used to treat cancer and in folk medicine for its cardiovascular properties. Clinical efficacy has not been established.

Side Effects: Mistletoe is a toxic plant, and side effects have been reported in clinical use. The use of preparations standardized to small doses of ML1 or depleted of lectins may reduce toxicity.

Dosing: Crude mistletoe fruit or herb is used to make a tea for hypertension at a dose of 10 g/day. There are a number of extracts of mistletoe used as adjuvant cancer therapies, including *Iscador*, a fermented product with different properties than unfermented mistletoe extracts, specifically, its low levels of mistletoe lectin-I. These extracts usually are given by IV or SC injection at doses of 0.1 to 30 mg several times/week.[1-4]

BOTANY: Mistletoe is a hemiparasitic plant that grows on a wide variety of host trees such as pine, oak, birch, and apple. The term hemiparasitic is used to indicate that the mistletoe plant carries out photosynthesis independently but obtains its water and minerals from the host. European mistletoe is dioecious, with male and female flowers on separate plants, which are pollinated by insects and bear small white berries on evergreen foliage. There are several subspecies and varieties of European mistletoe, which are defined by the host that they parasitize.[5]

HISTORY: Mistletoe preparations have been used medicinally in Europe for centuries for such varied indications as epilepsy, infertility, hypertension, and arthritis. The Celtic priests, known as Druids, revered the oak tree and the mistletoe that grew upon it, according to Pliny the Elder. At the winter celebration of Samhain, the sacred oaks were bare except for the green boughs of mistletoe, and this was taken as a sign of eternal fertility. The Celts placed a sprig of mistletoe above the door of their houses, and its sacred nature prohibited fighting beneath it. This evolved over centuries into the custom of kissing underneath mistletoe at Christmas.[6] In 1921, the anthroposophical spiritual leader Rudolf Steiner suggested that mistletoe might be used to treat cancer. Swiss and German clinics were founded to implement this idea and are still actively using a mistletoe preparation fermented with a strain of *Lactobacillus plantarum* for 3 days.[7]

PHARMACOLOGY:

Cardiovascular: A primary use of mistletoe in European folk medicine is for its cardiovascular properties. The viscotoxins have produced reflex bradycardia and possessed negative inotropic effects on the isolated cardiac muscle of cats. In higher doses, vasoconstriction also was observed.[8] Phoratoxin was less potent in the same model. In rabbit heart preparations, viscotoxins at 1 to 10 mg/mL reduced the isometric twitch and produced contracture and progressive depolarization of the muscle. These changes were reversed by addition of calcium to the tissue bath, suggesting that displacement of membrane-bound calcium might play a role in the cardiovascular mechanism.[9] Further studies with phoratoxin in frog skeletal muscle fibers attributed its activity to detergency; however, this may not be the primary cardiovascular mechanism.[10] Other investigators have proposed that phenylpropanoids might play a role in mistletoe's cardiovascular effects through a postulated inhibition of cAMP phosphodiesterase; however, it is unlikely that they are as pharmacologically important as the viscotoxins.[11,12]

Cancer: Despite the nonscientific, relatively recent origin of the use of mistletoe in cancer treatment, extensive scientific literature exists on the topic. Viscumin was initially isolated from mistletoe based on its cytotoxicity to mouse 3T3 cells and its lethality to mice.[13] Viscumin is a potent inhibitor of protein synthesis in cell-free and cellular systems.[14] The cytotoxic effect of mistletoe lectins was substantially reduced for cells grown in the presence of fetal calf serum, presumably caused by glycoproteins in serum that bind the lectin.[15] The viscotoxins also are cytotoxic to cultured cells, although generally less potently than the lectins.[16] It is likely that the galactose- or oligosaccharide-specific binding of the lectins targets only cells bearing the appropriate carbohydrates on the cell surface. The mechanism that renders cells (such as the Yoshida cell line) sensitive to the viscotoxins remains unknown.[17] Fermented mistletoe extracts such as *Iscador* have been found to be cytotoxic to tumor cells[7,18] despite the observations that ML1 content is greatly reduced.[19,20]

Mechanistic investigations of mistletoe lectins and viscotoxins have shown induction of apoptosis in lymphocytes most effectively by ML3, but also by ML2 and ML1, while the viscotoxins and carbohydrates had no apoptotic effects.[21] ML1 was further found to induce apoptosis in leukemic T- and B-cell lines through caspase-8 independently of death receptor signaling.[22] The galNAc-specific ML3 and ML2, on the other hand, appeared to operate through the death receptor.[23] ML2 was found to activate the c-Jun N-terminal kinase 1 in apoptotic death of U937 cells.[24] It remains to be seen whether induction of apoptosis is a primary event or a secondary result of ribosomal protein synthesis inhibition.

Several human clinical studies have attempted to measure changes in immunological status of cancer patients administered mistletoe preparations. Breast cancer patients given a single IV infusion of *Iscador* demonstrated a pronounced febrile reaction and increased natural killer cell activity and granulocyte phagocytosis. The presence of endotoxin in the preparation was ruled out as a cause of the response.[1,25] In the treatment of pleura carcinosis, intrapleural injection of *Iscador* had cytotoxic and immunostimulant activities.[26] The administration of lectin-depleted mistletoe extracts to breast cancer patients was compared with undepleted extracts, with the depleted extracts producing reduced immunological changes, thereby implicating the lectins in such effects.[2] Changes in cytokine levels (TNF-alpha, IL-1, and IL-6) after mistletoe extract injection were detected in 8 cancer patients in a further study by the same investigators.[27] Similar experiments measuring changes in DNA repair in lymphocytes of breast cancer patients found improved DNA repair after *Iscador*.[3] The difficulties of applying the observed changes in immunological status to practical cancer therapy have been reviewed.[28]

A retrospective study of 292 pancreatic cancer patients treated with *Iscador* showed a modest increase in survival time when compared with survival as reported in the literature; however, the absence of matched controls makes this result statistically weak.[4] A randomized clinical trial examined *Eurixor*, a preparation that is standardized for ML1 content, in head and neck cancer patients after treatment with surgery or radiotherapy. No treatment effect was detected for the mistletoe arm of the study, indicating that adjuvant use of mistletoe in this form was not effective.[29] A study on the use of mistletoe extract in melanoma was negative, although full details have not been published.[30] Earlier clinical studies of mistletoe have been reviewed, and it was determined that all of these studies

were weak and inconclusive.[31] Further studies are required to assess the appropriate use, if any, of mistletoe preparations in cancer therapy.[32]

TOXICOLOGY: Mistletoe has a reputation as a toxic plant, and its content of toxic lectins lends support to this opinion.[33] Nevertheless, poison center data from the US indicates that symptomatic poisoning by American mistletoe is infrequent.[34] Side effects from clinical use of mistletoe have been reported[32] although the use of preparations standardized to small doses of ML1 (1 ng/injection) or depleted of lectins by fermentation[19] may reduce toxicity.

1 Hajto T, Lanzrein C. *Oncology.* 1986;43:93-97.
2 Hajto T, Hostanska K, Gabius HJ. *Cancer Res.* 1989;49:4803-4808.
3 Kovacs E, Hajto T, Hostanska K. *Eur J Cancer.* 1991;27:1672-1676.
4 Schaefermeyer G, Schaefermeyer H. *Complement Ther Med.* 1998;6:172-177.
5 Becker H. *Oncology.* 1986;43(suppl 1):2-7.
6 Bryant VM, Grider S. *The World & I* 1991:613.
7 Ribereau-Gayon G, Jung ML, Di Scala D, Beck J. *Oncology.* 1986;43(suppl 1):35-41.
8 Rosell S, Samuelsson G. *Toxicon.* 1966;4:107-110.
9 Andersson KE, Johannsson M. *Eur J Pharmacol.* 1973;23:223-231.
10 Sauviat MP. *Toxicon.* 1990;28:83-89.
11 Wagner H, Feil B, Seligmann O, Petricic J, Kalogjera Z. *Planta Med.* 1986;2:102-104.
12 Deliorman D, Calis I, Ergun F, Dogan BSU, Buharahoglu CK, Kanzik I. *J Ethnopharmacol.* 2000;72:323-329.
13 Olsnes S, Stirpe F, Sandvig K, Pihl A. *J Biol Chem.* 1982;257:13263-13270.
14 Stirpe F, Legg RF, Onyon LJ, Ziska P, Franz H. *Biochem J.* 1980;190:843-845.
15 Ribéreau-Gayon G, Jung M, Beck J, Anton R. *Phytother Res.* 1995;9:336-339.
16 Urech K, Schaller G, Ziska P, Giannattasio M. *Phytother Res.* 1995;9:49-55.
17 Schaller G, Urech K, Giannattasio M. *Phytother Res.* 1996;10:473-477.
18 Ribéreau-Gayon G, Jung ML, Baudino S, Sallé G, Beck JP. *Experientia.* 1986;42:594-599.
19 Wagner H, Jordan E, Feil B. *Oncology.* 1986;43(suppl 1):16-22.
20 Jung ML, Baudino S, Ribéreau-Gayon G, Beck JP. *Cancer Lett.* 1990;51:103-108.
21 Büssing A, Suzart K, Bergmann J, Pfüller U, Schietzel M, Schweizer K. *Cancer Lett.* 1996;99:59-72.
22 Bantel H, Engels IH, Voelter W, Schulze-Osthoff K, Wesselborg S. *Cancer Res.* 1999;59:2083-2090.
23 Büssing A, Multani AS, Pathak S, Pfüller U, Schietzel M. *Cancer Lett.* 1998;130:57-68.
24 Park R, Kim MS, So HS, Jung BH, Moon SR, Chung SY, et al. *Biochem Pharmacol.* 2000;60:1685-1691.
25 Hajto T. *Oncology* 1986;43(suppl 1):51-65.
26 Salzer G. *Oncology* 1986;43 (suppl 1):66-70.
27 Hajto T, Hostanska K, Frei K, Rordorf C, Gabius HJ. *Cancer Res.* 1990;50:3322-3326.
28 Gabius HJ, Gabius S, Joshi SS, et al. *Planta Med.* 1994;60:2-7.
29 Steuer-Vogt MK, Bonkowsky V, Ambrosch P, Scholz M, Neiss A, Strutz J. *Eur J Cancer.* 2001;37:23-31.
30 McNamee D. *Lancet.* 1999;354:1101.
31 Kleijnen J, Knipschild P. *Phytomedicine.* 1994;1:255-260.
32 Ernst E. *Eur J Cancer.* 2001;37:9-11.
33 Stirpe F. *Lancet.* 1983;1:295.
34 Spiller HA, Willias DB, Gorman SE, Sanftleban J. *J Toxicol Clin Toxicol.* 1996;34:405-408.

SCIENTIFIC NAME(S): *Ptychopetalum olacoides* Benth. Olacaceae (Olax family). Less commonly *P. uncinatum* Anselm. and *Liriosma ovata* Miers

COMMON NAME(S): Muira puama, marapuama, potency wood, raiz del macho, potenzholz

❧❧❧❧ PATIENT INFORMATION ❧❧❧❧

Uses: *P. olacoides* is used as a tonic for neuromuscular problems. A root decoction is used externally in massages and baths for paralysis and beriberi. Tea made from the roots has been used for sexual impotence, rheumatism, and gastrointestinal problems. Muira puama is currently promoted as a male aphrodisiac or as a treatment for impotence.

Side Effects: Muira puama does not appear to have the serious side effect potential of yohimbine.

Dosing: Muira puama leaves, stem, and roots typically are used at a dose of 0.5 to 1.5 g/day, although there are no clinical studies supporting this dose.[1]

BOTANY: *P. olacoides* is a small tree native to the Brazilian Amazon where the stems and roots are used as a tonic for neuromuscular problems. A root decoction is used externally in massages and baths for paralysis and beriberi. Tea made from the roots has been used for sexual impotence, rheumatism, and gastrointestinal problems.[2]

HISTORY: Muira puama is currently promoted as a male aphrodisiac or as a treatment for impotence. However, there are few clinical studies to support these uses. This use can be traced back to the 1930s in Europe but has increased with the success of sildenafil (*Viagra*) and the concurrent promotion of "herbal *Viagra*" preparations. It is also a constituent of a popular Brazilian herbal tonic "catuama" consisting of guarana, ginger, *Trichilia catigua*, and *P. ola-*

coides. Muira puama was official in the Brazilian Pharmacopeia of 1956.

PHARMACOLOGY: Japanese patents have been issued that claim muira puama preparations are useful against stress-induced gastric ulceration[3] and stress-induced blood calcium elevation.[4]

Clinical studies to support the use of muira puama are sparse. Several promotional Web sites cite the work of a French clinician, Jacques Waynberg,[5] to support their claims; however, peer-reviewed publications are currently lacking. Muira puama has been contrasted favorably with yohimbine.[6] A German language review was published many years ago.[7]

TOXICOLOGY: Muira puama does not appear to contain yohimbine, nor to have the serious side effect potential of yohimbine.

[1] Gruenwald J, ed. *PDR for Herbal Medicines*, 2nd ed. Montvale, NJ: Thomson Medical Economics; 2000: 531-532.

[2] Schultes R, et al. *The Healing Forest: Medicinal and Toxic Plants of the Northwest Amazon.* Portland, OR: Dioscorides Press,1990, p. 343.

[3] Asano T, et al. *Oral compositions containing muira-puama for gastric mucosal lesions.* 1999; Japanese Patent No. 11343244.

[4] Sudo D, et al. Evaluation of tonic effects of bioactive substances based on stress-induced change in blood calcium. 2000; Japanese Patent No. 2000009717.

[5] Waynberg J. *J. Ethnopharmacol.* 1995.

[6] Murray M. *Am J Nat Med.* November 1994.

[7] Steinmetz E. Muira puama. *Quart J Crude Drug Res.* 1971;11:1787.

SCIENTIFIC NAME(S): *Urtica dioica* L. Family: Urticaceae

COMMON NAME(S): Stinging nettle, nettle

❧❧❧ PATIENT INFORMATION ❧❧❧

Uses: Proven as a diuretic, nettles are being investigated as treatment for hay fever and irrigation of the urinary tract.

Side Effects: External side effects result from skin contact and take the form of burning and stinging that persist for 12 hours or more. Internal side effects are rare and allergic in nature.

Dosing: The herb is used as a diuretic at doses of 8 to 12 g/day. In contrast, the root is used for urinary conditions such as benign prostate hypertrophy at 4 to 6 g/day.[1]

BOTANY: Nettles are perennial plants native to Europe and found throughout the US and parts of Canada. This plant has an erect stalk and stands up to 0.9 m. It has dark green serrated leaves that grow opposite each other along the stalk. The plant flowers from June to September. The leaves contain bristles that transmit irritating principles upon contact. The fruit of nettles is a small, oval, yellow-brown seed approximately 1 mm wide.[2]

HISTORY: This plant is known for its stinging properties. However, it has been used in traditional medicine as a diuretic, antispasmodic, expectorant, and treatment for asthma. The juice has been purported to stimulate hair growth when applied to the scalp. Extracts of the leaves have been used topically for the treatment of rheumatic disorders. The tender tips of young nettles have been used as a cooked pot herb in salads.

PHARMACOLOGY: Nettles mainly have diuretic actions. Treatment over 14 days increases urine volume and decreases systolic blood pressure.[2] Nettles claims against diabetes, cancer, eczema, rheumatism, hair loss, and aging have been reported[3,4] but are unsubstantiated. Other folk medicine applications include wound healing, treatment of scalp seborrhea and greasy hair, and gastric juice secretion.[2] A combination product includes nettles to treat hyposecretory gastritis.[5]

Nettles, in a combination product containing several other herbs, has been tested in 22 patients for bladder irrigation. Postoperative blood loss, bacteriuria, and inflammation were reduced following prostatic adenomectomy.[6] The German Commission E Monograph supports this indication by its similar listing for "irrigation in inflammation of the urinary tract and in the prevention and treatment of kidney gravel."[2] Nettles use in expelling bile has been studied.[7]

Nettles in a combined extract with pygeum (*Pygeum africanum*) was studied as a treatment of benign prostatic hyperplasia (BPH) in 134 patients. It was effective in reducing urine flow, nocturia, and residual urine. A 300 mg dose of the plant extract was as effective as 150 mg.[8] A possible mechanism may be a hydrophobic constituent (eg, steroidal), which inhibits the sodium-potassium ATP-ase activity of the prostate, leading to suppressed cell growth in this area.[9] Another report postulates a different mechanism but suggests the aqueous extract is the active component in BPH therapy to inhibit the sex hormone-binding globulin to its receptor.[10]

Freeze-dried nettles have been evaluated for allergic rhinitis. In a double-blind trial, 57% of 69 hay fever sufferers who completed the trial judged the nettles preparations to be moderately to highly effective in treatment vs placebo.[11]

When evaluated for its antidiabetic effect, nettles slightly increased glycemia, aggravating the condition in 2 reports.[12,13]

TOXICOLOGY: Nettles are known primarily for their ability to induce topical irritation following contact with exposed skin, accompanied by a stinging sensation lasting 12 hours or more. A report closely associates mast cells and dermal dendritic cells. Immediate reaction to nettles' sting is caused by histamine content, while the persistence of the sting may be caused by other substances directly toxic to nerves.[14]

The stinging hairs of the nettle plant comprise a fine capillary tube, a bladder-like base filled with the chemical irritant, and a minute spherical tip, which breaks off on contact, leaving a sharp point that penetrates the skin. The irritants are forced into the skin as the hair bends and constricts the bladder at the base.

Topical irritation is treated by gently washing the affected area with mild soapy water. Treatment with systemic antihistamines and topical steroids may be of benefit. Other side effects of nettles are rare but include allergic effects such as edema, oliguria, and gastric irritation.[2]

[1] Gruenwald J, ed. *PDR for Herbal Medicines*, 2nd ed. Montvale, NJ: Thomson Medical Economics; 2000: 729-733.

[2] Bisset N. *Herbal Drugs and Phytopharmaceuticals*, Stuttgart, Germany: CRC Press. 1994;502-7.

[3] Atasu E, et al. *Farmasotik Bilimler Dergisi*. 1984;9(2):73-81.

[4] Wichtl M. *Deutsche Apotheker Zeitung*. 1992 Jul 23;132:1569-1576.

[5] Krivenko V, et al. *Vrachebnoe Delo*. 1989;(3):76-78.

[6] Davidov M, et al. *Urologiia I Nefrologiia*. 1995;(5):19-20.

[7] Rossiiskaya G, et al. *Farmatsiia*. 1985;34(1):38-41.

[8] Krzeski T, et al. *Clin Ther*. 1993;15(6):1011-1020.

[9] Hirano T, et al. *Planta Med*. 1994;60(1):30-33.

[10] Hryb D, et al. *Planta Med*. 1995;61(1):31-32.

[11] Mittman P. *Planta Med*. 1990;56(1):44-47.

[12] Swanston-Flatt S, et al. *Diabetes Res*. 1989;10(2):69-73.

[13] Roman R, et al. *Arch Med Res*. 1992;23(1):59-64.

[14] Oliver F, et al. *Clin Exp Dermatol*. 1991;16(1):1-7.

SCIENTIFIC NAME(S): *Nigella sativa* L. Family: Ranunculaceae

COMMON NAME(S): Black seed, black cumin, charnushka, "black caraway" (not true caraway), baraka (the blessed seed), fitch (Biblical), "love in the mist"

ɪɐɪɐ PATIENT INFORMATION ɪɐɪɐ

Uses: *Nigella sativa* has been used for gastrointestinal disorders and respiratory problems. Studies have been performed researching its immune/protective or anticancer effects, anti-inflammatory actions, and antimicrobial and anthelmintic properties. More human studies are needed.

Side Effects: Contact allergic dermatitis can occur with topical use of the oil. Do not use *Nigella sativa* during pregnancy.

BOTANY: *Nigella sativa* (NS) is an annual herb with terminal, grayish-blue flowers reaching between 30 to 60 cm in height. The toothed seed pod contains the distinctive tiny (1 to 2 mm long), black, 3-sided seeds, that are the plant parts used for medicinal purposes.[1,2,3]

HISTORY: NS is said to have been used for 2000 years, with some recordings of traditional uses of the seed dating back 1400 years. Its use began in the Middle East and spread throughout Europe and Africa. NS was found in the tomb of King Tutankhamen. Ancient Egyptians believed that medicinal plants such as these played a role in the afterlife. In the 1st century AD, Greek physician Dioscorides documented that the seeds were taken for a variety of problems including headache, toothache, nasal congestion, and intestinal worms.[1,3]

PHARMACOLOGY: NS has been used to benefit the GI system, as it eases gas and colic.[1] It has been used for diarrhea (dysentery) and constipation (hemorrhoids).[2]

At least 2 references claim that the respiratory effects of NS make it beneficial for allergies, cough, bronchitis, emphysema, asthma, flu, and chest congestion.[2,3] Constituent nigellone, in low concentrations, inhibits the release of histamine from mast cells.[4] Another report discusses volatile oil of NS (with the thymoquinone component removed) to provide a centrally acting respiratory stimulant when tested in guinea pigs.[5]

There are many studies available discussing immune/protective or anticancer effects of certain preparations of NS. NS also enhances production of certain human interleukins and alters macrophages, suggesting changes in immune response in vitro.[6] Constituents thymoquinone and dithymoquinone have demonstrated cytotoxic actions in human cell lines, as well.[7]

Traditional use (ground seeds in poultice form) for inflammatory ailments such as rheumatism, headache, and certain skin conditions is proven by modern studies. A fixed oil preparation of NS demonstrated anti-eicosanoid and antioxidant activity, again supporting the seeds' use for anti-inflammatory actions.[8]

A mixture containing NS displayed hepatic gluconeogenesis in rats related to antidiabetic actions. This may be beneficial in non-insulin dependent diabetes mellitus patients.[9] However, NS was not proven to increase glucose tolerance as the other components of the investigational mixture.[10]

NS has been used as a vermifuge.[1] The essential oil of the seed has been reported as an effective antimicrobial and anthelmintic agent.[11] NS has displayed gram negative and gram positive antimicrobial actions, some of which are synergistic with other antibiotics.[12] NS traditionally has been used for conjunctivitis,[2] abscesses, parasites, and other infections.[3]

NS also plays a role in women's health, stimulating menstruation and increasing milk flow.[1,3]

NS may also possess the ability to decrease arterial blood pressure, suggesting possible use as an antihypertensive agent.[13]

NS has also been used as a flavoring or as a spice.[3]

TOXICOLOGY: One report discusses allergic contact dermatitis from topical use of the oil.[14]

[1] Chevallier A. *Encyclopedia of Medicinal Plants.*. New York, NY: DK Publishing, 1996, 237.

[2] Ghazanfar S. *Handbook of Arabian Medicinal Plants.*. Boca Raton, FL: CRC Press, 1994, 180-181.

[3] http://fisher.bio.umb.edu/pages/fatimah/fatimah.htm

[4] Chakravarty N. *Ann Allergy.* 1993;70:237-242.

[5] el Tahir K, et al. *Gen Pharmacol.* 1993;24(5):1115-1122.

[6] Haq A, et al. *Immunopharmacology.* 1995;30(2):147-155.

[7] Worthen D, et al. *Anticancer Res.* 1998;18(3A):1527-1532.

[8] Houghton P, et al. *Planta Med.* 1995;61(1):33-36.

[9] al-Awadi F, et al. *Diabetes Res.* 1991;18(4):163.

[10] al-Awadi F, et al. *Acta Diabetol Lat.* 1987;24(1):37.

[11] Agarwal R, et al. *Indian J Exp Biol.* 1979;17(11):1264-1265

[12] Hanafy M, et al. *J Ethnopharmacol.* 1991;34(2-3):275-278.

[13] el Tahir K, et al. *Gen Pharmacol.* 1993;24(5):1123-1131.

[14] Steinmann A, et al. *Contact Dermatitis.* 1997;36(5):268-269.

Olive Leaf

SCIENTIFIC NAME(S): *Olea europaea* L. Family: oleaceae.

COMMON NAME(S): Olive leaf

PATIENT INFORMATION

Uses: In traditional folk medicine, olive leaves have been used for hypertension (possibly only for mild cases) and also may have hypoglycemic, renal, and antimicrobial effects. More research and clinical trials are necessary.

Side Effects: Toxicity is not well known, but the leaf may cause gastric symptoms. Use in diabetic patients should be followed carefully because of the hypoglycemic effects of olive leaf.

Dosing: Olive leaves are used to make a tea for rheumatism, gout, and diabetes; however, there is no dosage information available on these uses.[1]

BOTANY: The olive tree is an evergreen, growing to approximately 10 m in height. Native to the Mediterranean regions, the trees also are cultivated in areas of similar climates in the Americas. The small, leatherly leaves are gray-green on top, and the underside contains fine, white, scale-like hairs. The leaves are gathered throughout the year.[2-4]

HISTORY: The olive tree was cultivated in Crete as far back as 3500 BC, where the leaves had been used to clean wounds. Symbolically, the olive branch stands for peace. The leaves were worn by athletes in ancient Olympic games.[2] Medicinal properties of the plant in the 1800s include malaria treatment. In the 1900s, the leaf constituent oleuropein was found to resist disease. The plant also has been reported to possess some hypotensive properties.[3]

PHARMACOLOGY: Documentation regarding olive leaf use as an antihypertensive is insignificant.[5] Other sources state no definite proof of the therapeutic efficacy in this area.[4,6] In contrast, Italian folk medicine employs dried olive leaf as a remedy for high blood pressure.[6] Other sources state that olive leaves do lower pressure and help to improve circulatory function, as well.[2] Another report mentions the hypotensive activity of olive leaves to be slight, but existent, and suggests their use only in mild cases of hypertension.[3]

Olive leaf is said to be mildy diuretic. It enhances renal and digestive elimination functions, along with renal excretion of water.[4] It may be used to treat cystitis, as well.[2] Oleuropein also was listed as a good antioxidant.[4] Many unsubstantiated claims and "cure-alls," except for "testimonial-type" proof, exist for olive leaf. Some of these claims include therapy for chronic fatigue syndrome, herpes and other viral infections, arthritis, yeast infection, skin conditions, and others. More research and clinical trials are necessary.

TOXICOLOGY: Potential toxicity of olive leaf is not well known.[4] *The German Commission E Monographs* list no known risks associated with the plant.[5] One source states the drug as causing gastric symptoms, and suggests that it be taken with meals because of this irritant effect.[3]

[1] Claus E, ed. *Pharmacognosy.* 3rd ed. Philadelphia, PA: Lea & Febiger; 1956.

[2] Chevallier A. *Encyclopedia of Medicinal Plants.* New York, NY: DK Publishing. 1996;239.

[3] Weiss R. *Herbal Medicine*. Beaconsfield, England: Beaconsfield Publ. Ltd. 1988;160-1.

[4] Bruneton J. *Pharmacognosy, Phytochemistry, Medicinal Plants*. Paris, France: Lavoisier Publishing. 1995;487-89.

[5] Blumenthal M, ed. *The Complete German Commission E Monographs*. Austin, TX: American Botanical Council. 1998;357.

[6] Schulz V, et al. *Rational Phytotherapy*. Verlin Heidelberg, Germany: Springer-Verlag. 1998;106.

SCIENTIFIC NAME(S): *Olea europaea* (fruit), *Oleum olivae* Family: Oleaceae

COMMON NAME(S): Olive oil, sweet oil, salad oil

❧❧❧ PATIENT INFORMATION ❧❧❧

Uses: Olive oil is used for cooking, as a salad oil, and as a vehicle for oily suspensions for injections. It is used to prepare soaps, plasters, ointments, and liniments, and is used as a demulcent and emollient. Olive oil is a mild laxative, and it lowers cholesterol.

Side effects: Olive oil has caused temporary mild diarrhea and allergic reactions from external use.

Dosing: Olive oil is used as a laxative at a typical dose of 30 mL.[1]

BOTANY: The olive is technically a fruit, ellipsoid and drupaceous in character, measuring 2 to 3 cm in length. The fruits grow from an evergreen tree, which seldom exceeds 10 or 12 m in height. The plants were first cultivated in Greece but are now widely grown in Mediterranean countries and the US. Many cultivated varieties are the result of its geographic diversity.

Olive oil is a fixed oil, expressed from ripe olive fruits. It is pale-yellow and may have a greenish tint, depending on the ratio of chlorophyll to carotene. Taste has been described as characteristic but slight or bland to faintly acrid. Olive oil is offered in several grades of purity, including "virgin" oil (initial unrefined oil from first fruit pressing) or "pure" (lower quality from subsequent pressings). Chemically, the difference between "extra virgin" and "virgin" oils involve the amount of free oleic acid (ie, virgin allows 4% free oleic acid, and extra virgin allows 1%).[2-5]

HISTORY: "Olea" comes from the Latin "oliva" meaning olive.[3] The fruit dates back to the 17th century BC and appears to be native to Palestine.[5] One source mentions that Ramses II, Egyptian ruler between 1300 and 1200 BC, used olive oil for every ailment.[6]

PHARMACOLOGY: Recent computer literature searches found more than 1800 citations on olive oil, hence the following is only a brief outline of some main points.

Olive oil is classed as a pharmaceutical acid.[3] It is used as a vehicle for oily injection suspensions.[4] Olive oil is also employed in the preparation of soaps, plasters, ointments, and liniments.[4,5] In addition, it is a good drug solvent.[4,7] Externally, olive oil is a demulcent and emollient. It is used to soften the skin in eczema and psoriasis.[4] It is useful as a lubricant for massage or for prevention of stretch marks. It also has been used as a wound dressing and for minor burns. In addition, olive oil softens ear wax and is helpful for ringing or pain in the ears. Effectiveness of certain applications is not documented.[8]

Olive oil is a nutrient, widely used as a salad oil and for cooking.[3] It is a common element in the Mediterranean diet.[9-11]

Olive oil is a mild laxative as an intestinal lubricant.[7] It is also claimed to be useful for gall bladder problems, including cholecystitis and cholelithiasis.[8]

A number of articles exist concerning olive oil's role against heart disease. Constituent oleic acid has been shown to lower blood cholesterol levels.[2] Monounsaturated fatty acids replacing saturated fatty acids in the diet decrease serum cholesterol as discussed in a review of population and clinical studies.[12] Olive oil supplementation in hypercholesterolemic patients was shown to reduce susceptibility of LDL to oxidation, which contributes to atherosclerotic processes.[13] Olive oil improves the good HDL-cholesterol ratios and combats arterial build-up of cholesterol as well. In middle-aged Americans, the oil decreased cholesterol by 13% and LDL-cholesterol by 21%. Four to 5 tablespoons/day of olive oil administered to heart surgery patients improved their blood profiles.[6] A comparative study of olive oil vs fish oil on blood lipids and atherosclerosis has been performed.[14]

A nutrition review of dietary fat and chronic disease risk finds monounsaturated oils, such as olive oil, to be a weak promoter of certain cancers (including breast and colon) as opposed to such strong promoters as n-6 polyunsaturated oils.[15] This author claims evidence for an enhancing effect of the latter strong promoters in increased breast cancers in western diets.

Other effects of olive oil include the reduction of blood pressure[6] and for antimicrobial properties including gram-negative bacteria, fungi, and enterotoxin B production by *Staphylococcus aureus*.[16,17]

TOXICOLOGY: Ingestion of excessive amounts of olive oil has resulted in temporary mild diarrhea.[6] In rare cases, topical use of olive oil has caused allergic reactions.[8]

[1] Claus E, ed. *Pharmacognosy.* 3rd ed. Philadelphia, PA: Lea & Febiger; 1956.

[2] Murray M. *The Healing Power of Foods.* Rocklin, CA: Prima Publishing. 1993;188.

[3] Robbers J, et al. *Pharmacognosy and Pharmacobiotechnology.* Baltimore, MD: Williams & Wilkins. 1996;70-71.

[4] Reynolds J, ed. *Martindale-The Extra Pharmacopoeia 31st ed..* London, England: Royal Pharmaceutical Society. 1996;1734.

[5] Evans W. *Trease and Evans' Pharmacognosy, 14th ed..* London, England: WB Saunders Co. Ltd. 1996;185-86.

[6] Carper J. *The Food Pharmacy.* New York, NY: Bantam Books. 1989;242-45.

[7] Bruneton J. *Pharmacognosy, Phytochemistry, Medicinal Plants.* Paris, France: Lavoisier. 1995;127-29.

[8] Blumenthal M, ed. *The Complete German Commission E Monographs.* Austin, TX: American Botanical Council. 1998;358.

[9] Maiani G, et al. *Eur J Cancer Prev.* 1997;(6 suppl)1:S3-9.

[10] Haber B. *Am J Clin Nutr.* 1997;66(4 suppl):1053S-1057S.

[11] Haas C. *Ann Med Interne.* 1998;149(5):275-79.

[12] Okolska G, et al. *Rocz Panstw Zakl Hig.* 1989;40(2):89-99.

[13] Aviram M. *Eur J Clin Chem Clin Biochem.* 1996;34(8):599-608.

[14] Mortensen A, et al. *Br J Nutr.* 1998;80(6):565-73.

[15] Weisburger J. *J Am Diet Assoc.* 1997;97(7 suppl):S16-23.

[16] Tranter H, et al. *J Applied Bacteriol.* 1993;74:253-59.

[17] Fleming H, et al. *Applied Microbiol.* 1973;26(5):777-82.

Onion

SCIENTIFIC NAME(S): *Allium cepa* Family: Liliaceae, Alliaceae

COMMON NAME(S): Onion

ᰠᰠᰠ PATIENT INFORMATION ᰠᰠᰠ

Uses: Onion is used as an antimicrobial, cardiovascular-supportive, hypoglycemic, antioxidant/anticancer, and asthma-protective agent, although some of these effects have not been clinically proven. In folk medicine, onion has been used for asthma, whooping cough, bronchitis, and similar ailments. Other uses include the treatment of stingray wounds, warts, acne, appetite loss, urinary tract disorders, and indigestion. Onion skin dye has been used as an egg and cloth coloring.

Side Effects: The toxicity of large doses of onion has been unresolved, but the stomach may be affected. Frequent contact with onion seeds has been reported as an occupational allergen.

Dosing: Fresh onion bulbs are used at daily doses of 50 g; dried onion is used at a dose of 20 g/day for dyspepsia.[1]

BOTANY: The onion plant is a perennial herb growing to about 1.22 m high, with 4 to 6 hollow cylindrical leaves. On top of the long stalk, greenish-white flowers are present in the form of solitary umbels growing up to 1-inch wide. The seeds of the plant are black and angular. The underground bulb, which is used medicinally, is made up of fleshy leaf sheaths forming a thin-skinned capsule. The onion is one of the leading vegetable crops in the world.[2-5]

HISTORY: Central Asia is believed to be the region of origin of the onion.[5] Onions were used as early as 5000 years ago in Egypt, as seen on ancient monuments. Ancient Greek and Roman recordings also refer to the onion. During the Middle Ages, onions were consumed throughout Europe. They were later thought to guard against evil spirits and the plague, probably because of their strong odor. Onion "skin" dye has been used for egg and cloth coloring for many years in the Middle East and Europe. Columbus was said to have brought the onion to America. Folk healers used the onion to prevent infection. The combination of onions and garlic cooked in milk is a European folk remedy used to clear congestion. Onions are also used in homeopathic medicine.[2,3,6,7]

PHARMACOLOGY: The main properties of onion include antimicrobial activity, cardiovascular support, hypoglycemic action, antioxidant/anticancer effect, and asthma protection.

Antimicrobial effects: Onion has had antibacterial,[4] antiparasitic,[8] and antifungal actions.[9,10] *Salmonella typhimurium* mutagenicity was reduced in hamburger when onions were added.[11] Growth of oral pathogenic bacteria, including *Streptococcus mutans*, *S. subrinus*, *Porphyromonas gingivalis*, and *Prevotella intermedia*, the main causes of dental caries and periodontitis, was prevented by onion extracts.[12] Either onion juice or onion oil also has been shown to inhibit growth of other gram-positive and gram-negative bacteria *Klebsiella pneumoniae*.[9,10,13] Antifungal actions of onion include certain yeasts,[9] *Microsporum canis*, *M. gypseum*, *Trichophyton simii*, *Chrysosporium queenslandicum*, *T. mentagrophytes*, *Aspergillus flavus*, and *Penicillium rubrum*.[10] One source identifies thiosulfinate principle in the onion as one of the main antimicrobial agents.[4]

Cardiovascular disease: Onion may benefit cardiovascular disease. One report evaluates hemostatic effects of onion in humans,[14] but certain lipid-reducing and blood pressure-lowering effects in humans have not yet been clinically proven.[5] Cardiovascular disease risk factors also involve blood coagulability. Several reports confirm the onion's inhibitory effects on platelet formation. Boiling onion may cause decomposition of the antithrombotic ingredient.[15] Certain onion genotypes containing higher contents of sulfur in the bulb correlated with greater antiplatelet activity.[16] Thiosulfinates dimethyl- and diphenylthiosulfinate, for example, are known to retard thrombocyte biosynthesis.[5,17] The least polar fraction of onion extract was associated with the most inhibitory activity toward platelet aggregation, thus a greater inhibition of thromboxane synthesis was reported.[18] Synthesis of thromboxanes and prostaglandins in vitro has been shown with onions, as well as with garlic and other liliaceae family members.[19] Onion's benefits relating to cardiovascular disease have been reviewed.[6,20]

Diabetes: Although more research is needed on the use of onion as a treatment for diabetes in humans, many articles describe onion's benefits in improving glucose levels.[21]

Cancer: Onion also has proven to be an antioxidant and may be beneficial in certain cancers. The organosulfur compounds contained in onion exert chemopreventive effects on chemical carcinogenesis. The constituent diallyl disulfide possesses inhibitory properties against colon and renal cancers.[22] People consuming diets high in allium vegetables, including onion, suffer from fewer incidences of stomach cancer.[2,23] Onion's protective factors for breast cancer have been evaluated in a French case-control study.[24] Another report compares the antioxidant activity of onion polyphenols with those of other fruits and vegetables.[25] The quercetin component in onion; however, was found to be absorbed by humans from dietary sources but provided no direct protective effect during LDL oxidation.[26]

Respiratory problems: Folk medicine has used the onion for treatment of asthma, whooping cough, bronchitis, and similar ailments.[5,21] The onion is used in homeopathic medicine.[6] An ethanol extract of onion reduced "allergy-induced" bronchial constriction in certain patients.[5] The thiosulfinates present in the onion are said to inhibit bronchoconstriction, but definite efficacy remains unproven in this area.[17]

Other uses: Onions have been used in the treatment of stingray wounds,[27] warts, acne,[3] appetite loss,[2,4] urinary tract disorders,[6] and indigestion.[2] Onion cell extract was ineffective in treating postsurgical scarring.[27] General reviews of therapeutic uses of onion are available.[29,30]

Dosage: The *German Commission E Monographs* lists the average daily dose as 50 g of fresh onion, the juice from 50 g of fresh onion, or 20 g dried onion. A maximum of 35 mg diphenylamine/ day is recommended if onion preparations are used over several months.[4]

TOXICOLOGY: Certain sulfur compounds (eg, propanethial-s-oxide) escape from the onion in vapor form and hydrolyze to sulfuric acid when it is cut, causing the familiar eye irritation and lacrimation.[2,7] Corneal swelling from onion exposure has been reported.[31] Using a sharp knife also minimizes the crushing of onion tissue and liberation of volatiles, and cutting an onion under running water avoids lacrimation. Ingestion of onion seems relatively safe, as the *German Commission E* lists no contraindications, side effects, or interactions from the plant.[4] With large intake, the stomach may be affected, and frequent contact with onion rarely may cause allergic reaction.[5] The onion seeds have been reported as an occupational allergen.[32] Onion toxicity is only accociated with high intake.

A review of onion discussing ingestion of large amounts of the bulb finds toxicity unresolved.[20]

[1] Blumenthal M, Brinckmann J, Goldberg A, eds. *Herbal Medicine: Expanded Commission E Monographs*. Newton, MA: Integrative Medicine Communications; 2000.

[2] Ensminger, A. et al. *Foods and Nutrition Encyclopedia*, 2nd ed. Vol. 2., CRC Press Inc., Boca Raton, FL. 1994;1684-88.

[3] Dwyer, J. Sr. Ed. et al. *Magic and Medicine of Plants*. The Reader's Digest Association, Inc. 1986;261.

[4] Blumenthal, M. Sr. Ed. et al. *The Complete German Commission E Monographs*, American Botanical Council, Austin, TX, 1998:176-7.

[5] Fleming, T. Ch. Ed. et al. *PDR for Herbal Medicines*. Medical Economics Company, Inc., Montvale, NJ. 1998;624-5.

[6] Reynolds J. ed. *Martindale, The Extra Pharmacopoeia*. Royal Pharmaceutical Society, London, England. 1996;1734.

[7] Schulz, V. et al. *Rational Phytotherapy*, Springer-Verlag Berlin. Heidelberg 1998;153.

[8] Guarrera, P. *J Ethnopharmacol*. 1999;68(1-3):183-92.

[9] Dankert, J. et al. *Zentralbl Bakteriol [Orig A]*. 1979;245(1-2):229-39.

[10] Zohri, A. et al. *Microbial Res*. 1995;150(2):167-72.

[11] Kato, T. et al. *Mutat Res*. 1998;420(1-3):109-14.

[12] Kim, J. et al. *J Nihon Univ Sch Dent*. 1997;39(3):136-41.

[13] Elnima, E. et al. *Pharmazie*. 1983;38(11):747-8.

[14] Doutremepuich, C. et al. *Ann Pharm Fr*. 1985;43(3):273-9.

[15] Bordia, T. et al. *Prostaglandins Leukot Essent Fatty Acids*. 1996;54(3):183-6.

[16] Goldman, I. et al. *Thromb Haemost*. 1996;76(3):450-2.

[17] Miller, L. et al. *Herbal Medicinals, A Clinician's Guide*. Pharmaceutical Products Press. Binghamton, NY. 1998;195-202.

[18] Makheja, A. et al. *Prostaglandins Med*. 1979;2(6):413-24.

[19] Ali, M. et al. *Gen Pharmacol*. 1990;21(3):273-6.

[20] Kendler, B. *Prev Med*. 1987;16(5):670-85.

[21] Bratman, S. et al. *Natural Health Bible*. Prima Publishing, 1999;62.

[22] Fukushima, S. et al. *J Cell Biochem Suppl*. 1997;27:100-5.

[23] Winter, R. *Medicines in Food*. Crown Trade Paperbacks. New York, NY. 1995;61-3.

[24] Challier, B. et al. *Eur J Epidemiol*. 1998;14(8):737-47.

[25] Paganga, G. et al. *Free Radic Res*. 1999;30(2):153-62.

[26] McAnlis, G. et al. *Eur J Clin Nutr*. 1999;53(2):92-6.

[27] Whiting, S. et al. *Med J Aust*. 1998;168(11):584.

[28] Jackson, B. et al. *Dermatol Surg*. 1999;25(4):267-69.

[29] Breu, W. et al. *Econ Med Plant Res*. 1994;6:115-47.

[30] Augusti, K. et al. *Indian J Exp Biol*. 1996;34(7):634-40.

[31] Chan, R. et al. *Am J Optom Arch Am Acad Optom*. 1972;49(9):713-5.

[32] Navarro, J. et al. *J Allergy Clin Immunol*. 1995;96(5 pt 1):690-3.

SCIENTIFIC NAME(S): *Petroselinum crispum* (Mill.) Mansfield, *P. hortense* Hoffman, and *P. sativum.* Family: Umbelliferae

COMMON NAME(S): Parsley, rock parsley, garden parsley

❧❧❧❧ PATIENT INFORMATION ❧❧❧❧

Uses: Parsley, in addition to being a source of vitamins and minerals, has been used in the treatment of prostate, liver, and spleen diseases, anemia, arthritis, and cancer.

Side Effects: Adverse effects from the ingestion of parsley oil include headache, giddiness, loss of balance, convulsions, and renal damage. Pregnant women should not take parsley because of its potential uterotonic effects.

Dosing: Parsley has been used at daily doses of 6 g; however, no clinical studies have been found that support this dose. Because of toxicity, do not use the essential oil.[1]

BOTANY: Parsley is an herb indigenous to the Mediterranean but is now cultivated worldwide. It is deep green, with divided, curled leaves.

HISTORY: Parsley leaves and roots are popular as condiments and garnish. In Lebanon, parsley is a major ingredient in a national dish called tabbouleh. An average adult may consume as much as 50 g parsley per meal.[2]

Parsley seeds were used traditionally as a carminative to decrease flatulence and colic pain. The root was used as a diuretic and the juice to treat kidney ailments. Parsley oil also was used to regulate menstrual flow in the treatment of amenorrhea and dysmenorrhea, and is purported to be an abortifacient. Bruised leaves were used to treat tumors, insect bites, lice and skin parasites, and contusions.[3,4] Parsley tea once was used to treat dysentery and gallstones.[2] Other traditional uses include the treatment of diseases of the prostate, liver, and spleen, anemia, and arthritis; as an expectorant, antimicrobial, aphrodisiac, hypotensive, laxative; and as a scalp lotion to stimulate hair growth.[3,5]

PHARMACOLOGY: Parsley is a good natural source of vitamins and minerals including calcium, iron, carotene, ascorbic acid, and vitamin A.[3,6]

Myristicin, a component of parsley oil, has been thought to be in part responsible for the hallucinogenic effect of nutmeg. It is not known whether parsley oil induces hallucinations, but smoking parsley as a cannabis substitute was common during the 1960s. Parsley may have been smoked for a euphoric effect or as a carrier for potent drugs such as phencyclidine.[7]

Apiol, another parsley component, is an antipyretic and, like myristicin, is a uterine stimulant. Apiol was once available in capsules for use as an abortifacient. Although the effectiveness of this compound as a uterotonic has not been quantitated, a Russian product called "Supetin" (which contains about 85% parsley juice) is used to stimulate uterine contractions during labor.[8] Data regarding the safety and efficacy of this drug are not readily available.

Apiol and myristicin may be responsible for the mild diuretic effect of the seeds and oil.[9]

TOXICOLOGY: Adverse effects from parsley are uncommon. People allergic to other members of the Umbelliferae family (eg, carrot, fennel, celery) may be sensitive to the constituents (especially in the flowers) of parsley. Because of the potential uterotonic effects, parsley oil, juice, and seeds should not be taken by pregnant women. Adverse effects from the ingestion of the oil have included headache, giddiness, loss of balance, convulsions, and renal damage.

The psoralen compounds found in parsley have been linked to a photodermatitis reaction found among parsley cutters. This skin reaction is usually only evident if the areas that have contacted the juice are exposed to strong sunlight; it can be minimized by the use of protective clothing and sunscreens.[10]

[1] Blumenthal M, Brinckmann J, Goldberg A, eds. *Herbal Medicine: Expanded Commission E Monographs.* Newton, MA: Integrative Medicine Communications; 2000.

[2] Zaynoun S, et al. *Clin Exp Dermatol.* 1985;10:328.

[3] Duke JA. *Handbook of Medicinal Herbs.* Boca Raton, FL: CRC Press, 1985.

[4] Meyer J. *The Herbalist.* Hammond, IN: Hammond Book Co., 1934.

[5] Hoffman D. *The Herbal Handbook.* Rochester, VT: Healing Arts Press, 1988.

[6] Tyler VE, et al. *Pharmacognosy,* 9th ed. Philadelphia, PA: Lea & Febiger, 1988.

[7] Cook CE, et al. *Clin Pharm Ther.* 1982;31:635.

[8] Chemical Abstracts. 90:115465, 1979.

[9] Marczal G, et al. *Acta Agron Acad Sci Hung.* 1977;26:7.

[10] Smith DA. *Practitioner.* 1985;229:673.

Passion Flower

SCIENTIFIC NAME(S): *Passiflora* sp. Most often *P. incarnata* is used medicinally. Family: Passifloraceae

COMMON NAME(S): Passion flower; passion fruit, granadilla (species with edible fruit); water lemon; Maypop, apricot vine, wild passion flower (*P. incarnatus*); Jamaican honeysuckle (*P. laurifolia*)

·:·:·:· PATIENT INFORMATION ·:·:·:·

Uses: Passion flower has been used to treat sleep disorders and, historically, in homeopathic medicine to treat pain, insomnia related to neurasthenia or hysteria, and nervous exhaustion.

Drug Interactions: Passion flower may interact with anticoagulants (eg, wafarin) and monoamine oxidase inhibitor therapy.[1]

Side Effects: Although no adverse effects of the passion flower have been reported, large doses may result in central nervous system (CNS) depression.

Dosing: No clinical trials of passion flower as a single agent have been reported; therefore, the daily dose of 4 to 8 g currently is not supported.

BOTANY: The term "passion flower" connotes many of the approximately 400 species of the genus *Passiflora*, which includes primarily vines. Some of the species are noted for their showy flowers, others for their edible fruit. Common species include *P. incarnata*, *P. edulis*, *P. alata*, *P. laurifolia*, and *P. quadrangularis*. Those with edible fruit include *P. incarnata*, *P. edulis*, and *P. quadrangularis*, the last being one of the major species grown for its fruit.[2] *Passiflora* species are native to tropical and subtropical areas of the Americas. In the US, *P. incarnata* is found from Virginia to Florida and as far west as Missouri and Texas. The flowers of *Passiflora* have 5 petals, sepals, and stamens, 3 stigmas, and a crown of filaments. The fruit is egg-shaped, has a pulpy consistency, and includes many small seeds.[2,3]

HISTORY: The passion flower was discovered in 1569 by Spanish explorers in Peru, who saw the flowers as symbolic of the passion of Christ, and therefore a sign of Christ's approval of their efforts. This is the origin of the scientific and common names.[4] The folklore surrounding this plant possibly dates further into the past. The floral parts are thought to represent the elements of the crucifixion (3 styles represent 3 nails; 5 stamens for the 5 wounds; the ovary looks like a hammer; the corona is the crown of thorns; the petals represent the 10 true apostles; and the white and bluish purple colors are those of purity and heaven).[3,5] In Europe, passion flower has been used in homeopathic medicine to treat pain, insomnia related to neurasthenia or hysteria, and nervous exhaustion. Other indications included bronchial disorders (particularly asthma), in compresses for burns, and for inflammation, inflamed hemorrhoids, climacteric complaints, pediatric attention disorders, and pediatric nervousness and excitability.[6]

PHARMACOLOGY: A report describes CNS-receptor binding sites of *P. incarnata*.[7]

Passion flower was researched for its sedative and anxiolytic effects.[3,8,9] A 1986 survey of British herbal sedatives revealed passion flower as the most popular species (*P. incarnata*). Other popular species included *Valeriana of-*

ficinalis, Humulus lupulus, and *Scutellaria lateriflora*.[10,11] Martindale also lists many multi-ingredient preparations from other countries.[12]

The pharmacological activity of *Passiflora* is attributed primarily to the alkaloids and flavonoids. The harmala alkaloids inhibit monoamine oxidase and this may account for part of their pharmacologic effect.[13]

Human studies in the sedative/anxiolytic areas of *Passiflora* species are reported. A case report using the plant in a combination natural product, "calmanervin," for successful sedation before surgery is discussed.[14] In 91 patients, *Passiflora* (in combination, "Euphytose") exhibited statistically significant differences when compared with placebo in the treatment of adjustment disorder with anxious mood, in a multicenter, double-blind trial.[15] *Passiflora* in the combination product *Compoz* contradicts these last 2 studies. It was not possible to differentiate from either aspirin or placebo when tested as a daytime sedative. However, this report was from the early 1970s and was only 2 weeks in duration.[16]

Other *Passiflora* species exhibit similar effects. *P. coerulea* has sedative actions.[17] Constituent chrysin, isolated from this same species (a central benzodiazepine [BDZ] ligand) has anxiolytic effects, due in part to this role as a partial agonist of central BDZ receptors.[18] Tranquilizing effects have been seen from alkaloids from the harman group in *P. edulis* species as well.[19]

Passion flower's ability to reduce anxiety makes it useful for asthma, palpitations, and other cardiac rhythm abnormalities, high blood pressure, insomnia, neurosis, nervousness, pain relief, and other related conditions.[3,8,9]

The antimicrobial activity of *Passiflora* disappears rapidly from dried plant residues and fades gradually in aqueous extracts. Addition of dextran, milk, or milk products has a stabilizing effect on dry *Passiflora*.[20,21] A later report discusses *P. tetrandra* component, "4-hydroxy-2-cyclopentenone," to exhibit antipseudomonal actions. This consituent was also found to be cytotoxic to P388 murine leukemia cells.[22]

Other uses of passion flower include herbal treatment for menopausal complaints[23] and as a flavored syrup to mask drug taste.[24]

INTERACTIONS: Because passion flower contains coumarins, the risk of bleeding may be increased in patients taking warfarin.[25]

TOXICOLOGY: Little information is available on the clinical toxicity of *Passiflora*. Cyanogenesis from species *P. edulis* has been suggested.[26] The plant's known depressant actions may reduce arterial pressure affecting circulation and increasing respiratory rate.[9] There are no controlled human trials on single herb preparations of *Passiflora* extracts since the mid 1990s.[27] Some cases report vasculitis[28] and altered consciousness in 5 patients taking the herbal product *Relaxir*, produced mainly from *P. incarnata* fruits.[29] *P. adenopoda* fruits may produce some toxic effect.[30]

Use of passion flower is contraindicated during pregnancy because of the uterine stimulant action of its alkaloids harman and harmaline, and the content of the cyanogenic glycoside gynocardin.[31]

[1] Newall C, et al. *Herbal Medicines: A Guide for Health Care Professionals*. London, England: The Pharmaceutical Press, 1996:206.

[2] Seymour E. *The Garden Encyclopedia*. New York: Wm. H. Wise, 1940.

3 Chevallier, A. *Encyclopedia of Medicinal Plants*. New York, NY: DK Publishing,1996;117.

4 *Encyclopedia Americana*. Danbury, CT: Grolier, 1987.

5 Tyler, V. *The New Honest Herbal*. Philadelphia, PA: G.F. Stickley Co, 1987.

6 Lutomski J, et al. *Pharm Unserer Zeit*. 1981;10:45.

7 Burkard W, et al. *Pharmaceutical & Pharmacological Letters*. 1997;7(1):25-26.

8 Bruneton, J. *Pharmacognosy, Phytochemistry, Medicinal Plants*. Paris, France: Lavoisier Publishing Inc., 1995:284-85.

9 Duke, J. *CRC Handbook of Medicinal Herbs*. Boca Raton, FL: CRC Press, 1989;347.

10 Tyler, V. *Herbs of Choice, The Therapeutic Use of Phytomedicinals*. Binghamton, NY: Pharmaceutical Products Press, 1994:119.

11 Ross M, et al. *International J Crude Drug Research*. 1986(Mar);24:1-6.

12 Panfitt K, ed. *Martindale, The Complete Drug Reference*. London, England: Pharmaceutical Press, 1999:1615.

13 Aoyagi N, et al. *Chem Pharm Bull*. 1974;22(5):1008-13.

14 Yaniv R, et al. *J Ethnopharmacology*. 1995;46(1):71-72.

15 Bourin M, et al. *Fundam Clin Pharmacol*. 1997;11(2):127-32.

16 Rickels K, et al. *JAMA*. 1973(Jan 1);223:29-33.

17 Medina J, et al. *Biochem Pharmacol*. 1990;40(10):2227-31.

18 Wolfman C, et al. *Pharmacol Biochem Behav*. 1994;47(1):1-4.

19 Lutomski J, et al. *Planta Medica*. 1975(Mar);27:112-21.

20 Nicolls J, et al. *Antimicrob Agents Chemother*. 1973;3:110-17.

21 Birner J, et al. *Antimicrob Agents Chemother*. 1973;3(1):105-09.

22 Perry N, et al. *Planta Med*. 1981;57(2):129-31.

23 Israel D, et al. *Pharmacotherapy*. 1997;17(5):970-84.

24 Puffer H, et al. *Am J Hosp Pharm*. 1971(Aug);28:633-35.

25 Heck A, et al. *Am J Health Syst Pharm*. 2000;57:1221.

26 Spencer K, et al. *J Agric Food Chem*. 1983;31(4):794-96.

27 Schulz V, et al. *Rational Phytotherapy, 3rd edition*. Berlin, Germany: Springer Verlag, 1998:83-84.

28 Smith G, et al. *Br J Rheumatol*. 1993;32(1):87-88.

29 Solbakken A, et al. *Tidsskr nor Laegeforen*. 1997;117(8):1140-41.

30 Saenz J, et al. *Rev Biol Trop*. 1972;20(1):137-40.

31 Brinker, F. *Herb Contraindications and Drug Interactions*. Sandy, OR: Eclectic Medical Publications, 1998:109-10.

Pau D' Arco

SCIENTIFIC NAME(S): *Tabebuia avellanedae* Lorentz ex Griseb. Family: Bignoniaceae (Trumpet creepers). This species is synonymous with *T. impetiginosa* Mart. ex DC., *T. heptaphylla* Vell. Toledo, and *T. ipé* Mart. ex Schum. The distinct related species *Tecoma curialis* Solhanha da Gama is sometimes marketed under the same names.

COMMON NAME(S): Taheebo, Pau d'Arco, Lapacho morado, Lapacho colorado, Ipé Roxo

---

⚘⚘⚘ PATIENT INFORMATION ⚘⚘⚘

Uses: Pau d' arco is widely used in alternative cancer therapy without sufficient scientific proof. It may be more useful in antifungal applications, although no clinical trials have been conducted for any indication.

Drug Interactions: Do not use pau d' arco with anticoagulants.

Side Effects: There are no reported serious side effects.

BOTANY: *Tabebuia* is a large genus of tropical trees that grows worldwide. According to a source, the correct name for the source species is *T. impetiginosa*;[1] however, the majority of biological and chemical studies of the plant refer to *T. avellaneda*. The commercial product is derived from the inner bark. The tree grows widely throughout tropical South America, including Brazil, Paraguay, and northern Argentina. It has a hard, durable, and attractive wood that is extremely resistant to insect and fungal attack.

HISTORY: Pau d' arco has been promoted for many years as an anticancer herb, and lay reports have claimed efficacy in a variety of cancers.[2] Antifungal and antibiotic properties are also claimed in promotional literature, with both topical and oral dosing for candidiasis.

PHARMACOLOGY: Lapachol was extensively evaluated as an anticancer agent by the US National Cancer Institute and the Pfizer Co. in the 1960s.[3,4] While oral absorption in humans was relatively poor, peak blood levels of 14 to 31 mcg/mL were attained with doses of 30 to 50 mg/kg.[3] Extensive modifications of the lapachol structure have been performed in pursuit of better

antitumor activity,[5] in the search for antimalarial drugs,[6] and for antipsoriatic drugs.[7] Lapachol has also been reported to have modest antifungal and antibacterial activity,[8] as well as anti-inflammatory activity[9] and weak estrogenic action.[10]

Active β-lapachone has been found in tumor models.[11] It inhibits murine leukemia virus reverse transcriptase and DNA polymerase-α, but not DNA polymerase-β and several other related enzymes.[12]

While having apparent potential for drug development, the biological activity of lapachol and β-lapachone is not relevant to the use of pau d' arco bark, because the bark contains little of these constituents. Instead, the furanonaphthoquinones are the important constituents, having cytotoxic,[13,14] antifungal, antibacterial,[15,16] and rather potent immunomodulatory activity.[17]

Despite the promising activity shown by the furanonaphthoquinone constituents, there do not appear to be clinical studies to support the use of pau d' arco for any of the indications mentioned.

TOXICOLOGY: Because of lapachol, human toxicity was seen at doses greater than 1.5 g/day, with an elevated prothrombin time that was reversed by administration of vitamin K.[3] Because lapachol is not a major constituent of pau d' arco bark, these studies are not entirely relevant to the commercial product. No toxicology has been reported for either the bark extract or its main constituents.

[1] Woodson R, et al. *Ann Missouri Bot Gard.* 1973;60:45.

[2] Hartwell J. *Lloydia.* 1968;31:71.

[3] Block J, et al. *Cancer Chemother Repts.* 1974;4:27.

[4] Rao K, et al. *Cancer Res.* 1968;28:1952.

[5] Linardi M, et al. *J Med Chem.* 1975;18:1159.

[6] Fieser L, et al. *J Amer Chem Soc.* 1948;70:3151.

[7] Müller K, et al. *J Nat Prod.* 1999;62:1134.

[8] Guirard P, et al.*Planta Med.* 1994;60:373.

[9] De Almeida E, et al. *J Ethnopharmacol.* 1990;29:239.

[10] Sareen V, et al. *Phytotherapy Res.* 1995;9:139.

[11] Schaffner-Sabba K, et al. *J Med Chem.* 1984;27:990.

[12] Schürch A, et al. *Eur J Biochem.* 1978;84:197.

[13] Diaz F, et al. *J Nat Prod.* 1996;59:423.

[14] Rao M, et al. *J Nat Prod.* 1982;45:600.

[15] Binutu O, et al. *Planta Med.* 1996;62:352.

[16] Gafner S, et al. *Phytochemistry.* 1996;42:1315.

[17] Kreher B, et al. *Planta Med.* 1988;54:562.

Pawpaw

SCIENTIFIC NAME(S): *Asimina triloba* (L.) Dunal. Family: Annonaceae (Sometimes confused with *Carica Papaya*.)

COMMON NAME(S): Pawpaw, custard apple, poor man's banana

ꜩꜩꜩ PATIENT INFORMATION ꜩꜩꜩ

Uses: Pawpaw has historically been used for food, fishing nets, and medicine. It exhibits cytotoxic and pesticidal activities.

Side Effects: May cause contact dermatitis in certain people.

Dosing: Pawpaw has been used in homeopathy. Higher doses run a substantial risk of toxicity; therefore, pawpaw cannot be recommended.

BOTANY: The pawpaw is a small, North American tree, which grows from about 3 to 12 m high. It is common in the temperate woodlands of the eastern US. Its large leaves are "tropical looking" and droopy in nature. The dark brown, velvety flowers (about 5 cm across) grow in umbrella-like whorls, similar to some magnolia species, and can bloom for up to 6 weeks. Pawpaw fruit is smooth-skinned, yellow to greenish-brown in color, measuring from about 8 to 15 cm long. It can reach up to 045 kg in weight. It resembles that of a short, thick banana, and also is similar in nutrient value. The yellow, soft, "custard-like" pulp is edible but sickly sweet in flavor and contains dark seeds.[1-4]

HISTORY: One source states that pawpaw was introduced to the US in 1736.[3] It was used as food for the Native Americans. The thin, fibrous, inner bark has been used to make fish nets.[1,3] The bark also was used as medicine because it contains useful alkaloids.[3]

PHARMACOLOGY: The pawpaw acetogenins have consistently exhibited cytotoxic (antitumor) and pesticidal (antimicrobial) activities.

Brine shrimp lethality bioassay or "test" (BSLT) is a screening tool used to predict cytotoxic and pesticidal activity. Tiny shrimp, *Artemia salina*, are placed in brine where their eggs hatch within 48 hours. Extracts of test-plant material are then put in shrimp-containing vials where survivors are microscopically counted. LC_{50} values are then calculated to determine the potential killing activity of, in this case, pawpaw extracts.[5]

In several studies performed in this manner, it was found that specific acetogenins exhibited potent cytotoxicities.[6-9] Examples include acetogenin's cytotoxic potential against lung carcinoma, breast carcinoma, and colon adenocarcinoma.[7] Certain seed extracts also possessed cytotoxic actions comparable with doxorubicin against 6 human solid tumor cell lines.[9]

Of all the acetogenins, the adjacent-bis-THF-ring compounds are the most potent, showing cytotoxic activity against human lung and breast tumor cell lines with up to a million times the potency of doxorubicin.[10] Compound asiminocin, a pawpaw acetogenin isolate from stem bark was highly inhibitory against 3 human cell lines, with over a billion times the potency of doxorubicin.[11] The mechanism of action is via potent inhibitors of mitochondrial NADH: ubiquinone oxidoreductase, thus causing a decrease in cellular ATP levels.[12,13]

Various pawpaw tree parts were tested for pesticidal potential. The small twigs yielded the most potent extract, while the leaves were the least potent. Unripe fruits, seeds, root wood and bark, and stem bark were also notably potent.[14] A caterpillar-laden tree was sprayed with a pawpaw bark extract and 30 minutes later the majority of insects had died and fallen from the tree. Phlox plants infested with mildew fungus also were sprayed with pawpaw preparation and 10 days later improvement was markedly observed. Pawpaw tree samplings were collected, expressing monthly variation in pesticidal activity. All of these are examples of the plant's beneficial (and natural) properties. The pawpaw tree is usually insect- or disease-resistant because of its acetogenin content, which prevents the feeding of many organisms.[12]

TOXICOLOGY: Handling the fruit may produce a skin rash in sensitive individuals.[3]

[1] Hocking G. *A Dictionary of Natural Products.* Medford, NY: Plexus Publishing Inc., 1997;80.

[2] Davidson A. *Fruit-A Connoisseur's Guide and Cookbook.* NY, NY: Simon and Schuster, 1991;123-24.

[3] NNGA library. http://www.icserv.com/nnga/pawpaw.htm

[4] Univ. of Kentucky. http://www.pawpaw.kysu.edu

[5] Colegate S, et al. *Bioactive Natural Products.* Boca Raton, FL: CRC Press, 1993;15-17.

[6] Zhao G, et al. *J Nat Prod.* 1992;55(3):347-56.

[7] Zhao G, et al. *Phytochemistry.* 1993;33(5):1065-73.

[8] He K, et al. *J Nat Prod.* 1996;59(11):1029-34.

[9] Woo M, et al. *J Nat Prod.* 1995;58(10):1533-42.

[10] He K, et al. *Bioorg Med Chem.* 1997;5(3):501-06.

[11] Zhao G, et al. *Bioorg Med Chem.* 1996;4(1):25-32.

[12] Johnson H, et al. *Progress in New Crops.* Arlington, VA: ASHS Press, 1996;609-14.

[13] Zhao G, et al. *J Med Chem.* 1994;37(13):1971-76.

[14] Ratnayake S, et al. *J Econ Entomol.* 1992;85(6):2353-56.

SCIENTIFIC NAME(S): *Hedeoma pulegeoides* (L) Persoom and *Mentha pulegium* L. Family: Labiatae

COMMON NAME(S): American pennyroyal, squawmint, mosquito plant, pudding grass

---

⚘⚘⚘ PATIENT INFORMATION ⚘⚘⚘

Uses: Pennyroyal may be used as an insect repellent, antiseptic, fragrance, flavoring, as an emmenagogue, carminative, stimulant, antispasmodic and for bowel disorders, skin eruptions, and pneumonia.

Side Effects: Pennyroyal can cause abdominal pain, nausea, vomiting, lethargy, increased blood pressure and increased pulse rate, dermatitis and, in large portions, abortion, irreversible renal damage, severe liver damage, and death. A small amount of oil can produce delirium, unconsciousness, shock, seizures, and auditory and visual hallucinations.

Dosing: Pennyroyal usually is used as the volatile oil as an abortifacient. Because of severe toxicity at doses of 5 g, it should not be used.[1]

BOTANY: Both plants are members of the mint family and are referred to as pennyroyal. *H. pulegeoides* (American pennyroyal) grows in woods through most of the northern and eastern US and Canada, while *M. pulegium* is found in parts of Europe. Pennyroyal is a perennial, creeping herb that possesses small, lilac flowers at the stem ends. It can grow to be 30 to 50 cm in height. The leaves are grayish green and, like other mint family members, are very aromatic.[2,3]

HISTORY: Pennyroyal has been recorded in history as far back as the 1st century AD, where it was mentioned by Roman naturalist Pliny and Greek physician Dioscorides. In the 17th century, English herbalist Nicholas Culpeper wrote about some uses for the plant, including its role in women's ailments, venomous bites, and digestion. European settlers used the plant for respiratory ailments, mouth sores, and female disorders.[2] The plant's oil has been used as a flea-killing bath, hence the name *pulegeoides* (from the Latin word meaning flea), and has been used externally as a rubefacient. In addition, the oil found frequent use among natural health ad-

vocates as an abortifacient and as a means of inducing delayed menses. The oil and infusions of the leaves have been used in the treatment of weakness and stomach pains.[4]

PHARMACOLOGY: Pennyroyal has been used as an insect repellent and antiseptic.[2,3,5,6] It has been employed as a flavoring agent for food and spice[6] and also as a fragrance in detergents, perfume, and soaps.[3,6]

The plant has been used for female problems such as an emmenagogue (to induce menstruation). It has also been used as a carminative, stimulant and antispasmodic, and for bowel disorders, skin eruptions, pneumonia, and other uses.[2,3,5,6]

TOXICOLOGY: Pennyroyal herb teas are generally used without reported side effects (presumably because of low concentration of the oil),[5] but toxicity for pennyroyal oil is well recognized, with many reports of adverse events and fatalities documented.

American or European pennyroyal can cause dermatitis and, in large doses, abortion, irreversible renal damage, severe liver damage, and death. A teaspoonful of the oil can produce delirium, unconsciousness, and shock.[6]

One case of pennyroyal oil ingestion resulted in generalized seizures and auditory and visual hallucinations following the ingestion of less than 1 teaspoonful (5 mL) of the oil; the patient recovered uneventfully.[7] Other symptoms of plant ingestion may include abdominal pain, nausea, vomiting, lethargy, and increased blood pressure and pulse rate.[5]

The major component, pulegone, is oxidized by hepatic cytochrome P450 to the hepatotoxic compound menthofuran.[8] Pulegone, or a metabolite, also is responsible for neurotoxicity and destruction of bronchiolar epithelial cells.[9,10]

Pulegone extensively depletes glutathione in the liver, and its metabolites are detoxified by the presence of glutathione in the liver. Hepatic toxicity has been prevented by the early administration of acetylcysteine following ingestion of pennyroyal oil.[11] Various metabolite studies are available regarding hepatotoxicity.[12,13]

Case reports are widely reported. One woman who ingested up to 30 mL of the oil experienced abdominal cramps, nausea, vomiting, and alternating lethargy and agitation. She later exhibited loss of renal function, hepatotoxicity, and evidence of disseminated intravascular coagulation. She died 7 days after ingesting the oil. Another woman ingested 10 mL of the oil and only experienced dizziness.[1] Two infants (8 weeks of age and 6 months of age) who ingested mint tea containing pennyroyal oil developed hepatic and neurologic injury. One infant died, the other suffered hepatic dysfunction and severe epileptic encephalopathy.[14] A review of 18 previous cases reported moderate to severe toxicity in patients exposed to at least 10 mL of the oil, concluding that pennyroyal continues to be an herbal toxin of concern to public health.[15] Another review concluded that pennyroyal oil is toxic as well.[16]

Pennyroyal is contraindicated in pregnancy. It possesses abortifacient actions (because of pulegone content) and irritates the genitourinary tract.[5] The abortifacient effect of the oil is thought to be caused by irritation of the uterus with subsequent uterine contraction. Its action is unpredictable and dangerous.[17] The dose at which the herb induces abortion is close to lethal, and in some cases it is lethal.[3,6] However, one letter does report a pregnancy unaffected by pennyroyal use.[18]

[1] Sullivan JB Jr., et al. *JAMA*. 1979;242:2873.

[2] Low T, et al. eds. *Pennyroyal. Magic and Medicine of Plants*. Sydney, Australia: Reader's Digest, 1994;278.

[3] Lawless J. Pennyroyal. *The Illustrated Encyclopedia of Essential Oils*. Rockport, MA: Element Books, Inc., 1995;176.

[4] Da Legnano LP. *The Medicinal Plants*. Rome, Italy: Edizioni Mediterranee, 1973.

[5] Newall C, et al. *Pennyroyal. Herbal Medicines*. London, England: Pharmaceutical Press, 1996;208.

[6] Duke J. *Hedeoma Pulegioides*. CRC Handbook of Medicinal Herbs. Boca Raton, FL: CRC Press Inc., 1989;223,307–308.

[7] Early DF. *Lancet*. 1961;2:580.

[8] Gordon WP, et al. *Drug Metab Disp*. 1987;15(5):589.

[9] Thomassen D, et al. *J Pharmacol Exp Ther*. 1990;253(2):567.

[10] Gordon WP, et al. *Toxicol Appl Pharmacol*. 1982;65:413.

[11] Buechel DW, et al. *J Am Osteopath Assn*. 1983;2:793.

[12] Thomassen D, et al. *J Pharmacol Exp Ther*. 1988;244(3):825–29.

[13] Carmichael P. *Ann Intern Med*. 1997;126(3):250–51.

[14] Bakerink J, et al. *Pediatrics*. 1996(Nov);98:944–47.

[15] Anderson I, et al. *Ann Intern Med*. 1996;124(8):726–34.

[16] Mack R. *NC Med J*. 1997;58(6):456–57.

[17] Allen WT. *Lancet*. 1897;2:1022.

[18] Black D. *J Am Osteopath Assoc*. 1985;85(5):282.

SCIENTIFIC NAME(S): *Plantago lanceolata* L., P. major L., *P. psyllium* L., *P. arenaria* Waldst. & Kit. (*P. ramosa* Asch.) (Spanish or French psyllium seed), *P. ovata* Forsk. (Blond or Indian plantago seed) Family: Plantaginaceae. (Not to be confused with *Musa paradisiacae*, or edible plantain.)

COMMON NAME(S): Plantain, Spanish psyllium, French psyllium, blond plantago, Indian plantago, psyllium seed, flea seed, black psyllium

♣♣♣♣ PATIENT INFORMATION ♣♣♣♣

Uses: The psyllium in plantain has been used as gastrointestinal (GI) therapy, to treat hyperlipidemia, as a topical agent to treat some skin problems, as an anti-inflammatory and diuretic, for anticancer effects, and for respiratory treatment.

Drug Interactions: Plantain may interact with lithium and carbamazepine, decreasing their plasma concentrations.

Side Effects: Adverse events include anaphylaxis, chest congestion, sneezing and watery eyes, occupational asthma, and a situation involving the occurence of a giant phytobezoar composed of psyllium seed husks.

Dosing: Plantain leaves have been given as a tea for cold and cough at 3 to 6 g/day.[1]

BOTANY: Plantain is a perennial weed with almost worldwide distribution. There are about 250 species, of which 20 have wide geographic ranges, 9 have discontinuous ranges, 200 are limited to one region, and 9 have narrow ranges. *P. lanceolata* and *P. major* have the widest distribution.[2] Plantain species are herbs and shrubby plants characterized by basal leaves and inconspicuous flowers in heads or spikes. They grow aggressively. Plantain is wind-pollinated, facilitating its growth where there are no bees and few other plantain plants. It is tolerant of viral infections. *P. major* produces 13,000 to 15,000 seeds per plant, and the seeds have been reported to remain viable in soil for up to 60 years. *P. lanceolata* produces 2500 to 10,000 seeds per plant and has a somewhat shorter seed viability. Plantain seeds can survive passage through the gut of birds and other animals, facilitating their distribution further.[2] Plantain, or psyllium seeds, are small (1.5 to 3.5 mm), oval, boat-shaped, dark reddish-brown, odorless, and nearly tasteless. They are coated with mucilage that aids in their transportation by allowing adhesion to various surfaces.[2,3]

HISTORY: Plantain has long been associated with man and with agriculture. Certain species were spread by human colonization, particularly that of Europeans. As such, North American Indians and New Zealand Maori refer to plantain as "Englishman's foot," because it spread from areas of English settlement. *P. lanceolata* and *P. major* were used in herbal remedies and sometimes carried to colonies intentionally for that purpose. Psyllium seed has been found in malt refuse (formerly used as fertilizer) and wool imported to England. It has been commonly used in birdseed.[2] Pulverized seeds are mixed with oil and applied topically to inflamed sites; decoctions have been mixed with honey for sore throats. The seeds and refined colloid are used commonly in commercial bulk laxative preparations.[2,4]

PHARMACOLOGY: The pharmacology of plantain involves gastrointestinal tract therapy, hyperlipidemia treatment, anticancer effects, respiratory and other actions.

GI: Psyllium seed is classified as a bulk laxative. Mixed with water, it produces a mucilaginous mass. The indigestible seeds provide bulk for treatment of chronic constipation, while the mucilage serves as a mild laxative comparable to agar or mineral oil. The usual dose is 0.5 to 2 g of husk (5 to 15 g of seeds) mixed in 8 oz of water. A study of 10 healthy volunteers examined the effects of a 3 g ispaghula mixture (dried psyllium seed husks) given 3 times daily. It decreased intestinal transit time.[5] Effectiveness of psyllium seed on 78 subjects with irritable bowel syndrome (IBS) also has been reported.[6] *P. ovata* fiber is effective in regulating colon motility in a similar set of patients.[7] A postcholecystectomy patient with chronic diarrhea was given a 6.5 g dose of a 50% psyllium preparation, and symptoms resolved in 2 days.[8,9] Plantago seed as a cellulose/pectin mixture was as effective as a bulk laxative in 50 adult subjects.[10] The effects of different dietary fibers on colonic function, including plantago seed were evaluated.[11] Gastroprotective action from plantago extract (polyholozidic substances) also has been reported.[12]

In a triple-blind, crossover study of 17 female patients, *P. ovata* seed preparation was investigated on appetite variables. The preparation was deemed useful in weight control diets where a feeling of fullness was desired. Total fat intake was also decreased, again, suggesting the product to be a beneficial weight control diet supplement.[13]

A trial involving 393 patients with anal fissures found conservative treatment with psyllium effective. After 5 years of follow-up, 44% of the patients were cured without surgery within 4 to 8 weeks. There were complications (abscesses and fistulas requiring surgery) in 8% of the cases. The recurrence rate was 27%, but about one-third of these were fistulas that responded to further conservative management.[14]

A double-blind study of 51 patients with symptomatic hemorrhoids showed *Vi-Siblin*, a psyllium-containing preparation, to be effective in reducing bleeding and pain during defecation: 84% of the patients receiving the preparation reported improvement or elimination of symptoms, compared to 52% taking placebo.[15]

Hyperlipidemia: Many reports on psyllium have concluded that it can be helpful in treating various hyperlipidemias.[16,17]

Attention has been focused on the cholesterol-lowering effects of psyllium preparations. Psyllium hydrophilic mucilloid (*Metamucil*, Procter & Gamble) was found to lower serum cholesterol in a study of 28 patients who took 3 doses (3.4 g/dose) per day compared with placebo for 8 weeks. After 4 weeks, the psyllium-treated patients showed decreases in total serum cholesterol levels compared with the placebo group. Decreases were also seen in LDL cholesterol and the LDL/HDL ratio. At the end of 8 weeks, values for total cholesterol, LDL cholesterol, and the LDL/HDL ratio were 14%, 20% and 15%, respectively below baseline (all, $P < 0.01$). This study suggested that high cholesterol levels could be managed safely and easily by including psyllium preparations in the diet.[18]

Similar results of cholesterol reduction have been reported including: psyllium colloid administration for 2 to 29 months, reducing cholesterol levels by 16.9% and triglycerides by 52%;[19] a trial of 75 hypercholesterolemic patients, evaluating adjunct therapy of psyllium seed to a low cholesterol diet;[20] a 16-week, double-blind trial, proving plantago seed improved in total and LDL cholesterol in 37 patients;[21] and increased tolerance of psyllium seed in combination with colestipol (rather than monotherapy alone) in 105 hyperlipidemic patients.[22]

Psyllium seed was more effective than *P. ovata* husk in reducing serum cholesterol in normal and ileostomy patients.[23] However, a report on 20 hypercholesterolemic pediatric patients on low-fat diets found psyllium seed to be ineffective in lowering cholesterol or LDL levels.[24]

Issues of cereal companies including plantago seed in their products and claims of "cholesterol reduction" have been addressed.[25]

A polyphenolic compound (from *P. major* leaves) was found to exhibit hypocholesterolemic activity,[26] but in addition, the mechanism by which plantago reduces cholesterol may also include enhancement of cholesterol elimination as fecal bile acids.[27]

Respiratory: Plantain has been effective for chronic bronchitis,[28] asthma, cough, and cold.[4]

Other actions: A report by a physician described the topical use of crushed plantain leaves to treat poison ivy in 10 people. Although the trial was not conducted scientifically, the treatment eliminated itching and prevented spread of the dermatitis in all cases, 1 to 4 applications being required.[29] Fresh leaves of the plant have been poulticed onto herpes, sores, ulcers, boils, and infections. Plantain has been used for insect bites and gout.[4]

Aqueous extracts of plantain leaves possess antimicrobial activity caused by aglycone and aucubigenin.[3]

Aerial parts of plantago were used as an anti-inflammatory and a diuretic in folk medicine.[30]

Psyllium administration had no effect on postprandial plasma glucose in one report.[31]

INTERACTIONS: Drug interactions reported with psyllium involve lithium and carbamazepine. Psyllium may inhibit absorption of lithium in the GI tract, decreasing blood levels of the lithium, as seen in a 47-year-old woman with schizoaffective disorder.[32] Plantago seed also has decreased the bioavailability of carbamazepine in 4 male subjects.[33]

TOXICOLOGY: Plantain pollen has been found to contain at least 16 antigens, of which 6 are potentially allergenic. The pollen contains allergenic glycoproteins that react with concanavalin A, as well as components that bind IgE.[34] Antigenic and allergenic analysis has been performed on psyllium seed. All three fractions, husk, endosperm and embryo, contained similar antigens.[35] Formation of IgE antibodies to psyllium laxative has been demonstrated.[36] In addition, IgE-mediated sensitization to plantain pollen has been performed, contributing to seasonal allergy.[37]

There are many reported incidences of varying degrees of psyllium allergy including: nurses experiencing symptoms such as anaphylactoid reaction, chest congestion, sneezing and watery eyes (some of these reactions taking several years to acquire);[38,39] a case report describing severe anaphylactic shock following psyllium laxative ingestion, linked occupational respiratory allergies in pharmaceutical workers exposed to the substance;[40] consumption of plantago seed in cereal, responsible for anaphylaxis in a 60-year-old female (immunoglobulin E-mediated sensitization was documented, and patient was successfully treated with oral diphenhydramine);[41] and a report on workers in a psyllium processing plant evaluated for occupational asthma and IgE sensitization to psyllium.[42]

Another unusual adverse situation involves the occurrence of a giant phytobezoar composed of psyllium seed husks. The bezoar, located in the right colon, resulted in complete blockage of gastric emptying.[43] All psyllium preparations must be taken with adequate volumes of fluid. The seeds contain a pigment that may be toxic to the kidneys,[44] but this has been removed from most commercial preparations.[45]

Economic significance: As a weed, plantain is important because of its competition with commercial crops and small fruits. The presence of plantain seeds can make adequate cleaning of crop seed difficult, especially with small-seed legumes. Plantain, because of its tolerance of viral infection, can serve as a reservoir for economically important infections of crops including beets, potatoes, tomatoes, tobacco, turnips, cucumbers, and celery. Commercially, plantain is grown for use in forage mixtures and, primarily, for use in bulk laxatives.[2]

[1] Gruenwald J, ed. *PDR for Herbal Medicines.* 2nd ed. Montvale, NJ: Thomson Medical Economics; 2000: 278-280.

[2] Hammond J. *Adv Vir Res.* 1982;27:103.

[3] Bisset N. *Herbal Drugs and Phytopharmaceuticals.* Stuttgart, Germany: CRC Press, Inc. 1994;378–83.

[4] Duke J. *CRC Handbook of Medicinal Herbs.* Boca Raton, FL: CRC Press, Inc. 1989;386.

[5] Connaughton J, McCarthy CF. *Ir Med J.* 1982;75:93.

[6] Arthurs Y, Fielding JF. *Ir Med J.* 1983;76:253.

[7] Soifer L, et al. *Acta Gastroenterol Latinoam.* 1987;17(4):317–23.

[8] Dorworth T, et al. *ASHP Annual Meeting.* 1989 Jun;46:P-57D.

[9] Strommen G, et al. *Clin Pharm.* 1990 Mar;9:206–8.

[10] Spiller G, et al. *J Clin Pharmacol.* 1979 May-Jun;19:313–20.

[11] Spiller R. *Pharmacol Ther.* 1994;62(3):407–27.

[12] Hriscu A, et al. *Rev Med Chir Soc Med Nat Iasi.* 1990;94(1):165–70.

[13] Turnbull W, et al. *Int J Obes Rel Metab Dis.* 1995;19(5):338–42.

[14] Shub HA, et al. *Dis Colon Rectum.* 1978;21:582.

[15] Moesgaard F, et al. *Dis Colon Rectum.* 1982;25:454.

[16] Generali J. *US Pharmacist.* 1989 Feb;14:16, 20–21.

[17] Chan E, et al. *Ann Pharmacother.* 1995 Jun;29:625–27.

[18] Anderson J, et al. *Arch Int Med.* 1988 Feb;148:292–96.

[19] Danielsson A, et al. *Acta Hepatogastroenterol.* 1979;26:148.

[20] Bell L, et al. *JAMA.* 1989 Jun 16;261:3419–23.

[21] Sprecher D, et al. *Ann Int Med.* 1993 Oct 1;119:545–54.

[22] Spence J, et al. *Ann Intern Med.* 1995 Oct 1;123:493–99.

[23] Gelissen I, et al. *Am J Clin Nutr.* 1994;59(2):395–400.

[24] Dennison B, et al. *J Pediatr.* 1993 Jul;123:24–29.

[25] Gannon K. *Drug Topics.* 1989 Oct 2;133:24.

[26] Maksyutina N, et al. *Farmat Zhurnal.* 1978;33(4):56–61.

[27] Miettinen T, et al. *Clin Chim Acta.* 1989;183(3):253–62.

[28] Newall C, et al. *Herbal Medicines.* London, England: Pharmaceutical Press. 1996;210–11.

[29] Duckett S. *N Engl J Med.* 1980;303:583.

[30] Tosun F. *Hacettepe U Eczacilik Fakultesi Dergisi.* 1995;15(1):23–32.

[31] Frape D, et al. *Brit J Nutr.* 1995;73(5):733–51.

[32] Perlman B. *Lancet.* 1990 Feb 17;335:416.

[33] Etman M. *Drug Devel Indus Pharm.* 1995;21(16):1901–6.

[34] Baldo BA, et al. *Int Arch Allergy Appl Immunol.* 1982;68:295.

[35] Arlian L, et al. *J Allergy Clin Immunol.* 1992;89(4):866–76.

[36] Rosenberg S, et al. *Ann Allergy.* 1982;48:294.

[37] Mehta V, et al. *Int Arch Allergy Appl Immunol.* 1991;96(3):211–17.

[38] Wray M. ASHP Midyear Clinical Meeting. 1989 Dec;24:P-90D.

[39] Ford M, et al. *Hosp Pharm.* 1992 Dec;27:1061–62.

[40] Suhonen R, et al. *Allergy.* 1983;38:363.

[41] Lantner R, et al. *JAMA.* 1990;264:2534–36.

[42] Bardy J, et al. *Am Rev Respir Dis.* 1987;135(5):1033–38.

[43] Agha FP, et al. *Am J Gastroenterol.* 1984;79:319.

[44] Kamoda Y, et al. *Tokyo Ika Shika Daigaku Iyo Kizai Kenkyusho Hokoku.* 1989;23:81–85.

[45] Morton JF. *Major Medicinal Plants.* Springfield IL: C.C. Thomas, 1977.

SCIENTIFIC NAME(S): *P. americana* L., *P. decandra* L., *P. rigida*. Family: Phytolaccaceae

COMMON NAME(S): American nightshade, cancer jalap, cancerroot, chongras, coakum, pokeberry, crowberry, garget, inkberry, pigeonberry, poke, red ink plant, scoke, poke salad

---

❧❧❧ PATIENT INFORMATION ❧❧❧

Uses: Young pokeweed leaves may be eaten and the berries used for food, only after being cooked properly.

Side Effects: Ingestion of poisonous parts of the plant causes severe stomach cramping, nausea with persistent diarrhea and vomiting, slow and difficult breathing, weakness, spasms, hypotension, severe convulsions, and death.

Dosing: At doses of 1 g, dried pokeweed root is emetic and purgative. At lower doses of 60 to 100 mg/day, the root and berries have been used for rheumatism and for immune stimulation; however, there are no clinical trials that support these uses or doses.[1-3]

BOTANY: Pokeweed is a ubiquitous plant found in fields, along fences, in damp woods, and in other undisturbed areas. This vigorous shrub-like perennial can grow to 3.6 m. The reddish stem has large pointed leaves, which taper at both ends.[4] The flowers are numerous, small, and greenish white and develop into juicy purple berries that mature from July to September.

HISTORY: Folk uses of pokeweed leaves have included the treatment of chronic rheumatism and arthritis and use as an emetic and purgative.[5] The plant has been used to treat edema,[6] skin cancers, rheumatism, catarrh, dysmenorrhea, mumps, ringworm, scabies, tonsillitis, and syphilis. Poke greens, the young immature leaves, are canned and sold under the name "poke salet." Berry juice has been used as an ink, dye, and coloring in wine.[7]

PHARMACOLOGY: The plant's pharmacologic activity has not been well defined. Small doses of all parts of the plant can cause adverse reactions (see Toxicology), but the mechanisms of these actions are generally unknown.[8] Several anti-inflammatory saponins were isolated from the root;[9] however, the root has no known medicinal value.

TOXICOLOGY: Pokeweed poisonings were common in eastern North America during the 19th century, especially from the use of tinctures as antirheumatic preparations, and from eating berries and roots collected in error for parsnip, Jerusalem artichoke, or horseradish.[1]

All parts of pokeweed are toxic except the above-ground leaves that grow in the early spring. The poisonous principles are in highest concentration in the rootstock, less in the mature leaves and stems, and least in the fruits. Young leaves collected before acquiring a red color are edible if boiled for 5 minutes, rinsed, and reboiled. Berries are toxic when raw but are edible when cooked.

Ingestion of poisonous parts of the plant causes severe stomach cramping, nausea with persistent diarrhea and vomiting, slow and difficult breathing, weakness, spasms, hypotension, severe convulsions, and death.[10] Fewer than 10 uncooked berries are generally harmless to adults. Several investigators have reported deaths in children following the ingestion of uncooked berries or pokeberry juice.[10,11]

Severe poisonings have been reported in adults who ingested mature pokeweed leaves[12] and following the ingestion of a cup of tea brewed from ½ teaspoonful of powdered pokeroot.[1]

In addition, the CDC reported a case of toxicity in campers who ingested *properly* cooked young shoots. Sixteen of the 51 cases exhibited case-definitive symptoms (vomiting followed by any 3 of the following: nausea, diarrhea, stomach cramps, dizziness, headache). These symptoms persisted for up to 48 hours (mean, 24 hours).[13]

Poisoning also may occur when the toxic components enter the circulatory system through cuts and abrasions in the skin.

Symptoms of mild poisoning generally last 24 hours. In severe cases, gastric lavage, emesis, and symptomatic and supportive treatment have been suggested.[10]

In an attempt to curb potential poisonings from the use of this commercially available plant, the Herb Trade Association (HTA) formulated a policy stressing that the poke root is toxic and "should not be sold as an herbal beverage or food, or in any other form that could threaten the health of the uninformed consumer." Further, the HTA recommended that products containing pokeroot be labeled clearly as to their toxicity.[14]

The FDA classifies pokeweed as an herb of undefined safety that has demonstrated narcotic effects.

[1] Lewis WH, et al. *JAMA*. 1975;242:2759.
[2] Claus E, ed. *Pharmacognosy*. 3rd ed. Philadelphia, PA: Lea & Febiger; 1956.
[3] Gruenwald J, ed. *PDR for Herbal Medicines*. 2nd ed. Montvale, NJ: Thomson Medical Economics; 2000: 602-603.
[4] Dobelis I, ed. *Magic and Medicine of Plants*. Pleasantville, NY: Reader's Digest Association, Inc., 1986.
[5] Bianchini F, et al. *Health Plants of the World*. New York, NY: Newsweek Books, 1975.
[6] Kang S, et al. *J Nat Prod*. 1980;43:510.
[7] Duke J. *CRC Handbook of Medicinal Herbs*. Boca Raton, FL: CRC Press, 1985.
[8] Barker BE, et al. *Pediatrics*. 1966;38:490.
[9] Woo WS, et al. *Planta Med*. 1978;34:87.
[10] Hardin JW, et al. *Human Poisoning from Native and Cultivated Plants*, 2nd ed. Durham, NC: Duke University Press, 1974.
[11] *Med Lett Drugs Ther*. 1979;21:29.
[12] Stein ZLG. *Am J Hosp Pharm*. 1979;36:1303.
[13] Plant poisonings - New Jersey. *MMWR*. 1981;30:65.
[14] Herb Trade Association Policy Statement #2. May 1979.

SCIENTIFIC NAME(S): *Opuntia tuna mill* (tuna) and *Opuntia ficus-indica* (barbary fig, Indian fig). Other species include: *Opuntia fragilis* (brittle prickly pear), *Opuntia streptacantha*

COMMON NAME(S): Prickly pear, Nopal

⋆⋆⋆⋆ PATIENT INFORMATION ⋆⋆⋆⋆

Uses: Prickly pear has been used to treat wounds, gastrointestinal (GI) complaints, lipid disorders, and diabetes.

Side Effects: Dermatitis may be the most common side effect from prickly pear. *O. megacantha* has been shown to be nephrotoxic in rat studies. Side effects may include exacerbation of hypoglycemia if combined with oral hypoglycemic agents.

Dosing: Used primarily as a food, prickly pear was given as a treatment for diabetes in a single published clinical trial, with 30 capsules/day reported to be an unrealistic level for good compliance.[1]

BOTANY: Prickly pear is a perennial cactus native to tropical America and Mexico, preferring a dry habitat and rocky soil. It can grow to approximately 3 m high. The round stems (pads) have a thorny skin covered in spines. Prickly pear flowers are yellow. The oval, pear-shaped, purplish fruit has prickly outer skin with a sweet inner pulp.[2-5]

HISTORY: Prickly pear was used as a food source (conserves) and for alcoholic drinks in Mexico for hundreds of years. Native Americans applied the pads to wounds and bruises.[3,6]

PHARMACOLOGY:

Nutrition: Prickly pear fruit is nutritious.[3,7] The cactus pads are used in a variety of cooking preparations, including soups and salads. The taste has been compared with green beans or asparagus, with the sticky mucilage similar to okra.[6] Prickly pear fruit liquid was studied as a natural sweetener.[8]

Dermatologic effects: Prickly pear cactus flowers were used as an astringent for wounds and for their healing effects on the skin.[4] The cactus pads were used for medicinal purposes (mainly by Indian tribes in Mexico and the southwestern US) as a poultice for rash, sunburn, burns, insect bites, minor wounds, hemorrhoids, earaches, and asthmatic symptoms.[9]

GI effects: The pectins and mucilage from the plant are beneficial to the digestive system. The flowers are used for GI problems such as diarrhea, colitis, and irritable bowel syndrome.[3] *Opuntia* has been studied as a dietary fiber source.[10] *O. ficus-indica* species extracts exhibit protective effects on gastric mucosa and exert an anti-inflammatory action.[11]

Lipid effects: In capsule form, *Opuntia* had only a marginal beneficial effect on cholesterol and glucose levels.[12]

Hypoglycemic effects: *Opuntia* species have been studied for hypoglycemic effects.[13-15] Several reports specifically demonstrate *O. streptacantha* species as having hypoglycemic actions.[1,16-18]

Antiviral actions: One study reports *O. streptacantha* as having antiviral actions.[19]

TOXICOLOGY: Dermatitis from the plant was the most common toxicity found in current literature searches on prickly pear. A case report of cactus

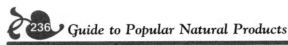

dermatitis in a 2-year-old child was described after contact with *O. microdasys*.[20] Two other patients were affected by this same species, both experiencing dermatitis, and one developing severe keratoconjunctivitis in the right eye.[21] A case of cactus granuloma in a 24-year-old male is described from contact with *O. bieglovii* thorns.[22] Granuloma formation also was seen from *O. acanthocarpa* spines embedded in the dermis, with onset occurring within several days and lasting several months. Treatment with topical corticosteroids is recommended.[23]

Side effects may include exacerbation of hypoglycemia if combined with oral hypoglycemic agents.

O. streptacantha is nontoxic in oral and IV preparations.[19]

[1] Frati-Munari A, et al. *Arch Invest Med (Mex)*. 1990;21(2):99-102.

[2] Hocking G. *A Dictionary of Natural Products*. Medford, NJ: Plexis Publishing, Inc., 1997:546-47.

[3] Chevallier A. *The Encyclopedia of Medicinal Plants*. New York, NY: DK Publishing, 1996:240.

[4] D'Amelio F. *Botanicals, A Phytocosmetic Desk Reference*. Boca Raton, FL: CRC Press, 1999:71.

[5] Ensminger A, et al. *Foods & Nutrition Encyclopedia*. Boca Raton, FL: CRC Press, 1994, 2nd ed, vol 2:1856.

[6] http://www.desertusa.com/magdec97/eating/nopales.html

[7] El Kossori R, et al. *Plant Foods Hum Nutr*. 1998;52(3):263-70.

[8] Saenz C, et al. *Plant Foods Hum Nutr*. 1998;52(2):141-49.

[9] http://www.arizonacactus.com/medicine.htm

[10] Rosado J, et al. *Rev Invest Clin*. 1995;47(4):283-99.

[11] Park E, et al. *Arch Pharm Res*. 1998;21(1):30-34.

[12] Frati Munari A, et al. *Gac Med Mex*. 1992;128(4):431-36.

[13] Roman-Ramos R, et al. *Arch Invest Med (Mex)*. 1991;22(1):87-93.

[14] Ibanez-Camacho R, et al. *Arch Invest Med (Mex)*. 1979;10(4):223-30.

[15] Frati-Munari A, et al. *Arch Invest Med (Mex)*. 1983;14(3):269-74.

[16] Frati A, et al. *Diabetes Care*. 1990;13(4):455-56.

[17] Frati A, et al. *Arch Invest Med (Mex)*. 1991;22(3-4):333-36.

[18] Roman-Ramos R, et al. *J Ethnopharmacol*. 1995;48(1):25-32.

[19] Ahmad A, et al. *Antiviral Res*. 1996;30(2-3):75-85.

[20] Vakilzadeh F, et al. *Z Hautkr*. 1981;56(19):1299-301.

[21] Whiting D, et al. *S Afr Med J*. 1975;49(35):1445-48.

[22] Suzuki H, et al. *J Dermatol*. 1993;20(7):424-7.

[23] Spoerke D, et al. *Vet Hum Toxicol*. 1991;33(4):342-44.

SCIENTIFIC NAME(S): *Portulaca oleracea* L. Family: Portulacaceae

COMMON NAME(S): Purslane, garden (common) purslane, pigweed, ma chi xian (Chinese), munyeroo, portulaca, "pusley"

ᘓᘓ PATIENT INFORMATION ᘓᘓ

Uses: Purslane is beneficial in urinary and digestive problems, has antifungal and antimicrobial effects, is high in vitamins and minerals, and has been used as a food source. It possesses marked antioxidant activity. These potential uses have not been verified by clinical studies.

Side Effects: Avoid use during pregnancy. Purslane is said to be safe, even in high dosages; however, individuals with a history of kidney stones should use purslane with caution.

Dosing: No dosing information is available on purslane. The leaves have been used widely as a potherb and, therefore, are known to be safe.

BOTANY: The purslane family includes several fleshy plants. *P. oleracea* is a herbaceous, succulent annual, cosmopolitan weed. Some consider it a weed because of its growth patterns. Purslane grows 10 to 30 cm tall and has reddish-brown stems, alternate wedge-shaped leaves, and clusters of yellow flowers containing 4 to 6 petals that bloom in summer. Its numerous seeds are black, shiny, and rough. The plant prefers sandy soil. The herb, juice, and seeds are mainly used. Golden purslane (*P. sativa*) is a similar, related species to purslane, with yellow leaves, but is a larger plant and is not weedy.[1-7]

HISTORY: In ancient times, purslane was considered one of the antimagic herbs used to protect against evil spirits.[6] Purslane's use as a medicinal herb dates back at least 2000 years, but it was used as food well before this period. Ancient Romans used purslane to treat dysentery, intestinal worms, headache, and stomachache.[2,3,6] The Zulu used the plant as an emetic.[6] Purslane was part of the Australian aborigines' diet as a salad green. The Chinese, French, Italians, and English also used purslane in salads. A folk use of purslane includes reducing fever.[5]

PHARMACOLOGY: Purslane is a versatile herb and has several culinary uses including "cooked greens" much like spinach or collards.[5] Its nutritive quality, especially the rich source of omega-3 fatty acids purslane provides, has a beneficial effect on cholesterol and triglyceride levels, in heart disease, and in strengthening the immune system.[3,4] Purslane is also high in vitamin and mineral content.[3] The plant possesses marked antioxidant activity.[8]

Purslane is valued in the treatment of urinary and digestive problems. The juice has diuretic effects.[2] Purslane is also considered to be a "cooling aid" and cleansing stimulant of the kidneys, helpful in the bladder for urinary tract infection.[3,6]

The plant's mucilagenous properties make it useful in GI problems.[2] Purslane, placed in animal feed, prevents diarrhea as well as provides immunostimulation in a report.[9] Other sources mention purslane as effective in treating hookworms and amoebic dysentery.[2,4] Besides having vermicidal properties, purslane has been reported to possess antifungal effects, with marked activity against the genus Trichophyton.[10] The phenolic constituents of the plant exhibit antimicrobial effects.[11] Purslane in a combination mouthwash also demonstrated antimicrobial as well as anti-inflammatory effects.[12] Skin conditions such as acne, psoriasis, or sunburn may benefit from purslane.[2] Other uses of the plant include the following: a poultice for backache/dysmenorrhea;[1] neuropharmacological actions;[13] and in cosmetics as a gamma-linolenic acid (GLA) source.[5]

TOXICOLOGY: Purslane is said to be safe, even in high dosages, as it is eaten as a vegetable.[4] Individuals with a history of kidney stones should use purslane with caution as it may increase kidney filtration, urine production, and possibly cause a stone to move.[6] Purslane injection induces powerful contractions of the uterus, but oral purslane is said to weaken uterine contractions. Avoid use during pregnancy.[2]

[1] Hocking, G. *A Dictionary of Natural Products.* Medford, NJ: Plexus Publishing, Inc., 1997;625.

[2] Chevallier, A. *The Encyclopedia of Medicinal Plants.* New York, NY: DK Publishing, 1996;253.

[3] Low T, Rodd T, eds. *Magic and Medicine of Plants.* Surry Hills, NSW: Reader's Digest, 1994;282.

[4] Reid, D. *Chinese Herbal Medicine.* Boston, MA: Shambhala Publications, Inc., 1986;56.

[5] D'Amelio, F. *Botanicals, A Phytocosmetic Desk Reference.* Boca Raton, FL: CRC Press, 1999;245-46.

[6] http://www.ann.com.au/herbs/Monographs/portulac.htm

[7] http://www.botanical.com/botanical/mgmh/p/prugol77.html

[8] Shang S, et al. *Tianran Chanwu Yanjiu Yu Kaifa.* 1994;6(1):36-39.

[9] Kato S, et al. *Jpn Kokai Tokkyo Koho.* 1994; appl. # JP 92-315865 19921030.

[10] Oh K, et al. *Phytother Res.* 2000;14(5):329-32.

[11] Awad N. *Bull Fac Pharm.* 1994;32(1):137-42.

[12] Wu W. *Faming Zhuanli Shenqing Gongkai Shuomingshu.* 1995; Chinese patent, appl. # CN 93-11712 19930908.

[13] Radhakrishnan R, et al. *J Pharm Pharmacol.* 1998;50(suppl. British Pharm. Conf. 1998):225.

۬۰۰۰ PATIENT INFORMATION ۰۰۰۰

Uses: Pycnogenol may provide chemoprotective actions and protect against Alzheimer disease. Pycnogenol is said to help with the treatment of attention deficit hyperactivity disorder (ADHD). Because the effectiveness, safety, and toxicity of pycnogenol for these disorders have not been tested adequately in clinical trials, contact your health care professional before discontinuing or adding to conventional ADHD or Alzheimer medications.[1]

Side Effects: Some children taking pycnogenol for ADHD became irritable and showed decreased energy.

SOURCE: The name "pycnogenol" is, in itself, a source of confusion. In product literature, this term is a trademark of a British company for a proprietary mixture of water-soluble bioflavonoids, derived from the bark of the European coastal pine, *Pinus maritima* (also known as *P. nigra* var. *maritima*, a widely planted variety of pine in Europe).

However, the term "pycnogenol" also has been assigned to a group of flavonoids termed the flavan-3-ol derivatives.[2] Numerous plants have been found to be sources for the class of compounds generally termed the flavonoids, and the chemical condensation of flavonoid precursors results in the formation of compounds known as condensed tannins. The broader term, bioflavonoid, has been used to designate those flavonoids with biologic activity.

HISTORY: Pycnogenol is available commercially OTC in the US in health food stores and pharmacies. Product literature indicates that pycnogenol, when taken as a dietary supplement, is a powerful free radical scavenger. The compound may improve circulation, reduce inflammation, and protect collagen from natural degradation. Pycnogenol has been available in Europe for some time, where it is taken as a supplement or incorporated into topical "anti-aging" creams.

PHARMACOLOGY: Pycnogenol is a mixture of bioflavonoids designated proanthocyanidins. A US patent for this material describes a mixture of proanthocyanidins that are effective in combating the deleterious effects of free radicals. The compound is said to assist in the treatment of hypoxia following atherosclerosis, cardiac or cerebral infarction, and to reduce tumor promotion, inflammation, ischemia, alterations of synovial fluid, and collagen degradation.[3]

An important property of flavonoid-containing mixtures in the modulation of nitric oxide (NO) metabolism is inflammation action, which may help explain the biological activity of pycnogenol in human conditions associated either with oxidative stress or dysfunction of NO production.[4,5] Neuropathological features of Alzheimer disease include intracellular neurofibrillary tangles and an amino acid residue peptide identified as amyloid β-protein.

Several studies have been conducted to evaluate the pharmacologic activity of pycnogenol. In 1 study, daily oral doses of pycnogenol were given for 30 days to patients with a variety of peripheral circulatory disorders. Pain, limb heaviness, and feeling of swelling decreased during therapy in most patients.[6] Similar results have been reported by other investigators.[7]

Results of a study comparing the response of human breast cancer cells (MCF-7) and normal human mammary cells (MCF-10) to apoptosis in the presence of pycnogenol suggest that pycnogenol selectively induced death in MCF-7 and not in MCF-10 cells. Further research is needed to evaluate the therapeutic value of pycnogenol as a chemoprotective agent.[8]

Another US patent for pycnogenol describes a method of inhibiting platelet aggregation with an agent that is able to normalize and enhance platelet reactivity without adversely affecting the bleeding time.[9] This was based on a study conducted in a group of smokers who were given a single dose of 100 to 120 mg pycnogenol or 500 mg aspirin. In this study, pycnogenol rapidly reduced smoking-induced platelet aggregation without increased bleeding.[10]

Another US patent was issued for a regimen and composition for treating ADHD by the use of proanthocyanidin with and without a heterocyclic antide-pressant and a citrus bioflavonoid.[11] A letter to the editor describes the treatment of over 100 patients with ADHD, using nutritional supplements similar to pycnogenol.[12] The author found that the most important improvements noted by patients were in the areas relating to sustained attention and distractibility.[12] A case report showed that a 10-year-old patient with ADHD demonstrated improvement when treated with pycnogenol.[13] In most cases of children with ADHD, the common practice is to combine pycnogenol with dextroamphetamine (eg, *Dexedrine*).[14]

TOXICOLOGY: No clinically important reports of adverse effects from pycnogenol have been published. Some children treated for ADHD with pycnogenol became irritable and showed decreased energy.[12]

[1] Chan E, et al. *Contemporary Ped Archive.* 2000.

[2] Masquelier J, et al. *Int J Vitam Nutr Res.* 1979;49:307.

[3] US Patent & Trademark Office. United States Patent #4,698,360.

[4] Packer L, et al. Abstract from the 1998 Oxygen Club of California World Congress.

[5] Fitzpatrick D, et al. *J Cardiovasc Pharmacol.* 1998;32:509-15.

[6] Sarrat L. *Bordeaux Medical.* 1981;14:685.

[7] Mollmann H, et al. *Therapiewoche.* 1983;33:4967.

[8] Huynh H, et al. *Anticancer Res.* 2000;20:2417-20.

[9] US Patent & Trademark Office. United States Patent #5,720,956.

[10] Putter M, et al. *Thrombosis Res.* 1999;95(4):155-61.

[11] US Patent & Trademark Office. United States Patent #5,719,178.

[12] Greenblatt J. *J Am Acad Child Adolesc Psychiatry.* 1999;38(10):1209-10.

[13] Heimann S. *J Am Acad Child Adolesc Psychiatry.* 1999;38(4):357-8.

[14] American Herbal Products Association. *American Herbal Products Association Botanical Safety Handbook.* CRC Press: Boca Raton, FL, 1997:41.

SCIENTIFIC NAME(S): Quassia is a collective term for 2 herbs: *Picrasma excelsa* and *Quassia amara* L. Family: Simaroubaceae.

COMMON NAME(S): Bitter wood, picrasma, Jamaican quassia (*Picrasma excelsa*), Surinam quassia (*Quassia amara*), Amara species, Amargo, Surinam wood, and ruda.

≈≈≈ PATIENT INFORMATION ≈≈≈

Uses: Quassia has a variety of uses including treatment for measles, diarrhea, fever, and lice. Quassia has antibacterial, antifungal, antifertility, antitumor, antileukemic, and insecticidal actions as well.

Drug Interactions: Quassia may interact with anticoagulants (eg, warfarin).

Side Effects: Quassia is used in a number of food products and is considered to be safe by the FDA. If taken in large doses, this product can irritate the gastrointestinal (GI) tract and cause vomiting. It is not recommended for women who are pregnant.

Dosing: Quassia wood has been used as a bitter tonic, with a typical oral dose of 500 mg of the wood. No recent studies have been performed to rationalize this dose. Several recent studies of topical quassia tincture for head lice have been reported.

BOTANY: Surinam quassia is a 2- to 5-m tall shrub or small tree native to northern South America, specifically Guyana, Colombia, Panama, and Argentina. Jamaican quassia is a taller tree, reaching 25 m, native to the Caribbean Islands, Jamaica, West Indies, and northern Venezuela. The pale yellow wood parts are used medicinally. Leaves also are used.[1-3]

HISTORY: Quassia has been used for malaria in the Amazon. It also has been used topically for measles, and orally or rectally for intestinal parasites, diarrhea, and fever. The plants, at one time, were also used as anthelmintics and insecticides. Central Americans have been known to build boxes to store clothing out of the quassia wood, which acts as a natural repellent.[1,3,4]

PHARMACOLOGY: Quassia has been used as an insecticide. Traditional use includes remedies for infestations of lice or worms, anorexia, and dyspepsia.[3] Certain tribes have used the plants for measles, fever, and as a mouthwash.[5-7]

Quassin, the extracts and purified mixtures of bitter principles of quassia, demonstrates antilarval activity, being effective at concentrations of 6 ppm.[8] A mechanism of this larvicidal activity may be caused by inhibition of cuticle development, as suggested in one report.[9] Quassia, as a tincture, has been used to successfully treat head lice in 454 patients. Canthin-6-1 possesses antibacterial and antifungal activity.[3]

Quassin have been used to give a bitter taste to various food products, especially alcoholic (eg, liqueurs, bitters) and nonalcoholic beverages, desserts, candy, baked goods, and puddings.[10]

TOXICOLOGY: Quassia is listed as generally regarded as safe (GRAS) by the FDA. No side effects were reported upon topical application of the scalp preparation in the 454 patients in the head lice study.[3] Large amounts, however, have been known to irritate the mucus membrane in the stomach and may lead to vomiting.[1] Excessive use may also interfere with existing cardiac and anticoagulant regimens. Because of the plant's cytotoxic and emetic properties, avoid its use during pregnancy.[3] Parenteral administration of quassin is toxic, leading to cardiac problems, tremors, and paralysis.[1]

[1] Bisset NG. *Herbal Drugs and Phytopharmaceuticals*. Stuttgart: CRC Press, 1994;400-1.

[2] Schulz V, et al. *Rational Phytotherapy*. Berlin: Springer, 1998;171.

[3] Newall CA, et al. *Herbal Medicines*. London: Pharmaceutical Press, 1996;223-4.

[4] Duke JA. *CRC Handbook of Medicinal Herbs*. Boca Raton, FL: CRC Press, Inc., 1989;399.

[5] Rutter R. *Catalogo de Plantas Utiles de la Amazonia Peruana*. Yarinacocha, Peru: Instituto Linguistico de Verano, 1990.

[6] Branch L, et al. *Folk Medicine of Alter do Chao*. Para, Brazil: Acta Amazonica 1983; 13(5/6):737-97.

[7] Duke JA, et al. *Amazonian Ethnobotanical Dictionary*. Boca Raton, FL: CRC Press, Inc., 1994.

[8] Evans DA, et al. *Indian J Med Res*. 1991; 93:324-7.

[9] Evans D, et al. *Indian J Biochem Biosphys*. 1992; 29(4):360-63.

[10] Raji Y, et al. *Life Sci*. 1997; 61(11):1067-74

SCIENTIFIC NAME(S): *Rubus idaeus* L. and *Rubus strigosus* Michx. Family: Rosaceae (roses)

COMMON NAME(S): Red raspberry

ᘯᘖᘯᘖ PATIENT INFORMATION ᘯᘖᘯᘖ

Uses: Raspberry leaves may be helpful for diarrhea or as a mouthwash because of their astringent action. They have been used historically in painful or profuse menstruation and in regulating labor pains during childbirth, but there is little evidence to support this use.

Side Effects: There is no evidence that raspberry leaf tea is toxic.

Dosing: Typical doses of raspberry leaf as a tea are 1.5 to 2.4 g/day. A clinical trial has been conducted to define its safety in labor.[1]

BOTANY: The cultivated red raspberries *R. idaeus* (Eurasian) or *R. strigosus* (North American, also known as *R. idaeus* var. *strigosus*) are 2 of many *Rubus* species worldwide. While the berries are cultivated as food items, it is the leaves that have been used medicinally. Raspberries grow as brambles with thorny canes bearing 3-toothed leaflets and stalked white flowers with 5 petals. The red berries detach easily from its cores when ripe. While some species of *Rubus* primarily reproduce clonally and commercial red raspberries are propagated as clones, DNA fingerprinting has indicated that wild *R. idaeus* populations exhibit substantial genetic diversity.[2]

HISTORY: The leaves of red raspberry were used for its astringent properties to treat diarrhea in the 19th century. A strong tea of raspberry leaves was used in painful or profuse menstruation and to regulate labor pains in childbirth.[3] The Eclectics used a decoction of the leaves to suppress nausea and vomiting. A gargle of raspberry leaf infusion has been used for sore throats and mouths and to wash wounds and ulcers.[4]

PHARMACOLOGY: The tannin components of the leaves have a definite astringent action,[5] which may be helpful in diarrhea or as a mouthwash; however, there is little pharmacologic evidence at present to support the use of raspberry leaf tea in pregnancy, menstruation, or childbirth.

TOXICOLOGY: There is no evidence that raspberry leaf tea is toxic.

A raspberry leaf monograph is included in the *British Herbal Pharmacopeia*, vol. 2.[6] It is listed as unapproved in the *German Commission E Monographs*.[7]

[1] Simpson M, et al. *J Midwifery Womens Health.* 2001;46:51-59.

[2] Antonius K, et al. *Mol Ecol.* 1994;3(2):177.

[3] Erichsen-Brown C. *Medicinal and Other Uses of North American Plants.*. Dover, NY. 1989:471-73.

[4] Grieve M. *A Modern Herbal.* London, England: Jonathan Cape, 1931:671-72.

[5] Haslam E, et al. *Planta Med.* 1989;55:1.

[6] *British Herbal Pharmacopoeia.* Bournemouth, Dorset: British Herbal Medicine Association, 1990.

[7] Blumenthal M, et al. *The Complete German Commission E Monographs.* Austin, TX: American Botanical Council, 1998.

Red Clover

SCIENTIFIC NAME(S): *Trifolium pratense* Family: Leguminosae

COMMON NAME(S): Cow clover, meadow clover, purple clover, trefoil

❧❧❧ PATIENT INFORMATION ❧❧❧

Uses: Red clover has been used in hormone replacement therapy and arterial compliance, and as a chemoprotective and expectorant.

Drug Interactions: Isoflavonoid properties may interfere with hormonal therapies. Do not take red clover with oral contraceptives, estrogen, progesterone compounds, anticoagulants, or aspirin.

Side Effects: Do not take during pregnancy, lactation, or in patients with a history of breast cancer. Avoid large doses. Coumarin activity may be problematic at high doses.

Dosing: Formerly used as a sedative at doses of 4 g of blossoms, red clover is now used primarily as a source of estrogenic and antioxidant isoflavones. Extracts standardized on isoflavone content (*Menoflavon, Rimostil*) have been given to perimenopausal women in several clinical studies at daily doses of 25 to 90 mg of isoflavones.[1-3]

BOTANY: The plant's medicinal value is found in its red and purple fragrant blossoms, dried for utilization. It is a perennial that flowers for a short duration. Several hairy-looking stems grow 0.3 to 0.6 m high from a single base. The leaves are ovate, nearly smooth, and end in a long point; the center is usually lighter in color. It is found most commonly in meadows of a light sandy nature in Britain and throughout Europe and Asia from the Mediterranean to the Arctic Circle. It also has been found in the mountains. Red clover is now naturalized in North America and Australia for hay and as a nitrogen-fixing crop.[4]

HISTORY: The flowers possess antispasmodic, estrogenic, and expectorant properties. Chinese medicine has used red clover in teas as an expectorant. Russians recommend the herb for bronchial asthma. Traditionally, the herb has been used in treating breast cancer.[5] Topically, it is used to accelerate wound healing and to treat psoriasis.[6] Research has indicated increased compliance of arterial vessels. In Australia, *Promensil* has been marketed for hormone replacement and *Trinivin* for benign prostatic hyperplasia.[7]

PHARMACOLOGY:

Hormone replacement: Isoflavones mimic estrogen effects in the body.[8] If an estrogen supplement is given, it binds to intracellular receptors and acts as an agonist to natural estrogen. Through negative feedback, production of GnRH, FSH, and LH is stopped, resulting in cessation of the production of estrogen.

Arterial compliance: In a placebo-controlled study of 17 women, arterial compliance, an index of elasticity of large arteries (eg, thoracic aorta) in which compliance diminishes with age and menopause, increased by 23% when 40 mg of red clover was given for 5 weeks followed by 80 mg for 5 more weeks. The hormonal effects of the isoflavonoids aid in arterial compliance, because arterial compliance decreases in postmenopausal women.[9]

Chemoprotective: Biochanin A, a composite of isoflavones, has been reported to inhibit carcinogenic activity in cell cultures.[10]

Expectorant: Saponins act as surfactants, reducing the surface tension in the lungs and creating a larger surface area for mucus to leave the bronchial tubes.[11]

INTERACTIONS: Isoflavonoids may interfere with hormonal therapies. Do not take red clover with oral contraceptives, estrogen, or progesterone compounds. Its coumarin effects may enhance anticoagulation. If possible, avoid red clover in patients receiving an anticoagulant or aspirin. If concurrent therapy is unavoidable, closely monitor prothrombin time or the International Normalized Ratio (INR).

TOXICOLOGY: Avoid doses greater than 40 to 80 mg daily. Do not take during pregnancy or lactation. Coumarin activity may also be problematic at high doses.[4]

Avoid use in patients with a history of breast cancer.

[1] Kelly G, et al. Standardized red clover extract clinical monograph. Seattle, WA: Natural Products Research Consultants; 1998.

[2] Clifton-Bligh PB, et al. *Menopause.* 2001;8:259-265.

[3] Hale GE, et al. *Menopause.* 2001;8:338-346.

[4] http://botanical.com/botanical/mgmh/c/clovrd75.html.

[5] Chevallier, A. *The Encyclopedia of Medicinal Plants.* NY, NY: DK Publishing Inc., 1996.

[6] Duke, James. *CRC Handbook of Medicinal Herbs.* Boca Raton, FL: CRC Press, Inc., 1985.

[7] http://www.healthcentral.com.

[8] Zava D, et al. *Proc Soc Exp Biol Med.* 1998 Mar;217(3):369-78.

[9] Nestel P, et al. *J Endocrinol Metab.* 1999 Mar;84(3):895-8.

[10] Newall C, et al. *Herbal Medicines.* London, Eng: The Pharmaceutical Press, 1996.

[11] http://bewell.com/vit/herb155.asp.

Reishi Mushroom

SCIENTIFIC NAME(S): *Ganoderma lucidum* (Leysser ex Fr.) Karst. Family: Polyporaceae

COMMON NAME(S): Reishi, ling chih, ling zhi, "spirit plant"

❧❧❧ PATIENT INFORMATION ❧❧❧

Uses: Reishi is high in polysaccharide content, which may be for anticancer and immunostimulatory effects. It also may have liver protectant actions, beneficial effects on the cardiovascular system, antiviral actions, and other effects.

Drug Interactions: Do not take with anticoagulants.

Side Effects: Side effects are mild and may include dizziness, gastrointestinal (GI) upset, or irritated skin. Do not use reishi with pregnant or lactating women.

Dosing: The effective dose for reishi has not been well established by human clinical trials, although a wide variety of animal studies have been carried out. A dose of 6 to 12 g/day of powdered fungus has been recommended.[1]

BOTANY: The reishi mushroom is a purplish-brown fungus with a long stalk and fan-shaped cap. It has a shiny, "varnish"-coated appearance, with spores resembling brown powder that can sometimes be seen. The reishi grows on decaying wood or tree stumps. It prefers the Japanese plum tree but also grows on oak. The fruiting body is the part of the plant used for medicinal purposes. This mushroom grows in China, Japan, and North America and is cultivated throughout other Asian countries. Cultivation of reishi is a long, complicated process. The reishi grows in 6 colors, each having its own characteristics: *Aoshiba* (blue reishi), *Akashiba* (red reishi), *Kishiba* (yellow reishi), *Shiroshiba* (white reishi), *Kuroshiba* (black reishi), and *Murasakishiba* (purple reishi).[2]

HISTORY: Reishi has been used in traditional Chinese medicine for over 4000 years to treat problems such as fatigue, asthma, cough, and liver ailments, and to promote longevity.[2] The Chinese name *ling zhi* means "herb of spiritual potency."[2] A Japanese name for the reishi is *mannentake*, meaning "10,000-year-old mushroom." Reishi's use is documented in what is said to be the oldest Chinese medical text, which is over 2000 years old. This book contains information on about 400 medicines but lists the reishi as the most superior.[3] Cultivation of reishi began in the 1980s.[4]

PHARMACOLOGY:

Anticancer immunostimulant effects:
Older texts mention reishi's immunostimulatory and anticancer effects.[3] Modern research confirms these indications, attributing the polysaccharide components to be responsible for these properties. Polysaccharides beta-d-glucan and GL-1 have been found to inhibit sarcoma.[5] Reishi has been shown to be of benefit in myeloblastic leukemia and nasopharyngeal carcinoma in combination with other chemotherapeutic agents, demonstrating tumor shrinkage, significant changes in hemoglobin counts, and overall quality-of-life markers.[4] In another report, extract of reishi shows radioprotective ability and protective ability against hydroxyl radical-induced DNA strand breaks.[6] Reishi has demonstrated positive effects on cytokine release from human macrophages and T-lymphocytes, confirming its role in immunopotentiation.[7] Reishi's antican-

cer properties are almost certainly "host-mediated" through stimulation of the immune system.

Hepatitis: The reishi mushroom also has been beneficial in the treatment of hepatitis.[7] Another report shows improvement in 92% of 355 hepatitis patients taking reishi.[8]

Cardiovascular effects: Positive effects on the cardiovascular system have been demonstrated by reishi. Decreases in high blood pressure have been affected by the ganoderic acids.[2,4] ACE-inhibiting triterpenes from reishi have been discussed.[9] The risk of coronary artery disease also may be decreased by reishi, which was found to decrease platelet adhesion.[2] In one report, ganodermic acid was found to exert inhibitory effects on platelets, leading to decreased thromboxane formation.[10] Reduction of cholesterol from reishi has been addressed, including decreases in triglycerides and LDL.[2]

Antiviral effects: Certain polysaccharides isolated from reishi have been proven effective against herpes simplex virus types 1 and 2.[11] Certain reishi isolates also have been tested against other viral strains including influenza A and demonstrated effectiveness against their growth.[12]

Other effects: There are numerous claims for reishi (some unconfirmed) including the following: treatment of diabetic ulcers,[4] altitude sickness,[2] and headaches.[4]

TOXICOLOGY:

Side effects: Side effects from reishi may include dizziness, dry mouth, stomach upset, nose bleed, sore bones, irritated skin, diarrhea, or constipation from initial use, which may disappear with continued use or may develop from use over 3 to 6 months.[2] Because reishi may increase bleeding time, it is not recommended for use with anticoagulants. Pregnant or lactating women should consider these issues and consult a doctor before taking reishi.[2]

[1] *American Herbal Pharmacopeia.* Santa Cruz, CA: American Herbal Pharmacopeia; 2000.

[2] Lininger S, et al, eds. *The Natural Pharmacy.* Rocklin, CA: Prima Publishing, 1998;303-04.

[3] Matsumoto, K. *The Mysterious Reishi Mushroom.* Santa Barbara, CA: Woodbridge Press Publishing, 1979.

[4] http://www.kyotan.com/lectures/lectures/lecture6.html.

[5] Miyazaki T, et al. *Chem Pharma Bull.* (Tokyo) 1981;29:3611-16.

[6] Kim K, et al. *Int J Mol Med.* 1999;4(3):273-77.

[7] Wang S, et al. In: Program and Abstracts of the 1994 International Symposium on Ganoderm Research.

[8] Chang H, et al. *Pharmacology and Applications of Chinese Materia Medica.* Vol. 1 Singapore: World Scientific, 1986.

[9] Morigiwa A, et al. *Chem Pharm Bull.* (Tokyo) 1986;34:3025-28.

[10] Su C, et al. *Biochem Pharmacol.* 1999;58(4):587-95.

[11] Eo S, et al. *J Ethnopharmacol.* 1999;68(1-3):175-81.

[12] Eo S, et al. *J Ethnopharmacol.* 1999;68(1-3):129-36.

SCIENTIFIC NAME(S): *Rosmarinus officinalis* L. Family: Labiatae or Lamiaceae. Bog rosemary (*Andromeda* species) and wild or marsh rosemary (*Ledum palustre* L.) are members of the family Ericaceae and are not related to rosemary.

COMMON NAME(S): Rosemary, Old Man

❧❧❧❧ PATIENT INFORMATION ❧❧❧❧

Uses: Rosemary has decreased capillary permeability and fragility, and extracts have been used in insect repellents. The plant may have anticancer properties.

Side Effects: Ingestion of large quantities of rosemary can result in stomach and intestinal irritation and kidney damage.

Dosing: Rosemary leaf was approved for dyspepsia, high blood pressure, and rheumatism by the German Commission E at doses of 4 to 6 g/day. The essential oil has been used at doses of 0.1 to 1 mL.[1]

BOTANY: Rosemary grows as a small evergreen shrub with thick aromatic leaves.[2] The plant has small pale blue flowers that bloom in late winter and early spring.[3,4] Although rosemary is native to the Mediterranean, it is now cultivated worldwide.

HISTORY: Rosemary is a widely used culinary herb. Tradition holds that rosemary will grow only in gardens of households where the "mistress" is truly the "master."[5] The plant has been used in traditional medicine for its astringent, tonic, carminative, antispasmodic, and diaphoretic properties. Extracts and the volatile oil have been used to promote menstrual flow and as abortifacients.[5,6] Rosemary extracts are commonly cosmetic ingredients, and a rosemary lotion is said to stimulate hair growth and prevent baldness.[7]

PHARMACOLOGY: The clinical value of rosemary is difficult to establish because of the lack of studies. Diosmin, the flavonoid pigment in the leaves, has been reported to decrease capillary permeability and fragility.[5] Rosemary extracts are reported to have antioxidant properties comparable to those of butylated hydroxytoluene and butylated hydroxy-anisole. Carnosic acid and labiatic acid are reported to be the active compounds.[2] The plant may have anticancer properties.[3] Extracts have been used as insect repellents.[3]

TOXICOLOGY: Although the oil is used safely as a flavoring and the whole leaves are used as a potherb, ingestion of large quantities of the oil can be associated with toxicity.[8] Toxicity is characterized by stomach and intestinal irritation and kidney damage.[4] There is no valid role for rosemary oil as an abortifacient. Bath preparations containing the oil may cause erythema, and toiletries can cause dermatitis in sensitive individuals.[7]

[1] Blumenthal M, Brinckmann J, Goldberg A, eds. *Herbal Medicine: Expanded Commission E Monographs.* Newton, MA: Integrative Medicine Communications; 2000.

[2] Leung AY. *Encyclopedia of Common Natural Ingredients Used in Food, Drugs and Cosmetics.* New York, NY: John Wiley and Sons, 1980.

[3] Simon JE. *Herbs: An Indexed Bibliography, 1971-1980.* Hamden, CT: Shoe String Press, 1984.

[4] Osol A, et al, eds. *The Dispensatory of the United States of America,* 25th ed. Philadelphia, PA: JB Lippincott, 1955.

[5] Tyler VE. *The New Honest Herbal.* Philadelphia, PA: G.F. Stickley Co., 1987.

[6] Dobelis IN, ed. *Magic and Medicine of Plants.* Pleasantville, NY: Reader's Digest, 1986.

[7] Duke JA. *Handbook of Medicinal Herbs.* Boca Raton, FL: CRC Press, 1985.

[8] Spoerke DG. *Herbal Medications.* Santa Barbara, CA: Woodbridge Press, 1980.

Sage

SCIENTIFIC NAME(S): *Salvia officinalis* L. (Dalmatian sage), *S. lavandulaefolia* Vahl. (Spanish sage). Family: Labiatae or Lamiaceae

COMMON NAME(S): Garden sage, true sage, scarlet sage, meadow sage

---

ꤍꤍꤍ PATIENT INFORMATION ꤍꤍꤍ

Uses: Sage has no proven medical effects but may be antispasmodic and carminative.

Side Effects: The only side effects reported with the ingestion of sage include cheilitis, stomatitis, dry mouth, or local irritation.

Dosing: Sage leaves, apart from their culinary uses, have been recommended for dyspepsia, excessive sweating, and as a gargle in coughs and colds. Typical dosage is 4 to 6 g/day of the leaf.[1]

BOTANY: Sage is a small, evergreen perennial plant with short woody stems that branch extensively and can attain heights of 0.6 to 0.9 m.[2] Its violet-blue flowers bloom from June to September. The plant is native to the Mediterranean region and grows throughout much of the world. Do not confuse the plant with red sage or the brush sage of the desert.

HISTORY: Dried sage leaf is used as a culinary spice and as a source of sage oil, which is obtained by steam distillation. Traditionally, sage and its oil have been used for the treatment of a wide range of illnesses; the name *Salvia* derives from the Latin word meaning "healthy" or "to heal."[3,4] Extracts and teas have been used to treat digestive disorders, as a tonic, and as an antispasmodic. The plant has been used topically as an antiseptic and astringent and to manage excessive sweating.[5] Sage has been used internally as a tea for the treatment of dysmenorrhea, diarrhea, gastritis, and sore throat. The dried leaves have been smoked to treat asthma. Despite these varied uses, there is little evidence that the plant exerts any significant pharmacologic activity. The plant's fragrance is said to suppress fish odor. Sage oil is used as a fragrance in soaps and perfumes. It is a widely used food flavoring, and sage oleoresin is also used in the culinary industry.

PHARMACOLOGY: Sage extracts have strong antioxidative activities, with labiatic acid and carnosic acid reported to be the active compounds.[2] The phenolic acid salvin and its monomethyl ether found in sage have antimicrobial activity, especially against *Staphylococcus aureus*.[2] There is some evidence that sage oil may exert a centrally mediated antisecretory action; the carminative effect likely is because of the irritating effects of the volatile oil.[6]

TOXICOLOGY: Although sage oil contains thujone, the oil does not have a reputation for toxicity. The oil is nonirritating and nonsensitizing when applied topically to human skin in diluted concentrations.[2] Cheilitis and stomatitis have been reported in some cases following sage tea ingestion.[5] Others have reported that ingestion of large amounts of the plant extract may cause dry mouth or local irritation.

---

[1] Blumenthal M, Brinckmann J, Goldberg A, eds. *Herbal Medicine: Expanded Commission E Monographs*. Newton, MA: Integrative Medicine Communications; 2000.

[2] Leung AY. *Encyclopedia of Common Natural Ingredients Used in Food, Drugs, and Cosmetics*. New York, NY: John Wiley and Sons, 1980.

[3] Dobelis IN, ed. *Magic and Medicine of Plants*. Pleasantville, NY: Reader's Digest Association, Inc., 1986.

[4] Simon JE. *Herbs: an indexed bibliography*, 1971-1980. Hamden, CT: Shoe String Press, 1984.

[5] Duke, JA. *Handbook of Medicinal Herbs*. Boca Raton, FL: CRC Press, 1985.

[6] Spoerke DG, Jr. *Herbal Medications*. Santa Barbara, CA: Woodbridge Press, 1980.

SAMe

SCIENTIFIC NAME(S): *S-adenosylmethionine, S-adenosyl-L-methionine, ademetionine, ademetionine 1,4-butanedisulfonate, ADE-SD4.*

COMMON NAME(S): SAMe, SAM

♦♦♦♦ PATIENT INFORMATION ♦♦♦♦

Uses: SAMe has been used in the treatment of depressive disorders, osteoarthritis, fibromyalgia, liver disorders, migraine headaches, and for sleep modulation.

Side Effects: Other than occasional nausea and gastrointestinal disturbances, no side effects have been reported. Bipolar disorder patients should not use SAMe.

Dosing: SAMe has been studied in clinical trials for depression and Parkinsonism at oral doses of 800 to 3600 mg/day. It has been administered IV in a fibromyalgia trial at 600 mg/day.[1,2,3]

BOTANY: SAMe is found in all living cells. It is a naturally occurring molecule produced by a reaction between the amino acid methionine and ATP. SAMe acts as a substrate in many biological reactions and is the precursor of certain essential amino acids.[4,5] The commercial product is not a botanical, but a supplement or biochemical compound produced in yeast cell cultures. One manufacturing process describes its preparation through fermentation of yeast *Saccharomyces cerevisiae,* enriched by the Schlenk method in the presence of methionine.[4]

HISTORY: SAMe was discovered in Italy in 1952. Since that time, numerous clinical studies have been performed on its efficacy.[6] SAMe has been used in Europe, where it has been available by prescription since 1975, to treat arthritis and depression. It is available in the US as a supplement by several companies (eg, Natural Made, Pharmavite, GNC).[5,6]

PHARMACOLOGY: The properties of SAMe have been studied in a variety of areas including the CNS, osteoarthritis, fibromyalgia, liver disorders, and others.

CNS: SAMe's uses in depressive disorders were first seen in the early 1970s. Shortcomings from trials around this time (varied dosages of SAMe, small number of patients enrolled, severity of depression variation, etc) eventually led to improvement in consistency, specifically the Hamilton rating scale, grouping similar patients.[7]

Studies indicate the importance of the methylation process in the brain. SAMe is known to be an important methyl donor for a wide range of substrates (eg, proteins, lipids, hormones, nucleic acids). SAMe has shown some value in psychiatry, particularly in depressive disorders. A meta-analysis of all studies comparing SAMe with either placebo or standard tricyclic antidepressants has shown SAMe to have greater efficacy than placebo and efficacy comparable to that of tricyclics.[8] An adequate supply of SAMe must be attained for normal CNS function. Vitamin B_{12} or folate deficiency decreases the levels of SAMe, which lowers serotonin levels associated with depression.[9] Low SAMe levels in the cerebrospinal fluid (CSF) of patients with neurological and psychiatric disorders (eg, Alzheimer disease, spinal cord degeneration, HIV-type neuropathies) suggest that supplementation with this compound may be beneficial in treating these disorders.[10,11] Similarly, increased plasma concentrations of SAMe were associated with mood improvement in depressed patients.[12] In another report, disruption of methylation by low SAMe levels was found to cause structural and functional abnormalities including myelopathy and depression.[13] Nerve regeneration requires the presence of SAMe.[14]

These findings support the hypothesis that in the CNS, SAMe has modulating effects on mood, with adequate amounts needed to maintain normal mood and remission of symptoms in patients with major depressive disorders. Dosage ranges for depression have been reported as 400 mg 3 to 4 times daily. If nausea and GI upset occur, the dosage can be tapered.[5]

Osteoarthritis: SAMe appears to enhance native proteoglycan synthesis and secretion in chondrocyte cultures in the cartilage of patients with osteoarthritis.[15] It possesses analgesic properties similar to NSAIDs but with no or minimal GI side effects.[16]

Clinical trials involved a total of greater than 21,000 patients who received SAMe treatment, 458 patients who were given different NSAIDs (ibuprofen, indomethacin, naproxen, and piroxicam), and 279 who received placebo. The periods of treatment ranged from 3 weeks to 2 years. These controlled clinical trials demonstrated that SAMe improved subjective and objective symptoms of osteoarthritis more than placebo and showed the same efficacy as the NSAIDs.[4,17,18] Maintenance dosage of SAMe for osteoarthritis is 200 mg twice daily.[5]

Fibromyalgia: Fibromyalgia is a disorder that is a common cause of chronic musculoskeletal pain and fatigue. At least 3 clinical trials found SAMe to be beneficial. Subjects given 200 mg SAMe per day parenterally demonstrated reductions in certain trigger points and painful areas, as well as mood improvements. The other reports confirmed SAMe's benefits in pain relief, morning stiffness, and mood enhancement.[5]

Liver disorders: Through methylation, SAMe regulates liver cell membrane lipid composition and fluidity, and by activation of the transsulfuration pathway, promotes endogenous detoxification processes in the liver. Further, it is the main source of glutathione, a major compound involved in several detoxification reactions in this organ.[19] SAMe restores normal hepatic function in conditions such as cirrhosis and cholestasis and aids in reversing hepatotoxicity.[7] Its liver-protectant actions are apparent in experimentation where high concentrations of SAMe were associated with reduced liver injury.[20-24] SAMe can be considered an important nutrient in alcoholic subjects.[25]

Others: Other beneficial effects of SAMe include treatment of migraine headaches (200 to 400 mg twice daily),[26] alteration of the aging process,[27-29] and sleep modulation.[30]

TOXICOLOGY: Other than occasional nausea and GI disturbances, no side effects, drug interactions, or disease contraindications have been found in recent literature reviews. Patients with bipolar disorder should not take SAMe, as it may lead to the manic phase.[5] In a field trial involving greater than 20,000 patients, the overall withdrawal rate caused by adverse effects was about 5%, mainly during the first 2 weeks of treatment when the oral dose of SAMe was the highest (800 to 1200 mg daily).[7]

Toxicological studies of SAMe by parenteral and oral administration performed in different animal species recommended and commonly utilized in preclinical research labs included mutagenicity and carcinogenicity studies. They concluded that SAMe is completely safe even at the highest dosages.[4]

1 Di Rocco A, et al. *Mov Disord.* 2000;15:1225-1229.

2 Salmaggi P, et al. *Psychother Psychosom.* 1993;59:34-40.

3 Volkmann H, et al. *Scand J Rheumatol.* 1997;26:206-211.

4 *Am J Med* 1987;Nov 20:83(5A):1-110.

5 Murry M. *Encyclopedia of Nutritional Supplements.* Rocklin, CA: Prima Publ., 1996;365-73.

6 http://www.mothernature.com/articles/sam-e/about_sam-e.stm.

7 *Drugs* 1989;38(3):390-416.

8 Bressa G. *Acta Neurol Scand.* 1994(Suppl. 154):7-14.

9 Young S. *J Psychiatry Neurosci.* 1993;18(5):235-44.

10 Bottigueri T, et al. *Acta Neurol Scand.* 1994(Suppl. 154):19-26.

11 Lesley D, et al. *J Neurochem.* 1999;67(3):1328.

12 Bell K, et al. *Acta Neurol Scand.* 1994;(Suppl. 154):15-18.

13 Scott J, et al. *Acta Neurol Scand.* 1994;(Suppl. 154):27-31.

14 Cestaro B. *Acta Neurol Scand.* 1994;(Suppl. 154):32-41.

15 Harmand, et al. *Am J Med.* 1987;83(5A):48-54.

16 Di Padova C. *Am J Med.* 1987;83(5A):60-65.

17 Montrone F, et al. *Clin Rheumatol.* 1985;4:484-85.

18 Caruso I, et al. *Am J Med.* 1987;83(5A):66-71.

19 Kaplowitz N. *Yale J Biol Med.* 1981;54:407-502.

20 Shivapurkar N, et al. *Carcinogenesis.* 1982;3(5):589-91.

21 Poirier L. *Adv Exp Med Biol.* 1986;206:269-82.

22 Barak A, et al. *Alcohol Clin Exp Res.* 1993;17(3):552-55.

23 Dausch J, et al. *Nutr Cancer.* 1993;20(1):31-39.

24 Barak A, et al. *Alcohol.* 1994;11(6):501-03.

25 Chawla R, et al. *Drug Invest.* 1992;4(4):41-45.

26 Gatto G, et al. *Int J Clin Pharmacol Res.* 1986;6:15-17.

27 Baldessarini R, et al. *J Neurochem.* 1966;13;769-77.

28 Stramentinoli G, et al. *J Gerontology.* 1977;32(4):392-94.

29 Bohuon C, et al. *Clinica Chimica Acta.* 1971;33:256.

30 Stramentinoli G. *Scandinavica.* 1994;(Suppl. 154), vol. 59:5-41.

SCIENTIFIC NAME(S): *Smilax* species including *Smilax aristolochiifolia* Mill. (Mexican sarsaparilla), *S. officinalis* Kunth (Honduras sarsaparilla), *Smilax regelii* Killip et Morton (Honduras, Jamaican sarsaparilla), *Smilax febrifuga* (Ecuadorian sarsaparilla), *Smilax sarsaparilla*, *Smilax ornata*. Family: Liliaceae

COMMON NAME(S): Sarsaparilla, smilax, smilace, sarsa, khao yen

---

⋘ PATIENT INFORMATION ⋙

Uses: Sarsaparilla has been used for treating syphilis, leprosy, psoriasis, and other ailments.

Side Effects: No major contraindications, warnings, or side effects have been documented; avoid excessive ingestion. In unusually high doses, the plant possibly could be harmful, including gastrointestinal (GI) irritation.

Dosing: Typical doses of sarsaparilla for a variety of uses range from 0.3 to 2 g/day of the powdered root.[1,2]

BOTANY: Sarsaparilla is a woody, trailing vine that can grow to 50 m in length. It is grown in Mexico, Honduras, Jamaica, and Ecuador. Many *Smilax* species are similar in appearance regardless of origin. The part of the plant used for medicinal purposes is the root. Although this root has a pleasant fragrance and spicy sweet taste, and has been used as a natural flavoring agent in medicines, foods, and nonalcoholic beverages.[3,4]

HISTORY: The French physician Monardes described using sarsaparilla to treat syphilis in 1574. In 1812, Portuguese soldiers suffering from syphilis recovered faster if sarsaparilla was taken to treat the disease vs mercury, the standard treatment at the time.[5] Sarsaparilla has been used by many cultures for ailments including skin problems, arthritis, fever, digestive disorders, leprosy, and cancer.[3,5] Late 15th century accounts explaining the identification and the first descriptions of American drugs include sarsaparilla.[6] Sarsaparilla's role as a medicinal plant in American and European remedies in the 16th century is also evident.[7]

PHARMACOLOGY: Sarsaparilla has been used for treating syphilis and other sexually transmitted diseases (STDs) throughout the world for 40 years and was documented as an adjuvant for leprosy treatment in 1959.[8]

The ability of sarsaparilla to bind to endotoxins may be a probable mechanism of action as to how the plant exerts its effects. Problems associated with high endotoxin levels circulating in the blood stream such as liver disease, psoriasis, fevers, and inflammatory processes, all seem to improve with sarsaparilla.[5]

Antibiotic actions of sarsaparilla also are seen but are probably secondary to its endotoxin-binding effects.[5] Antibiotic properties of the plant[3] are shown by its treatment of leprosy and its actions against leptosirosis, a rare disease transmitted by rats.[9]

Other positive effects of sarsaparilla on the skin have been demonstrated. The endotoxin-binding sarsaponin from the plant has improved psoriasis in 62% of patients and has completely cleared the disease in 18%.[10] Antidermatophyte activity from the species *S. regelii* has been demonstrated in a later report.[11] In addition, sarsaparilla has been used as an herbal or folk remedy for other skin conditions including eczema, pruritus, rashes, and wound care.[4,9]

Sarsaparilla's anti-inflammatory actions are useful for treating arthritis, rheumatism, and gout.[5,7] *S. sarsaparilla* inhibited carrageenan-induced paw inflammation in rats, as well as cotton pellet-induced exudation.[12]

Advertising claims of sarsaparilla being a "rich source of testosterone," are unsubstantiated as there is no testosterone present in the plant.[5] However, some sources state that sarsaparilla exhibits testosterogenic actions on the body, increasing muscle bulk and estrogenic actions as well to help alleviate female problems. In Mexico, the root is used for its alleged aphrodisiac properties.[9] A recent review addresses *Smilax* compounds (among others) present in bodybuilding supplements said to "enhance performance." Results of the study of over 600 commercial supplements determined that there was no research to validate these claims.[13]

Other documented uses of sarsaparilla include the following: improvement in appetite and digestion,[3] adaptogenic effects from *S. regelii*,[14] sarsaparilla in combination as an herbal remedy and mineral supplement,[15] and haemolytic

activity of steroidic saponins from *S. officinalis*.[16] An overview of medicinal uses of sarsaparilla is available.[17] One report evaluating fracture healing finds sarsaparilla to have insignificant effects on tensile strength and collagen deposition.[18] Other species of smilax have been evaluated for antimutagenic actions (*S. china*)[19] and GI disorders (*S. lundelii*).[20] The species *S. glabra* exhibits wormicidal effects,[21] improves hepatitis B in combination,[22] had marked therapeutic effects (in combination) in the treatment of intestinal metaplasia and atypical hyperplasia,[23] and has hepatoprotective effects.[24]

TOXICOLOGY: No major contraindications, warnings, or toxicity data have been documented with sarsaparilla use. No known problems exist regarding its use in pregnancy or lactation either; however, avoid excessive ingestion.[3] In unusually high doses, the saponins present in the plant could possibly be harmful, resulting in GI irritation.[4] The fact that sarsaparilla binds bacterial endotoxins in the gut, making them unabsorbable, greatly reduces stress on the liver and other organs.[5]

One report describing occupational asthma caused by sarsaparilla root dust exists in the literature.[25]

[1] Claus E, ed. *Pharmacognosy*, 3rd ed. Philadelphia, PA: Lea & Febiger; 1956.
[2] Gruenwald J, ed. *PDR for Herbal Medicines*, 2nd ed. Montvale, NJ: Thomson Medical Economics; 2000: 661-662.
[3] Newall C, et al. *Herbal Medicines*. London, England: Pharmaceutical Press, 1996;233-34.
[4] Duke J. *CRC Handbook of Medicinal Herbs*. Boca Raton, FL: CRC Press, Inc., 1989;446.
[5] Murray M. *The Healing Power of Herbs*, 2nd ed. Rocklin, CA: Prima Publishing, 1995;302-5.
[6] Estes J. *Pharmacy in History*. 1995;37(1):3-23.
[7] Elferink J. *Pharmaceutica Acta Helvitiae*. 1979;54(9-10):299-302.
[8] Rollier R. *Int J Leprosy*. 1959;27:328-40.
[9] Chevallier A. *Encyclopedia of Medicinal Plants*. New York, NY: DK Publishing 1996;268.
[10] Thurman F. *New Engl J Med*. 1942;227:128-33.
[11] Caceres A, et al. *J Ethnopharmcol*. 1991 Mar;31(3):263-76.
[12] Ageel A, et al. *Drugs Exp Clin Res*. 1989;15(8):369-72.
[13] Grunewald K, et al. *Sports Med*. 1993;15(2):90-103.
[14] Di Pasquale M. *Drugs in Sports*. 1993 Feb;2:2-4.
[15] Hamlin T. *Matol. Can J Hosp Pharm*. 1991;44(1):39-40.
[16] Santos W, et al. *Vaccine*. 1997;15(9):1024-29.
[17] Osborne F, et al. *Can Pharm J*. 1996 Jun;129:48-51.
[18] Ahsan S, et al. *Int J Crude Drug Res*. 1989 Dec;27:235-39.
[19] Lee H, et al. *Mutat Res*. 1988;204(2):229-34.
[20] Caceres A, et al. *J Ethnopharmacol*. 1990;30(1):55-73.

[21] Rhee J, et al. *Am J Chin Med.* 1981;9(4):277-84.

[22] Chen Z. *Chung Hsi I chieh Ho Tsa Chih.* 1990;10(2):71-74, 67.

[23] Liu X, et al. *Chung Kuo Chung Hsi I chieh Ho Tsa Chih.* 1992;12(10):602-3, 580.

[24] Chen T, et al. *Planta Med.* 1999;65(1):56-59.

[25] Vandenplas O, et al. *J Allergy Clin Immunol.* 1996;97(6):1416-18.

Sassafras

SCIENTIFIC NAME(S): *Sassafras albidum* (Nuttal) Nees, synonymous with *S. officinale* Nees et Erbem. and *S. variifolium* Kuntze. Family: Lauraceae

COMMON NAME(S): Sassafras, saxifras, ague tree, cinnamon wood, saloop

---

❧❧❧ PATIENT INFORMATION ❧❧❧

Uses: Sassafras has been used for eye inflammation, insect bites and stings, lice, rheumatism, gout, sprains, swelling, and cutaneous lesions but is now banned in the US, even for use as a flavoring or fragrance.

Side Effects: Besides containing a cancer-causing agent, sassafras can induce vomiting, stupor, and hallucinations. It can also cause abortion, diaphoresis, and dermatitis.

Dosing: Sassafras root bark has been used as an aromatic and carminative at doses of 10 g; however, the carcinogenicity of its constituent safrole has limited its use.[1]

BOTANY: Sassafras is the name applied to 3 species of trees: 2 native to eastern Asia and 1 native to eastern North America. Fossils show that sassafras was once widespread in Europe, North America, and Greenland. The trees grow up to about 30 m in height and 1.8 m in diameter, though they are usually smaller. Sassafras bears leaves 10 to 15 cm long that are oval on older branches but mitten-shaped or three-lobed on younger shoots and twigs. All parts of the tree are strongly aromatic. The drug is obtained by peeling the root (root bark).[2]

HISTORY: American Indians have used sassafras for centuries and told early settlers that it would cure a variety of ills. The settlers exported it to Europe, where it was found to be ineffective.[3]

Over the years, the oil from the roots and wood has been used as a scent in perfumes and soaps. The leaves and pith, when dried and powdered, have been used as a thickener in soups. The roots are often dried and steeped for tea, and sassafras was formerly used as a flavoring in root beer. Its use as a drug or food product has been banned by the FDA as carcinogenic; however, its use and sale persist throughout the US.

Medicinally, sassafras has been applied to insect bites and stings to relieve symptoms.[4]

PHARMACOLOGY: Sassafras has been used as an agent to induce sweating,[4] a flavoring agent for dentifrices, root beers, and tobaccos, and for treatment of eye inflammation.[5] Extracts of the root and bark have been found to mimic insect juvenile hormone in *Oncopeltus fasciatus*.[6] The oil has been applied externally for relief of insect bites and stings and for lice. Other external uses include treatment of rheumatism, gout, sprains, swelling, and cutaneous eruptions.[5,6]

The plant has been reported to have antineoplastic activity[8] and to induce cytochrome P488 and P450 enzymes.[7] Sassafras is said to antagonize certain alcohol effects.[5]

TOXICOLOGY: Sassafras oil and safrole have been banned for use as flavors and food additives by the FDA because of their carcinogenic potential. Based on animal data and a margin-of-safety factor of 100, a dose of 0.66 mg safrole per kg body weight is considered hazardous for humans; the dose obtained from sassafras tea may be as high as 200 mg (3 mg/kg).[2,9] One study showed that even a safrole-free extract produced malignant mesenchymal tumors in more than 50% of black rats treated. These tumors corresponded to malignant fibrous histiocytomas in humans.[10]

Oil of sassafras is toxic in doses as small as 5 mL in adults.[11] Ingestion of 5 mL produced shakes, vomiting, high blood pressure and high pulse rate in a 47-year-old female.[12] Another case of a 1 tsp dose of sassafras oil in a young man also caused vomiting, along with dilated pupils, stupor, and collapse.[5] There have been additional reports of the oil causing death,[7] abortion,[5] and liver cancer.[2,5,7] Safrole is a potent

inhibitor of liver microsome hydroxylating enzymes; this effect may result in toxicity caused by altered drug metabolism.[10] Symptoms of sassafras oil poisoning in humans may include vomiting, stupor, lowering of body temperature, exhaustion, tachycardia, spasm, hallucinations, paralysis, and collapse.[2,7]

Additionally, sassafras can cause diaphoresis[13] and contact dermatitis in certain individuals.[4] A case study reported oil of sassafras in combination as a teething preparation, which resulted in false-positive blood tests for diphenylhydantoin in a 4-month-old child.[14]

[1] Kapadia GJ, et al. *J Natl Cancer Inst.* 1978;60:683-686.

[2] Bisset N. *Herbal Drugs and Phytopharmaceuticals.* Stuttgart, Germany: CRC Press, 1994;455–56.

[3] Winter R. *The People's Handbook of Allergies and Allergens.* Chicago, IL: Contemporary Books, 1984.

[4] *Merck Index,* 10th ed. Rahway, NJ: Merck and Co. 1983.

[5] Duke J. *CRC Handbook of Medicinal Herbs.* CRC Press:Boca Raton, FL. 1989;430-31.

[6] Jacobson M, et al. *Lloydia.* 1975;38:455.

[7] Newall C, et al. *Herbal Medicine.* London, England: Pharmaceutical Press, 1996;235-36.

[8] Hartwell JL. *Lloydia.* 1969;32:247.

[9] Segelman AB. *JAMA.* 1976;236:477.

[10] Benedetti MS, et al. *Toxicology.* 1977;7:69.

[11] Spoerke DG. *Herbal Medications.* Santa Barbara, CA: Woodridge Press Publishing Co. 1980.

[12] Grande G, et al. *Vet Hum Toxicol.* 1987 Dec;29:447.

[13] Haines J. *Postgrad Med.* 1991;90(4):75-76.

[14] Jones M, et al. *Am J Dis Child.* 1971 Sep;122:259-60.

Saw Palmetto

SCIENTIFIC NAME(S): *Serenoa repens* (Bartram) Small. Also referred to as *Sabal serrulata* (Michx.) Nicholson or *Sabal serrulatum* Schult. Family: Palmae (Palms)

COMMON NAME(S): Saw palmetto, sabal, American dwarf palm tree, cabbage palm, fan palm, scrub palm

---

≈≈≈≈ PATIENT INFORMATION ≈≈≈≈

Uses: Saw palmetto is used to treat symptoms of benign prostatic hyperplasia, including reduction of urinary frequency, increase of urinary flow, and decrease of nocturia. Saw palmetto may delay the need for prostate surgery.

Drug Interactions: May interact with hormones, including oral contraceptives, and hormone replacement therapy.

Side Effects: Saw palmetto is generally well tolerated, with occasional reports of adverse gastrointestinal (GI) effects; do not use in pregnancy.

Dosing: The crude saw palmetto berries usually are administered at 1 to 2 g/day; however, lipophilic extracts standardized to 85% to 95% fatty acids in soft native extract or 25% fatty acids in a dry extract are more common. Some of the brand name products include *Permixon* (Pierre Fabre Medicament), *Prostaserene* (Indena) SCF extract, *Prostagutt* (WS 1473, Schwabe), *Remigeron* (Schaper & Brummer), *IDS 89* (Strathmann AG), *Quanterra Prostate* (Warner Lambert), and *LG 166/S* (Lab. Guidotti). Typical doses of standardized extracts range from 100 to 400 mg given twice daily for benign prostatic hypertrophy.[1,2,3,4,5,6]

BOTANY: The saw palmetto is a low, scrubby palm that grows in the coastal plain of Florida and other southeastern states. Its fan-shaped leaves have sharp saw-toothed edges that give the plant its name. Dense clumps of saw palmetto can form an impenetrable thicket. The abundant 2 cm long berries are harvested from the wild in the fall and are dried for medicinal use. They also serve as a source of nutrition for deer, bears, and wild pigs.[7]

HISTORY: Native tribes of Florida relied on saw palmetto berries for food; however, Europeans often found the taste of the berries objectionable.[7] While native medicinal use of saw palmetto is not recorded, it was introduced into Western medical practice in the 1870s and was a favorite of Eclectic medical practitioners for prostate and other urologic conditions. Saw palmetto berries were official in the US Pharmacopeia in

1906 and 1916, and in the National Formulary from 1926 to 1950. While use in the US declined after that time, saw palmetto has long been a staple phytomedicine in Europe. Recent interest has been rekindled, and saw palmetto is currently ranked in the top 10 herbal products in the US.[8] It is primarily used for its activity in benign prostatic hyperplasia (BPH).

PHARMACOLOGY:

BPH: Saw palmetto's mechanism of action in suppressing the symptoms of BPH is poorly understood. The leading hypothesis involves the inhibition of testosterone 5-alpha reductase, an enzyme that converts testosterone to 5-alpha-testosterone in the prostate. Hexane extracts of saw palmetto were found to inhibit the enzyme from human foreskin fibroblasts, while they had no direct effect on androgen receptor binding.[9] Serum levels of dihydrotestosterone

(DHT) were reduced markedly by the synthetic drug finasteride, but not by saw palmetto.[10]

Further studies using both known 5-alpha reductase isozymes found that finasteride inhibited only type 1 reductase, while saw palmetto inhibited formation of all testosterone metabolites in both cultured prostate epithelial cells and fibroblasts.[11] A different saw palmetto extract, IDS 89, dose dependently inhibited 5-alpha reductase in both the stroma and epithelium of human BPH tissue. This inhibition was related to the free fatty acids present in the extract.[12] Studies in a coculture model of human prostate epithelial cells and fibroblasts found that saw palmetto inhibited both type 1 and type 2 isoforms of 5-alpha reductase without altering the secretion of prostate-specific antigen.[13] Structure-activity studies of pure fatty acid inhibition of steroid 5-alpha reductase have found gamma-linolenic acid to be the most potent and specific inhibitor of the enzyme.[14] It is possible that the C_{18} monounsaturated fatty oleic acid found in saw palmetto is partly responsible for the observed effects on 5-alpha reductase, though more extensive analysis of saw palmetto fatty acids is required.

There is less support for other hormonal mechanisms. One study found 5-alpha reductase inhibition and inhibition of DHT binding to androgen receptors,[15] and another study demonstrated inhibition of DHT and testosterone receptor binding.[16] Administration of saw palmetto extract over 30 days led to no changes in plasma levels of testosterone, follicle stimulating hormone, or luteinizing hormone.[1] In the prostate cancer line LNCaP, saw palmetto induced a mixed proliferative/differentiative effect that was not seen in the nonhormone-responsive PC3 prostate cancer cell line.[17] Treatment of patients for 3 months with saw palmetto preceding prostatectomy caused a reduction in DHT levels in BPH tissue along with a corresponding rise in testosterone levels. A marked reduction in epidermal growth factor concentration was also observed in the periurethral region of the prostate.[18]

Although the mechanism of action of saw palmetto is not completely understood, clinical trials in BPH have shown convincing evidence of moderate efficacy. A 6-month, double-blind, head-to-head study vs finasteride in 1098 men found equivalent efficacy and a better side effect profile for saw palmetto.[19] Likewise, a 3-year study of IDS 89 in 435 BPH patients found clear superiority to placebo in reduction of BPH symptoms.[20] A 1-year study of 132 patients comparing 2 dose levels of saw palmetto demonstrated efficacy in symptom reduction but little difference between dose levels.[3] The general consensus has been that saw palmetto extracts reduce BPH symptoms without reducing prostate size, therefore delaying surgical intervention.[21] A meta-analysis that included a total of 18 clinical trials in BPH concluded that saw palmetto was better tolerated than finasteride and equivalent in efficacy.[22] A clinical trial in BPH of the saw palmetto constituent beta-sitosterol showed similar efficacy to that seen with saw palmetto itself.[23]

Other observations of saw palmetto extracts include shown by others to be noncompetitive in nature[24] and interference with 5-lipoxygenase metabolites in neutrophils.[25]

INTERACTIONS: Because of possible antiandrogen and antiestrogenic activity, avoid taking with any hormone therapy including oral contraceptive and hormone replacement therapy. Saw palmetto also has shown immunostimulant and anti-inflammatory activity; hence, watch for patients taking drugs that may increase or decrease these effects. For reproducible effects, it is recommended that the fat-soluble saw palmetto extracts standardized to contain 85% to 95% fatty acids and sterols be taken at the recommended dosage of 160 mg twice daily. Effects occur in 4 to 6 weeks. There have been no demonstrated effect on serum prostate-specific antigen levels.

TOXICOLOGY: Saw palmetto products are generally well tolerated, with occasional reports of adverse GI effects. Its antiandrogenic activity suggests that it should not be used in pregnancy.

[1] Casarosa C, et al. *Clin Ther.* 1988;10:585-88.

[2] Di Silverio F, et al. *Prostate.* 1998;37:77-83.

[3] Braeckman J, et al. *Phytother Res.* 1997;11:558.

[4] Gerber GS, et al. *Urology.* 1998;51:1003-1007.

[5] Marks LS, et al. *J Urol.* 2000;163:1451-1456.

[6] Redecker W. *Extracta Urol.* 1998;21:24-26.

[7] Bennett B, et al. *Econ Bot.* 1998;52:381.

[8] Winston, D. *Saw Palmetto for Men & Women.* Pownal, VT: Storey Books, 1999.

[9] Düker E, et al. *Planta Med.* 1989;55:587.

[10] Strauch G, et al. *Eur Urol.* 1994;26:247-52.

[11] Délos S, et al. *J Steroid Biochem Mol Biol.* 1995;55:375.

[12] Weisser H, et al. *Prostate.* 1996;28:300-06.

[13] Bayne C, et al. *Prostate.* 1999;40:232-46.

[14] Liang T, et al. *Biochem.* J 1992;285:557-62.

[15] Sultan C, et al. *J Steroid Biochem.* 1984;20:515-19.

[16] el-Sheikh M, et al. *Acta Obstet Gynecol Scand.* 1988;67:397-99.

[17] Ravenna L, et al. *Prostate.* 1996;29:219-30.

[18] Gutiérrez M, et al. *Planta Med.* 1996;62:507-11.

[19] Carraro J, et al. *Prostate.* 1996;29:231-40.

[20] Bach D, et al. *Phytomedicine.* 1996;3:105.

[21] Marandola P, et al. *Fitoterapia.* 1997;68:195.

[22] Wilt T, et al. *JAMA.* 1998;280:1604–09.

[23] Berges R, et al. *Lancet.* 1995;345:1529-32.

[24] Goepel M, et al. *Prostate.* 1999;38:208-15.

[25] Paubert-Braquet M, et al. *Prostaglandins Leukot Essent Fatty Acids.* 1997;57:299-304.

SCIENTIFIC NAME(S): *Schisandra chinensis* Baillon, *S. arisanensis* Hayata, *S. sphenanthera* Rehd, *S. rubriflora* Franch. Family: Schizandraceae

COMMON NAME(S): Schisandra, schizandra, gomishi, hoku-gomishi, kita-gomishi (Japanese); wu-wei-zu (Chinese)

ᴀᴀᴀᴀ PATIENT INFORMATION ᴀᴀᴀᴀ

Uses: Schisandra has been used as a tonic and restorative, as well as for liver protection, nervous system effects, respiratory treatment, and gastrointestinal therapy.

Side Effects: Research indicates that side effects are infrequent, although schisandra has the ability to produce profound central nervous system depression and may interfere with the metabolism of other concurrently administered drugs.

Dosing: Schisandra fruit is used as an adaptogen at doses of 1.5 to 6 g/day. A standardized extract containing 3.4% schisandrin has been used in a clinical trial for improved athletic performance at 91 mg/day of extract.[1,2]

BOTANY: The family Schizandraceae (Schisandraceae) comprises 2 genera (*Schisandra* and *Kadsura*). *Schisandra* spp are climbing, aromatic trees with white, pink, yellow, or reddish male or female flowers. The fruits are globular and red with several kidney-shaped seeds. The fruit is harvested in autumn when fully ripened.[3] *S. chinensis* is native to northeastern and north central China and is found in eastern Russia.

HISTORY: Schisandra is one of the many traditional Chinese medicines that are recommended for coughs and various nonspecific pulmonary diseases.[4] It has been studied extensively in Chinese and Japanese literature. Schisandra had been used for healing purposes for more than 2000 years. It is often used as an ethanolic tincture. The Chinese name for the plant, "wu-wei-zu," means "5-flavored herb" because of the flavor of the 5 main "elemental energies" of the plant. The fruit has a salty, sour taste.[3]

PHARMACOLOGY: Besides serving as a tonic and restorative, schisandra has other reported uses, such as liver protection, nervous system effects, res-

piratory treatment, GI therapy, adaptogenic properties, and others.

Liver: The lignan components in schisandra possess definite liver protectant effects. The active principles appear to be lignans such as wu-wei-zu C, shisantherin D, deoxygomisin A, gomisin N, and gomisin C. Active hepatoprotective constituents all appear to share 1 or 2 methylene dioxy group.[4,5] Animal studies on gomisin A offer convincing evidence of liver protection, including protective actions against halothane-induced hepatitis,[6] carbon tetrachloride, d-galactosamine, and dl-ethionine toxicity,[7,8] hepatic failure induced by bacteria,[9] and preneoplastic hepatic lesions.[10-13] Gomisin A's mechanism for tumor inhibition may be a result of its ability to improve bile acid metabolism.[14]

Nervous System: Schisandra is a nervous system stimulant, increasing reflex responses and improving mental alertness. In China, the berries are used to treat mental illnesses such as depression. It is also used for irritability and memory loss.[3] There is a possible use in treating age-related memory deficits in humans.[15] Schisandra (also in combination with *Zizyphus spinosa* and *Angelica sinensis*) has accelerated neurocyte growth and may prevent atrophy of neurocyte process branches.[16]

Schisandra has been evaluated for its inhibitory effects on the CNS as well. In Chinese medicine, it is used as a sedative for insomnia.[3] This inhibition mechanism has been evaluated and may be related to effects on dopaminergic receptors.[17]

Respiratory: Schisandra is used to treat respiratory ailments such as shortness of breath, wheezing, and cough.[3]

GI: Experiments show that it increases the activity of glutathione S-transferase. In the intestine, schisandra shifts BaP metabolism in favor of diols and 3-hydroxybenzopyrene and away from BaP- 4,5-epoxide and the mutagenic BaP quinones. Schisandra does not increase intestinal cytochrome P450 activity.[18] Schisandra has been used for treatment of diarrhea and dysentery.[3]

One report found schisandra extract to have no significant effects on gastric secretory volume, gastric pH, and acid output.[19] Metabolism of schisandra has been reported.[20-22] It has been used to balance fluid levels, improve sexual stamina, treat rashes, stimulate uterine contractions, and improve failing senses.[3] One report found antibacterial effects in alcohol and acetone extracts of the fruit.[5]

TOXICOLOGY: Schisandra has the capability to produce profound CNS depression. Because of its documented effects on hepatic and gastric enzyme activity, it is possible that schisandra may interfere with the metabolism of other concurrently administered drugs. The full spectrum of the clinical effects of the plant on the liver are not well documented, and the safety of the plant has not been established scientifically. However, research does not report any incidence of toxic side effects.

[1] Panossian AG, et al. *Phytomed.* 1999;6:17-26.
[2] *American Herbal Pharmacopeia.* Santa Cruz, CA: American Herbal Pharmacopeia; 1999.
[3] Chevallier A. *Encyclopedia of Medicinal Plants.* New York, NY: DK Publishing, 1996.
[4] Hikino H, et al. *Planta Med.* 1984;50:213.
[5] Maeda S, et al. *Yakugaku Zasshi.* 1982;102(6):579–88.
[6] Jiaxiang N, et al. *J Appl Toxicol.* 1993;13(6):385-88.
[7] Ko K, et al. *Planta Med.* 1995;61(2):134-37.
[8] Takeda S, et al. *Nippon Yakurigaku Zasshi.* 1986;87(2):169-87.
[9] Mizoguchi Y, et al. *Planta Med.* 1991;57(4):320-24.
[10] Nomura M, et al. *Cancer Lett.* 1994;76(1):11-18.
[11] Ohtaki Y, et al. *Biol Pharm Bull.* 1994;17(6):808-14.
[12] Nomura M, et al. *Anticancer Res.* 1994;14(5A):1967-71.

[13] Miyamoto K, et al. *Biol Pharm Bull.* 1995;18(10):1443-45.
[14] Ohtaki Y, et al. *Anticancer Res.* 1996;16(2):751-55.
[15] Nishiyama N, et al. *Biol Pharm Bull.* 1996;19(3):388-93.
[16] Hu G, etal. *Chin Pharm J.* 1994 Jun;29:333-36.
[17] Zhang L, et al. *Chung Kuo I Hsueh Ko Hsueh Yuan Hsueh Pao.* 1991;13(1):13-16.
[18] Salbe AD, et al. *Food Chem Toxicol.* 1985;23:57.
[19] Hernandez D, et al. *J Ethnopharmacol.* 1988 May/Jun;23:109-14.
[20] Hendrich S, et al. *Food Chem Toxicol.* 1936;24(9):903-12.
[21] Chi Y, et al. *Yao Hsueh Hsueh Pao.* 1992;27(1):57-63.
[22] Chi Y, et al. *Eur J Drug Metab Pharmacokinet.* 1993;18(2):155-60.

SCIENTIFIC NAME(S): *Scutellaria laterifolia* L. Family: Labiatae

COMMON NAME(S): Scullcap, skullcap, helmetflower, hoodwort, mad-dog weed

---

❧❧❧ PATIENT INFORMATION ❧❧❧

Uses: Scullcap is not recognized as having therapeutic activity although recent studies suggest that it might have anti-inflammatory activity.

Side Effects: If taken in a normal dose, scullcap does not seem to exhibit any adverse effects.

Dosing: Scullcap traditionally has been used in doses of 1 to 2 g for hysteria, epilepsy, and as a bitter tonic and febrifuge; however, there are no clinical studies to support these uses or the dosage.[1]

BOTANY: Scullcap, a member of the mint family, is native to the US where it grows in moist woods. Scullcap is an erect perennial that grows to 0.6 to 0.9 m in height. Its bluish flowers bloom from July to September. Official compendia (eg, NF VI) recognized only the dried overground portion of the plant as useful; however, some herbal texts listed all parts as medicinal.[2] The aerial parts of the plant are collected during the flowering period, typically August and September. A number of species have been used medicinally, and the most common European species has been *S. baicalensis* Georgii, a native of East Asia.

HISTORY: Scullcap appears to have been introduced into traditional American medicine toward the end of the 1700s as a treatment for the management of hydrophobia. It was later used as a tonic, particularly in proprietary remedies for "female weakness."[3] The plant was reputed to be an herbal tranquilizer, particularly in combination with valerian but has since fallen into disuse.

PHARMACOLOGY: Over the past 15 years, Japanese researchers have investigated the activity of the related plant *S. baicalensis*. Animal studies indicate that extracts of the plant have a demonstrable anti-inflammatory effect. Although the mechanism of action is not well understood, it is believed that hot water extracts of *Scutellaria* and the active metabolites of the flavonoids baicalin and wogonin glucuronide (baicalein and wogonin, respectively) are potent inhibitors of the enzyme sialidase.[4] In another study, isoscutellarein-8-*O*-glucuronide from the leaf was found to be a potent inhibitor of the enzyme.[5] Serum sialic acid increases cancers, rheumatic diseases, infections, and inflammations, and a sialidase inhibitor, such as scullcap extract, may have a therapeutic application. Teas prepared from *Scutellaria* species have demonstrable in vitro antibacterial and antifungal activity.[6]

TOXICOLOGY: There is no evidence to indicate that *Scutellaria* is toxic when ingested at "normal" doses. According to the FDA, overdose of the tincture causes giddiness, stupor, confusion, twitching of the limbs, intermission of the pulse, and other symptoms similar to convulsions.[7]

---

[1] Claus E, ed. *Pharmacognosy.* 3rd ed. Philadelphia, PA: Lea & Febiger; 1956.

[2] Meyer JE. *The Herbalist.* Hammond, IN: Hammond Book Co., 1934.

3 Tyler VE. *The New Honest Herbal*. Philadelphia, PA: G.F. Stickley Co., 1987.

4 Nagai T, et al. *Planta Med*. 1989;55:27.

5 Nagai T, et al. *Biochem Biophys Res Comm*. 1989;163:25.

6 Franzblau SG, et al. *J Ethnopharmacol*. 1986;15:279.

7 Duke JA. *Handbook of Medicinal Herbs*. Boca Raton, FL: CRC Press, 1985.

SCIENTIFIC NAME(S): *Polygala senega* L. Family: Polygalaceae (Milkworts)

COMMON NAME(S): Seneca snakeroot, rattlesnake root, milkwort, mountain flax

---

≈≈≈ PATIENT INFORMATION ≈≈≈

Uses: Senega has been used as an antitussive.

Side Effects: High doses of powdered senega root or tincture are emetogenic and irritating to the GI tract.

Dosing: Antitussive dosage of senega root is 1 to 3 g/day.[1]

BOTANY: Senega root is an uncommon perennial herb about 30 cm high that grows throughout eastern North America. The leaves are small, alternate, and narrowly tapered to a point at the apex. Numerous pinkish-white or greenish-white flowers are crowded on a terminal spike. The root is twisted and has an irregular, knotty crown with a distinctive ridge. The variety *P. senega* var. *latifolia* Torr. & Gray has been distinguished, but occurs throughout the same habitat and differs from *P. senega* only in the size of leaves and flowers and in having a slightly later flowering period. The related species *P. tenuifolia* Willd., *P. reinii* Franch., *P. glomerata* Lour., and *P. japonica* Houtt. are used in Asia for similar purposes.

HISTORY: Senega root was used by eastern Native American tribes. Snakeroot refers to the purported use in snakebite. However, the early European observers gave little credence to this use. The Europeans and colonists used senega root as an emetic, cathartic, diuretic, and diaphroetic in a variety of pulmonary diseases (eg, pneumonia, asthma, pertussis) and also in gout and rheumatism.[2] It was also used as an expectorant cough remedy.

PHARMACOLOGY: The antitussive effect of senega root has been attributed to the saponin content of the plant, which is consistent with the general detergent property of saponins in breaking up phlegm. In addition, senega is thought to act by irritation of the gastric mucosa, leading by reflex to an increase in bronchial mucous gland secretion.

The senega saponins were found to reduce alcohol absorption when given orally 1 hour before alcohol.[3-5]

Substance P and lipopolysaccharide-induced production of tumor necrosis factor and interleukin-1 was blocked by the saponin-containing extract at low concentration.[6] It is possible that a systemic anti-inflammatory effect may be the result of a similar mechanism.

TOXICOLOGY: High doses of powdered senega root (more than 1 g) or tincture were reported as emetogenic and irritating to the GI tract. Senega root is contraindicated in pregnancy and patients with peptic ulcer disease or inflammatory bowel disease.[7]

[1] Claus E, ed. *Pharmacognosy.* 3rd ed. Philadelphia, PA: Lea & Febiger; 1956.

[2] Erichsen-Brown C. *Medicinal and Other Uses of North American Plants.* Dover, NY. 1979;359-362.

[3] Yoshikawa M, et al. *Chem Pharm Bull.* (Tokyo) 1995;43(12):2115.

[4] Yoshikawa M, et al. *Chem Pharm Bull.* (Tokyo) 1996;44(7):1305.

[5] Yoshikawa M, et al. *Chem Pharm Bull.* (Tokyo) 1995;43(2):350.

[6] Kim HM, et al. *J Ethnopharmacol.* 1998;61(3):201.

[7] Grieve M. *A Modern Herbal.* London: Jonathan Cape. 1931;733-734.

Senna

SCIENTIFIC NAME(S): *Cassia acutifolia* Delile, syn. with *Cassia senna* L. and *C. angustifolia* Vahl. Family: Fabaceae

⋙ PATIENT INFORMATION ⋘

Uses: Senna is most commonly used as a laxative.

Side Effects: The chronic use of senna has resulted in pigmentation of the colon, reversible finger clubbing, cachexia, and a dependency on the laxative.

Dosing: Senna leaves or pods have been used as a cathartic laxative at doses of 0.6 to 2 g/day, with a daily dose of sennoside B from 20 to 30 mg. Senna should not be used at higher doses or for extended periods of time.[1]

BOTANY: *C. acutifolia* is native to Egypt and the Sudan while *C. angustifolia* is native to Somalia and Arabia. Plants known as "wild sennas" (*C. hebecarpa* Fern. and *C. marilandica* L.) grow on moist banks and woods in the eastern US. Do not confuse this plant with "cassia," a common name for cinnamon. Senna is a low branching shrub, growing to about 0.9 m in height. It has a straight woody stem and yellow flowers.[2] The top stems are harvested, dried, and graded. The hand-collected senna is known as Tinnevally senna. Leaves that have been harvested and graded mechanically are known as Alexandria senna. There are more than 400 known species of *Cassia*.[2]

HISTORY: Senna was first used medicinally by Arabian physicians in the ninth century AD.[2] It was used in traditional Arabic and European medicine as a cathartic. The leaves have been brewed and the tea administered for its strong laxative effect. Because it is often difficult to control the concentration of the active ingredients in the tea, an unpredictable effect may be obtained. Therefore, standardized commercial dosage forms have been developed, and these concentrates are available as liquids, powders, and tablets in *otc* laxatives. The plant derives its name from the Arabic "sena" and from the Hebrew word "cassia," which means "peeled back," a reference to its peelable bark.

PHARMACOLOGY: Senna is a potent laxative. Its cathartic effects can be obtained from a tea prepared from 5 or 10 mL of dried leaves.

Senna's use in treating constipation is well documented. It is a popular laxative, especially in the elderly.[3] Many reports are available discussing senna's role in constipation,[4,5] its use in the elderly,[6-10] in psychiatric patients,[11] in spinal cord injury patients,[12] and in pregnancy, where it is the stimulant laxative of choice.[13] In cancer treatment protocols, senna also has reversed the constipating effects of narcotics and may prevent constipation if given with the narcotic.[14] However, it may cause more adverse effects than other laxatives, primarily abdominal pain.[15] Castor oil was superior to senna for chronic constipation sufferers in another report.[15]

Senna may affect intestinal transit time.[17-19] Its effectiveness as part of a cleansing regimen to evacuate the bowels in preparation for such tests as colonoscopies or barium enemas is documented.[20-30] Results from these studies include reduced ingestion of commercial *Golytely* solution and simethicone when given with senna[25] and more effective colon cleansing with senna in combination with polyethylene glycol electrolyte lavage solution, compared with the solution alone.[26] Senna also has been studied in chronic constipation[31] and as long-term laxative treatment.[32] Several mechanisms are postulated as to how senna acts as an effective laxative. Sennosides irritate the lining of the large intestine, causing contraction, which results in a bowel movement about 10 hours after the dose is taken.[2] The anthraquinone glycosides are hydrolyzed by intestinal bacteria to yield the active, free anthraquinones. Alternately, it has been suggested that the glycosides are absorbed in small quantities from the small intestine, hydrolyzed in the liver, and the resultant anthraquinones are secreted into the colon.[33] One report using human intestinal flora showed sennoside A converts to rheinanthrone, the active principle causing peristalsis of the large intestines. Sennosides A and B also play a role in inducing fluid secretion in the colon.

Prostaglandins also may be involved in the laxative actions.[34] One report suggests prostaglandin-mediated action of sennosides.[35] Indomethacin can partly inhibit the actions of sennosides A and B.[34] However, conflicting reports argue that prostaglandins do not contribute to the laxative effect.[36,37]

Metabolism of anthranoid laxatives has been reported,[38,39] as has the metabolism of sennosides.[40-42] The kinetics of senna constituents rhein and aloe-emodin have been investigated.[43]

TOXICOLOGY: Chronic use of any laxative, in particular irritant laxatives such as senna, often results in a "laxative-dependency syndrome" characterized by poor gastric motility in the absence of repeated laxative administration. Other reports of laxative abuse include laxative-induced diarrhea,[44,45] osteomalacia, and arthropathy associated with prolonged use.[46]

The chronic use of anthroquinone glycosides has been associated with pigmentation of the colon (*Melanosis coli*). Several cases of reversible finger clubbing (enlargement of the ends of the fingers and toes) have been reported following long-term abuse of senna-containing laxatives.[47-49] One report described a woman who developed finger clubbing following ingestion of 4 to 40 *Senokot* tablets per day for about 15 years.[50] Clubbing reversed when the laxative was stopped. The mechanism may be related to either increased vascularity of the nail beds or a systemic metabolic abnormality secondary to chronic laxative ingestion.

Senna abuse has been associated with the development of cachexia and reduced serum globulin levels after chronic ingestion.[51]

Risk assessment for senna's use during pregnancy has been addressed.[52] One review suggests senna to be the "stimulant laxative" of choice during pregnancy and lactation.[13] None of the breastfed infants experienced abnormal stool consistency from their mothers' ingestion of senna laxatives. The constituent rhein, taken from milk samples varied in concentration from 0 to 27 ng/mL, with 89% to 94% of values less than 10 ng/mL.[53,54] Nonstandardized laxatives are not recommended during pregnancy.[34]

Generally, senna may cause mild abdominal discomfort such as cramping. Prolonged use may alter electrolytes. Patients with intestinal obstruction should avoid senna.[34]

Various case reports of senna toxicity are available and include coma and neuropathy after ingestion of a senna-combination laxative,[55] hepatitis after chronic use of the plant,[56] occupational asthma and rhinoconjunctivitis from a factory worker exposed to senna-containing hair dyes,[57] and asthma and allergy symptoms from workers in a bulk laxative manufacturing facility.[58]

[1] Blumenthal M, Brinckmann J, Goldberg A, eds. *Herbal Medicine: Expanded Commission E Monographs.* Newton, MA: Integrative Medicine Communications; 2000.

[2] Chevallier A. *Encyclopedia of Medicinal Plants.* New York, NY: DK Publishing, 1996;72.

[3] Heaton K, et al. *Dig Dis Sci.* 1993;38(6):1004-8.

[4] Marlett J, et al. *Am J Gastroenterol.* 1987;82(4):333-37.

[5] Godding E. *Pharmacology.* 1988;36(Suppl)1:230-36.

[6] Maddi V. *J Am Geriatr Soc.* 1979 Oct;27:464-68.

[7] Passmore A, et al. *BMJ.* 1993;307(6907):769-71.

[8] Kinnunen O, et al. *Pharmacology.* 1993;47(Suppl)1:253-55.

[9] Passmore A, et al. *Pharmacology.* 1993;47(Suppl)1:249-52.

[10] Pahor M, et al. *Aging.* 1995;7(2):128-35.

[11] Georgia E. *Curr Ther Res.* 1983 Jun;33(Sec 1);1018-22.

[12] Cornell S, et al. *Nurs Res.* 1973 Jul-Aug;22:321-28.

[13] Gattuso J, et al. *Drug Saf.* 1994;10(1):47-65.

[14] Cameron J. *Cancer Nurs.*1992;15(5):372-77.

[15] Sykes N. *J Pain Sympt Manage.* 1996; 11(6):363-69.

[16] Pawlik A, et al. *Herba Polonica.* 1994;40(1-2):64-67.

[17] Rogers H, et al. *Br J Clin Pharmacol.* 1978 Dec;6:493-97.

[18] Sogni P, et al. *Gastroenterol Clin Biol.* 1992;16(1):21-24.

[19] Ewe K, et al. *Pharmacology.* 1993;47(Suppl)1:242-48.

[20] Staumont G, et al. *Pharmacology.* 1988;36(Suppl)1:49-56.

[21] Han R. *Chung Hua Hu Li Tsa Chih.* 1989;24(5):273-75.

[22] Hangartner P, et al. *Endoscopy.* 1989;21(6):272-75.

[23] Labenz J, et al. *Med Klin.* 1990;85(10):581-85.

[24] Borkje B, et al. *Scand J Gastroenterol.* 1991;26(2):162-66.

[25] Wildgrube H, et al. *Bildgebung.* 1991;58(2):63-66.

[26] Ziegenhagen D, et al. *Gastrointest Endosc.* 1991;37(5):547-49.

[27] Bailey S, et al *Clin Radiol.* 1991;44(5):335-37.

[28] Fernandez S, et al. *Rev Esp Enferm Dig.* 1995;87(11):785-91.

[29] Tooson J, et al. *Postgrad Med.* 1996;100(2):203-4, 207-12, 214.

[30] Ziegenhagen D, et al. *Z. Gastroenterol.* 1992;30(1):17-19.

[31] Mishalany H. *J Pediatr Surg.* 1989;24(4):360-62.

[32] Ralevic V, et al. *Gastroenterology.* 1990;99(5):1352-57.

[33] Bowman WC, et al. *Textbook of Pharmacology,* 2nd ed. Blackwell Scientific Publications, 1980.

[34] Newall C, et al. *Herbal Medicines.*, London, England: Pharmaceutical Press, 1996;243-44.

[35] Beubler E, et al. *Pharmacology.* 1988;36(Suppl)1:85-91.

[36] Mascolo N, et al. *Pharmacology.* 1988;36(Suppl)1:92-97.

[37] Mascolo N, et al. *J Pharm Pharmacol.* 1988;40(12):882-84.

[38] deWitte P, et al. *Hepatogastroenterology.* 1990;37(6):601-5.

[39] deWitte P. *Pharmacology.* 1993;47(Suppl)1:86-97.

[40] Lemli J. *Pharmacology.* 1988;36(Suppl)1:126-28.

[41] Hietala P, et al. *Pharmacology.* 1988;36(Suppl)1:138-43.

[42] Lemli J. *Ann Gastroenterol Hepatol (Paris).* 1996;32(2):109-12.

[43] Krumbiegel G, et al. *Pharmacology.* 47(Suppl)1:120-24.

[44] Cummings J, et al. *BMJ.* 1974 Mar 23;1:537-41.

[45] Morris A, et al. *Gastroenterology.*1979 Oct;77:780-86.

[46] Frier B, et al. *Br J Clin Pract.* 1977 Jan-Feb-Mar;31:17-19.

[47] Prior J, et al. *Lancet.*1978;ii:947.

[48] Malmquist J, et al. *Postgrad Med.* 1980 Dec;56:862-64.

[49] Armstrong R, et al. *BMJ.* 1981 Jun 6;282:1836.

[50] FitzGerald O, et al. *Ir J Med Sci.* 1983:152:246.

[51] Levin D, et al. *Lancet.* 1981;1:919.

[52] Anonymous. *Pharmacology.* 1992;44(Suppl)1:20-22.

[53] Faber P, et al. *Pharmacology.* 1988;36(Suppl)1:212-20.

[54] Faber P, et al. *Geburtshilfe Frauenheilkd.* 1989;49(11):958-62.

[55] Dobb G, et al. *Med J Aust.* 1984 Apr 14;140:495-96.

[56] Beuers U, et al. *Lancet.* 1991;337(8737):372-73.

[57] Helin T, et al. *Allergy.* 1996;51(3):181-84.

[58] Marks G. *Am Rev Respir Dis.* 1991;144(5):1065-69.

SCIENTIFIC NAME(S): *Ulmus rubra* Muhl. Also known as *U. fulva* Michx. Family: Ulmaceae

COMMON NAME(S): Slippery elm, red elm, Indian elm, moose elm, sweet elm

---

✿✿✿ PATIENT INFORMATION ✿✿✿

Uses: Parts of slippery elm have been used as an emollient and in lozenges. It protects irritated skin and intestinal membranes in such conditions as gout, rheumatism, cold sores, wounds, abscesses, ulcers, and toothaches.

Side Effects: Extracts from slippery elm have caused contact dermatitis, and the pollen has been reported to be allergenic. The FDA has declared slippery elm to be a safe and effective oral demulcent.

Dosing: Slippery elm inner bark has been used for treatment of ulcers at doses of 1.5 to 3 g/day. It is commonly decocted with ethyl alcohol. No formal clinical studies support this dosage.

BOTANY: The genus *Ulmus* contains 18 species of deciduous shrubs and trees.[1]

The slippery elm tree is native to eastern Canada and eastern and central US, where it is found most commonly in the Appalachian mountains. The trunk is reddish brown with gray-white bark on the branches. The bark is rough with vertical ridging. The slippery elm can grow to 18 to 20 m in height.[2] In the spring, dark brown floral buds appear and open into small, clustered flowers at the branch tips.[3] White elm (*U. americana*) is a related species and is used in a similar manner.[2]

HISTORY: North American Indians and early settlers used the inner bark of the slippery elm not only to build canoes, shelter, and baskets, but as a poultice or as a soothing drink.[2,4,5] Upon contact with water, the inner bark, collected in spring, yields a thick mucilage or demulcent that was used as an ointment or salve to treat urinary tract inflammation and applied topically for cold sores and boils. A decoction of the leaves was used as a poultice to remove discoloration around blackened or bruised eyes. Surgeons during the American Revolution treated gun-shot wounds in this manner.[3] Early settlers boiled bear fat with the bark to prevent rancidity.[1,4] Late in the 19th century, a preparation of elm mucilage had been recognized as an official product by the *US Pharmacopoeia.*[6]

PHARMACOLOGY: Slippery elm prepared as a poultice coats and protects irritated tissues such as skin or intestinal membranes. The powdered bark has been used in this manner for local application to treat gout, rheumatism, cold sores, wounds, abscesses, ulcers, and toothaches.[4,7] It has also been known to "draw out" toxins, boils, splinters, or other irritants.[2]

Powdered bark is incorporated into lozenges to provide demulcent action (soothing to mucous membranes) in the treatment of throat irritation.[8] It also is used for its emollient and antitussive actions, to treat bronchitis and other lung afflictions, and to relieve thirst.[1-3,5,7]

When slippery elm preparations are taken internally, they cause reflex stimulation of nerve endings in the GI tract, leading to mucus secretion.[2] This may be the reason they are effective for protection against stomach ulcers, colitis, diverticulitis, gut inflammation, and acidity. Slippery elm is also useful for diarrhea, constipation, hemorrhoids, irritable bowel syndrome, and to expel tapeworms. It also has been used to treat cystitis and urinary inflammations.[2-4,7]

The plant is also used as a lubricant to ease labor,[3,4] as a source of nutrition for convalescence or baby food preparations,[2] and for its activity against herpes and syphilis.[4] The tannins present are known to possess astringent actions.[7]

TOXICOLOGY: The FDA has declared slippery elm to be a safe and effective oral demulcent.[5] An oleoresin from several *Ulmus* species has been reported to cause contact dermatitis[6] and the pollen is allergenic.[4] Preparations of slippery elm had been used as abortifacients, a practice that has not remained popular.[1,7] Generally, there are no known problems regarding toxicity of slippery elm or its constituents.[7]

[1] Hocking G. *A Dictionary of Natural Products.* Medford, NJ: Plexus Publishing Inc. 1997;826-27.

[2] Chevallier A. *Encyclopedia of Medicinal Plants.* New York, NY: DK Publishing. 1996;144.

[3] Low T, et al, eds. *Magic and Medicine of Plants.* Surry Hils, NSW:Reader's Digest Assoc. Inc. 1994;385.

[4] Duke J. CRC *Handbook or Medicinal Herbs.* Boca Raton, FL: CRC Press, Inc. 1989;495-96.

[5] Tyler V. *Herbs of Choice, The Therapeutic Use of Phytomedicinals.* Binghamton, NY: Pharmaceutical Products Press. 1994;93,94.

[6] Lewis W, Elvin-Lewis MPF. *Medical Botany.* New York, NY: J. Wiley and Sons, 1977.

[7] Newall C, et al. *Herbal Medicines.* London, England: Pharmaceutical Press. 1996;248.

[8] Morton J. Major Medicinal Plants. Springfield, IL:C.C. Thomas, 1977.

SCIENTIFIC NAME(S): *Aristolochia serpentaria* L., *Aristolochia reticulata* Nuttall. Family: Aristolochiaceae (birthwort family)

COMMON NAME(S): Snakeroot, Virginia snakeroot, snakeweed, sangree root, sangrel, birthwort, pelican flower, Texas snakeroot, Red River snakeroot

---

·ᴥ·ᴥ· PATIENT INFORMATION ·ᴥ·ᴥ·

Uses: Do not use snakeroot because of its toxicity. Snakeroot stimulates gastric secretions and smooth muscle contractions. In small doses, snakeroot can promote appetite and tone digestive organs, and larger doses promote arterial action, diaphoresis, and diuresis.

Side Effects: Aristolochic acid, a component of snakeroot, can affect the kidneys and irritate the GI tract, and may also cause genetic mutations. Do not use snakeroot, especially in those with diseases of the GI tract and in women who are pregnant or breastfeeding.

Dosing: While *Aristolochia* formerly was used as a bitter tonic at 1 g dosage, in view of the nephrotoxicity of aristolochic acid derivatives, it cannot be recommended at any dose.[1]

BOTANY: Aristolochia is a genus comprising approximately 300 species of herbs and vines. *A. serpentaria* is a low-growing perennial (up to 0.6 m tall) found primarily in the rich woods of central and southern US, including Connecticut to Florida, Michigan, Missouri, Louisiana, Arkansas, and Texas. Snakeroot possesses a foul, fruit-like odor that attracts insects. Its exotic, brownish-purple flowers are tube-like and lined with hairs. Insects caught in this area become covered with pollen while struggling to escape and carry it to pollinate other flowers. The leaves of the plant are heart-shaped. The medicinal parts of the plant are the dried rhizome and the roots.[2-5] *A. reticulata* differs from *A. serpentaria* in having a larger rhizome with fewer, thicker rootlets and thicker leaves with more prominent reticulations and petioles.[2]

HISTORY: Snakeroot was used as a cure for snakebite, hence the common name. Native Americans chewed the root and also applied it to wounds. Colonial and European doctors were said to have used snakeroot for infectious fevers, malaria, and rabies. The heart-shaped leaves of the plant promoted its use as a heart tonic. Modern herbalists employ snakeroot as an aphrodisiac, to treat convulsions, and to promote menstruation. However, none of these claims have been scientifically validated.[4,6] One source mentions that *A. serpentaria* was grown in England as far back as 1632.[5]

PHARMACOLOGY: Snakeroot has been used as an aromatic bitter.[2] Its known effects include stimulation of gastric secretions and smooth muscle contractions of the GI tract and heart.[7] In small doses, snakeroot can promote appetite and tone digestive organs. Larger doses promote arterial action, diaphoresis, and diuresis. It is also said to be helpful in amenorrhea.[6] Unproven effects of the plant include increased circulation, heart stimulation, fever reduction, and in the treatment of dyspepsia and skin sores.[7] Folk uses of snakeroot include treatment of fever, prevention of convulsions, promotion of menstruation, and as an aphrodisiac. Snakeroot's effectiveness as an antidote for snakebite and rabies remains unproven.[4]

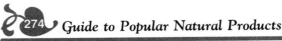

A. clematitis, a related species, is used to stimulate the immune system and to treat wounds.[8] Taliscanine, a component of *A. taliscana*, has been reported to treat Parkinson and related diseases.[9] Tumor inhibiting properties are clearly because of aristolochic acids.[10]

TOXICOLOGY: Do not use snakeroot in humans. Aristolochic acid is a known kidney toxin in rodents.[11] Several articles confirm aristolochic acid's nephrotoxic and carcinogenic effects in humans as well. Aristolochic acids from *A. fangchi*, *A. clematitis*, and others have been found to cause kidney damage or "Chinese herb nephropathy." Cases of interstitial renal fibrosis, urothelial lesions, malignancy, Fanconi syndrome, and end-stage renal failure all

have been extensively reported.[1,8,12-29] A review with 108 references discusses this further.[30]

The structural basis for mutagenicity of aristolochic acid has been reported.[31] In large doses, constituent aristolochine also can affect the kidneys and irritate the GI tract, leading to coma and death from respiratory paralysis.[6,10]

No one should take snakeroot, especially those with any disease of the GI tract, including ulcer, reflux, or colitis, as well as those who are pregnant or breastfeeding.[7] Aristolochic acid also may cause genetic mutations; some countries ban the plant's sale.[4] A case report explains acute hepatitis from a tea mixture (including *A. debilis*) containing toxic aristolochic acids.[32]

[1] Vanhaelen M, et al. *Lancet.* 1994;343(8890):174.

[2] Youngken H. *Textbook of Pharmacognosy*, 6th ed. Philadelphia, PA: Blakiston Co., 1950:287-90.

[3] Hocking G. *A Dictionary of Natural Products.* Medford, NJ: Plexus Publishing, 1997:69-70.

[4] Dwyer J, Rattray D, eds. *Magic and Medicine of Plants.* Pleasantville, NY: The Reader's Digest Association, 1986:324.

[5] http://www.botanical.com/botanical/mgmh/s/snaker56.html

[6] Duke J. *CRC Handbook of Medicinal Herbs.* Boca Raton, FL: CRC Press, Inc., 1985:63.

[7] http://search1.healthgate.com/vit/herb171.shtml

[8] Fleming T, ed. *PDR for Herbal Medicines.* Montvale, NJ: Medical Economics Company, Inc., 1998:660-61.

[9] De la Parra J. US Patent 1988. Application: US 87-8743219870820.

[10] Evans W. *Trease and Evans' Pharmacognosy*, 14th ed. London: WB Saunders Company Ltd., 1996:373-74.

[11] Mengs U. *Arch Toxicol.* 1987;59(5):328-31.

[12] Cosyns J, et al. *Kidney Int.* 1994;45(6):1680-88.

[13] Vanherweghem J, et al. *Am J Kidney Dis.* 1996;27(2):209-15.

[14] Zhu M, et al. *Int J Pharmacogn.* 1996;34(4):283-89.

[15] Tanaka A, et al. *Nippon Jinzo Gakkai Shi.* 1997;39(4):438-40.

[16] Tanaka A, et al. *Nippon Jinzo Gakkai Shi.* 1997;39(8):794-97.

[17] Sekita S, et al. *Kokuritsu Iyakuhin Shokuhin Eisei Kenkyusho Hokoku.* 1998;116:195-96.

[18] Stengel B, et al. *Nephrologie.* 1998;19(1):15-20.

[19] Cosyns J, et al. *Arch Toxicol.* 1998;72(11):738-43.

[20] Motoo T. *Nippon Naika Gakkai Zasshi.* 1999;88(2):368-69.

[21] Cosyns J, et al. *Am J Kidney Dis.* 1999;33(6):1011-7.

[22] De Broe M. *Am J Kidney Dis.* 1999;33(6):1171-73.

[23] Stiborova M, et al. *Exp Toxicol Pathol.* 1999;51(4-5):421-27.

[24] Lord G, et al. *Lancet.* 1999;354(9177):481-82.

[25] But P, et al. *Lancet.* 1999;354(9191):1731-32.

[26] Okada M. *Lancet.* 1999;354(9191):1732.

[27] Yang C, et al. *Am J Kidney Dis.* 2000;35(2):313-18.

[28] Tanaka A, et al. *Clin Nephrol.* 2000;53(4):301-06.

[29] Kessler D. *N Engl J Med.* 2000;342(23).

[30] Violon C. *J Pharm Belg.* 1997;52(1):7-27.

[31] Pfau W, et al. *Cancer Lett.* 1990;55(1):7-11.

[32] Levi M, et al. *Pharm World Sci.* 1998;20(1):43-44.

SCIENTIFIC NAME(S): *Prunus cerasus* L. (*Cerasus vulgaris* Mill.) Family: Rosaceae

COMMON NAME(S): Sour cherry, morello cherry, tart cherry, pie cherry, red cherry

---

৯ঽৡৡ PATIENT INFORMATION ৯ঽৡৡ

Uses: A study has been done on the anti-inflammatory and antioxidant properties of sour cherries. Tart cherry's anthocyanins have the potential to inhibit tumor growth, slow cardiovascular disease, and possibly retard the aging process. Tart cherry juice is used to mask the unpleasant taste of some drugs.

Side Effects: Little information exists; one document reports the contamination percentages of the mycotoxin, patulin, in sour cherry.[1]

Dosing: There is no dosage information available for sour cherry.

BOTANY: There are about 270 varieties of sour cherries, a handful of which are of commercial importance (eg, Montmorency, Richmond, English morello). The sour cherry tree is smaller than the sweet cherry tree (*Prunus avium*) and is more tolerant of extreme temperatures.[2] The sour cherry originated in Europe but is widely cultivated in America. The trees may reach about 11.89 m in height, with a trunk diameter of 30 to 45 cm. The bark is a grayish-brown, flowers are white to pale pink, and leaves are ovate with serrated edging.[3,4] Sour cherry fruits can grow to 20 mm in length and 18 mm in width. They are heart-shaped drupes by nature, with color ranging from light to dark red. This fruit envelops a light brown seed.[5]

HISTORY: The Greek botanist Theophrastus described the cherry circa 300 BC; although, it is believed to have been cultivated even earlier than this time. In 70 AD, Pliny indicated locations of cherry trees to be in Rome, Germany, England, and France. By the mid 1800s, cherries were being cultivated in Oregon. The first commercial cherry orchard was planted in the late 1800s. By the early 1900s, the sour cherry industry was flourishing. As of the late 1900s, 100,000 tons of sour cherries are produced in the US each year.[2,6]

PHARMACOLOGY: Cherries were traditionally used by Cherokee Indians as a remedy for arthritis and gout. Today, components of the plant responsible for this anti-inflammatory and antioxidant activity have been identified.[7] Michigan State University studies indicate tart cherry compounds (eg, cyanidin) to be 10 times more active than aspirin, without the side effects. Antioxidant activity has been studied as well. Tart cherry's anthocyanins have the potential to inhibit tumor growth, slow cardiovascular disease, and possibly retard the aging process.[6]

The juice of tart cherries is used in the formulation of cherry syrup, USP, as a vehicle for unpleasant-tasting drugs.[4,5]

TOXICOLOGY: Little information concerning the toxicology of tart cherry was found in recent literature searches. One document reports in an analysis of fruits and vegetables, the contamination percentages of the mycotoxin, patulin, in sour cherry.[1]

---

[1] Thurm V, et al. *Nahrung.* 1979;23(2):131-34.

[2] Ensminger A, et al. *Foods and Nutrition Encyclopedia, 2nd ed.* Boca Raton, FL: CRC Press, 1994;386-89.

[3] http://www.gypsymoth.ento.vt.edu/vagm/Tree-images/cherry.html

[4] Youngken, H. *Textbook of Pharmacognosy, 6th ed*. Philadelphia, PA: The Blakiston Co., 1950;414-15.

[5] Osol A, et al. *The Dispensatory of the United States of America, 25th ed*. Philadelphia, PA: JB Lippincott Co., 1960;272-73.

[6] http://www.cherrymkt.org/mediinfo.html

[7] Wang H, et al. *J Nat Prod*. 1999;62(1):86-88.

SCIENTIFIC NAME(S): *Hypericum perforatum* L. Family: Hypericaceae

COMMON NAME(S): St. John's wort, klamath weed, John's wort, amber touch-and-heal, goatweed, rosin rose, millepertuis

---

ꙮ PATIENT INFORMATION ꙮ

Uses: St. John's wort has been primarily studied for its potential antidepressant and antiviral effects. There is information to show that St. John's wort is more effective than placebo, but evidence is still lacking regarding its efficacy compared with the standard antidepressants, partially due to ineffective dosing. In addition, at least 3 studies have shown that commercially available St. John's wort products vary considerably in content and may be standardized to the wrong component (hypericin instead of hyperforin). St. John's wort is still in the early stages of clinical trials investigating its effects against certain viruses, including HIV.

Drug Interactions: St. John's wort has been reported to decrease the efficacy of theophylline, warfarin, and digoxin and reduce AUC of indinavir (and potentially other protease inhibitors). Known interactions with cyclosporine have occurred. Concomitant use with prescription antidepressants is not recommended. Use with oral contraceptives may cause breakthrough bleeding but has not been reported to result in unexpected pregnancy. See Potential Drug Interactions with St. John's Wort in appendix.

Side Effects: Side effects are usually mild. Potential side effects include the following: dry mouth, dizziness, constipation, other GI symptoms, and confusion. Photosensitization also may occur. In clinical trials, side effects and medication discontinuation with St. John's wort were usually less than that observed with standard antidepressants. Other possible rare side effects include induction of mania and effects on male and female reproductive capabilities.

Dose: The majority of clinical trials for the treatment of depression administered St. John's wort 300 mg tid standardized to 0.3% hypericin, but research has shown that products should contain 2% to 4% or more of hyperforin.

BOTANY: St. John's wort is a perennial native to Europe but is found throughout the US and parts of Canada. The plant is an aggressive weed found in the dry ground of roadsides, meadows, woods, and hedges. It generally grows to 0.3 to 0.61 m, except on the Pacific coast where it has been known to reach heights of 1.52 m.[1] The plant has oval-shaped leaves and yields golden-yellow flowers that bloom from June to September. The petals contain black or yellow glandular dots and lines. Some sources say that the blooms are at their brightest coincidental with the birthday of John the Baptist (June 24).[2] There are about 370 species in the genus *Hypericum*, which is derived from the Greek words, *hyper* and *eikon* meaning "over an apparition," alluding to the plant's ancient use to "ward off" evil spirits. *Perforatum* refers to the leaf's appearance; when held up to light, the translucent leaf glands resemble perforations.[3,4] Harvest of the plant for medicinal purposes occurs in July and August; the plant must be dried immediately to avoid loss of potency.[5] The dried herb consists of the plant's flowering tops.[3]

HISTORY: This plant has been used as an herbal remedy for its anti-inflammatory and healing properties since the Middle Ages.[2,5] Many noteworthy ancient herbalists, including Hippocrates and Pliny, recorded the medicinal properties of St. John's wort. It was noted for its wound-healing and diuretic properties, as well as for the treatment of neuralgic conditions such as back pain. In 1633, Gerard recorded the plant's use as a balm for burns. The oil of the plant was also popular during this time.[3] An olive oil extract of the fresh flowers that acquires a reddish color after standing in the sunlight for several weeks has been taken internally for the treatment of anxiety but also has been applied externally to relieve inflammation and promote healing. Its topical application is believed to be particularly useful in the management of hemorrhoids. Although it is often listed as a folk treatment for cancer, there is no scientific evidence to document an antineoplastic effect.[2,5]

Although it fell into disuse, a renewed interest in St. John's wort occurred during the past decade, and it is now a component of numerous herbal preparations for the treatment of anxiety and depression. The plant has been used in traditional medicine as an antidepressant and diuretic and for the treatment of gastritis and insomnia. Since 1995, St. John's wort has become the most prescribed antidepressant in Germany. Sales have increased from $10 million to over $200 million in the past 8 years in the US. Since 1997, St. John's wort has been one of the leading herbal products; estimated sales of St. John's wort worldwide total $570 million.[6]

PHARMACOLOGY:

Depression: Early research focused on the hypericin constituents in St. John's wort. Originally, hypericin was thought to exert its tranquilizing effect by increasing capillary blood flow.

Many reports have postulated certain mechanisms and behavioral characteristics of *H. perforatum*, concentrating mostly on hypericin as the active ingredient. The following are major findings: inhibition of serotonin uptake by postsynaptic receptors has been confirmed in a number of reports; neuroblastoma cells treated with the extract demonstrated reduced expression of serotonin receptors;[7] *H. perforatum* extract inhibited both serotonin and norepinephrine uptake in astrocytes, the cells surrounding synaptic terminals that regulate neurotransmission by their uptake systems;[8] and *H. perforatum* also has increased brain dopamine function.[9] St. John's wort extract has been found to modulate interleukin-6 (IL-6) activity, linking the immune system with mood. IL-6 is involved in cell communication within the immune system and in modulating the hypothalamic-pituitary-adrenal (HPA) axis. St. John's wort has the ability to reduce IL-6 levels that reduce HPA axis elevations and certain hormones, which if elevated, are associated with depression.[10] Sigma receptor binding of hypericin has been demonstrated.[11] *H. perforatum* does not act as a classical serotonin inhibitor but resembles reserpine's properties. Its antidepressant effects are unlikely to be associated with serotonin, benzodiazepine, or GABA receptors.[12] In addition, *H. perforatum* differs from other selective serotonin reuptake inhibitors (SSRIs) by failing to enhance natural killer cell activity (NKCA).[13] Other effects on neurotransmitters from hypericin include inhibition of dopamine-beta-hydroxylase[14] and inhibition of metekephaline and tyrosine dimerization.

Hyperforin is the major lipophilic constituent in the plant and a potent inhibitor of serotonin, noradrenaline, and dopamine uptake, increasing their concentrations in the synaptic cleft. Some identify it as the major active principle for its efficacy as an antidepressant.[15-18] Hyperforin's spectrum of central activity is affected by other constituents, as proven by alteration of serotonergic effects using different extracts of the plant.[19,20] Hyperforin is a major neuroactive component of *H. perforatum* extracts; modulating neuronal ionic conductances is only one of many mechanisms of action it possesses.[21] Hyperforin inhibits serotonin uptake by elevating free intracellular sodium, not seen with conventional SSRIs.[22] In a clinical trial involving 147 patients with mild-to-moderate depression, subjects given *H. perforatum* extract containing greater concentrations of hyperforin exhibited the largest Hamilton Rating Scale for Depression (HAMD) reduction compared with those given lower concentrations or placebo, confirming that the therapeutic effects of St. John's wort depend on its hyperforin content.[23]

St. John's wort continues to be a topic of interest because of its antidepressant effects.[24,25] Reports from 1994 to 1996, including a study using the HAMD, evaluate St. John's wort as clinically effective in treating depression,[26-28] rating close to 70% in treatment response.[29] A meta-analysis evaluating 23 randomized trials was conducted to investigate St. John's wort (vs placebo and other conventional antidepressants). Results found St. John's wort to be superior to placebo. Side effects occurred in about 20% of patients on *H. perforatum* and 53% of patients on standard antidepressants.[30] Other reviews described similar outcomes; lower doses of standard antidepressants were used.[5,26,31]

Review articles and meta-analyses concerning *H. perforatum*'s antidepressive effects have become available from 1998 to 2000,[32-40] the most notable are the following: question and answer format in common language containing tables summarizing clinical trials;[41] a review of clinical studies, most commonly using 300 mg 3 times daily of 0.3% hypericin (600 mg in severe depression); a review of *H. perforatum*'s equiva-

lence in efficacy to numerous antidepressants with fewer incidences of side effects;[42] meta-analyses on *H. perforatum* finding a response rate of 60% to 70% (estimate of pooled data) in patients with mild-to-moderate depression,[43] and its use resulting in 1.5 times the likelihood to observe antidepressant response than placebo, along with equivalence in efficacyto tricyclic antidepressants (TCAs);[44] a clinical trial review confirming greater efficacy vs placebo and equal efficacy to TCAs, MAO inhibitors, and SSRIs, with superior side-effect profile;[38] a review of 20 clinical trials including 1787 patients, describing similar outcomes;[45] and a broad-based literature search from 1980 to 1998, yielding about 1300 records confirming St. John's wort's increased efficacy over placebo in treating mild-to-moderate depressive disorders.[46] Some opposing views mention a lack of information regarding long-term effects, use in other depressive states, the use of different preparations,[47] and the exact mechanism of action being unknown with more definitive data being needed.[48] Mechanisms of action similar to SSRIs or MAO inhibitors are seen in *H. perforatum*, but its clinical efficacy is probably attributable to the combined contribution of several mechanisms.[49]

Other literature concerning the antidepressant effects of St. John's wort include the following: ongoing confirmation of *H. perforatum*'s benefits for depression; dose-dependent response rates were seen using 3 different standardized extracts;[50] different population-type trials, including adolescents with psychiatric problems,[51] elderly patients experiencing dementia such as Alzheimer disease,[52] and mild-to-moderate depression;[53] *H. perforatum* compared with conventional antidepressant medications was found to have effects similar to the antidepressant properties of TCAs, imipramine, and fluoxetine;[54]

800 mg of a certain St. John's wort extract compared with 20 mg fluoxetine proved to be equally effective in about 150 depressed elderly patients (both groups experiencing adverse reactions);[55] certain dosages of St. John's wort significantly increased latency to REM sleep without affecting other sleep patterns, consistent with other antidepressants' mechanisms of action;[56] and seasonal affective disorder (SAD), a type of depression in which symptoms occur in fall/winter and resolve in spring/summer, benefited from St. John's wort, in combination with light therapy.[57]

There are limitations to the studies, which make drawing conclusions about St. John's wort's efficacy in treating depression difficult. In most of the studies, the antidepressant doses were low, the diagnosis of depression was not uniformly documented, and the trials were short (average: 4 to 6 weeks). In addition, the studies standardized St. John's wort to hypericin that varied widely among studies, and there is evidence that hyperforin might be the active ingredient, which was not quantified in the studies.[23]

Pharmacokinetic studies of hypericin and pseudohypericin found that, while similar in structure, they possess substantial pharmacokinetic differences.[58] Single-dose and steady-state pharmacokinetics also have been evaluated.[59] A daily dose of *H. perforatum*, as determined by trials and studies, is 200 to 900 mg of alcohol extract,[5] or 300 mg 3 times daily of a 0.3% hypericin-containing, standardized extract.[41]

HIV: Hypericin is still in the early stages of clinical trials investigating its effects against certain viruses, including HIV. One study found 16 of 18 patients had improved CD4 cell counts over a 40-month period. CD4/CD8 ratios also improved in the majority of patients. Hypericin and pseudohypericin inhibit a variety of encapsulated viruses, including HIV.[3]

The FDA sanctioned hypericin as an investigational new drug, making it eligible to be tested on humans. It is in phase 1/phase 2 clinical trial testing and is being developed under the name *VIMRxyn*. In late 1996, its developers (VIMRx Pharmaceuticals, Inc.) announced "a well tolerated oral dose with no untoward toxicity or cutaneous photosensitivity." Viral load measured in a 12-patient population ranged from no change to 97% reduction.[60,61] Another report in 1999 of a phase 1 study evaluating hypericin's effects concluded hypericin had no antiretroviral activity (in a 30-patient trial), with phototoxicity being observed.[62]

Antiviral: Hypericin and pseudohypericin exert effects against a wide spectrum of other viruses, including influenza virus, herpes simplex virus types 1 and 2, Sindbis virus, poliovirus, retrovirus infection in vitro and in vivo, murine cytomegalovirus, and hepatitis C.[3,5,63,64] Hypericin and pseudohypericin have been found to exert unique and uncommonly effective antiviral actions, possibly because of nonspecific association with cellular and viral membranes. It has been reported more than once that the antiviral activity involves a photoactivation process.[3] Recent reports find that exposure of hypericin to fluorescent light markedly increases its antiviral activity.[5] *H. perforatum* has been considered as a photodynamic agent and may be helpful in future therapeutics and diagnostics.[65]

Antibacterial: Extracts of the plant have been active against gram-negative and gram-positive bacteria in vitro.[66] Reports have documented antimicrobial effects against such organisms as *S. equinus*, *K. pneumoniae*, *E. coli*, *B. lichteniforms*, and *S. flexneri*.[67] Antibacterial activity of constituent hyperforin against *S. aureus* and other gram-positive bacteria also has been reported.[68] In another study, *H. perforatum* extract showed bacteriostatic activity at a dilution of 1:200,000 and bactericidal action at 1:20,000.[5] St. John's wort has also been used in a 20% tincture form to treat otitis. The tannin component of the plant probably exerts an astringent action that contributes to the plant's traditional use as a wound-healing agent.[4]

Other uses: Other uses of the plant include the following: wound-healing effects, including burn treatment;[3,5,69] oral and topical administration of hypericin for treatment of vitiligo (failure of skin to form melanin)[70] and other skin diseases;[71] anti-inflammatory and anti-ulcerogenic properties from the component amentoflavone (a biapigenin derivative);[4,72] treatment for hemorrhoids,[5] alcoholism,[54] bedwetting,[4] glioblastoma brain cancer,[73] and menopausal symptoms of psychological origin.[74] St. John's wort can increase and suppress immunity.[75] Hypericin has inhibited T-type calcium channel activity.[76] *H. perforatum* enhances coronary flow and also may be useful in treating certain headaches.[3] Fibromyalgia also may benefit from St. John's wort extracts by keeping serotonin levels high and decreasing pain sensations. Other neuralgias may also benefit from the plant.[4,41]

INTERACTIONS: Several recent articles concerning drug interactions with *H. perforatum* include the following: a meta-analysis of St. John's wort and other herbs possessing potentially unsafe effects;[77] reviews regarding similar issues;[78-81] and a letter.[82] More specific reports include drug interactions with St. John's wort and theophylline,[83] digoxin[84] (decreasing bioavailability in both), and indinavir. St. John's wort reduced the AUC of this HIV-1 protease inhibitor 57% in 16 patients, indicating possible treatment failure or drug resistance issues.[85] An interaction between St. John's wort and cyclosporine caused acute rejection in 2 heart transplant patients.[86] At least 7 cases of a decrease in the anticoagulant effects of warfarin have been reported.[87] Central serotonergic syndrome was reported among elderly patients combining St. John's wort with other prescription antidepressants.[88] The use of St. John's wort with SSRIs, venlafaxine HCl, and various TCAs (with close monitoring of symptoms) has been successfully undertaken. Avoidance of tyramine-containing foods during coadministration of St. John's wort and MAO inhibitors has been recommended; recent information proving lack of MAO inhibition does not justify this.[41]

Since St. John's wort may induce the isozymes cytochrome P450 1A2, 2C9, and 3A4 in addition to inducing p-glycoprotein transporter, numerous other drug interactions with St. John's wort are possible.[81] Research is needed to determine the magnitude and clinical importance of these potential drug interactions.

Women taking oral contraceptives and St. John's wort have experienced breakthrough bleeding.[89]

TOXICOLOGY: Phototoxic activity by *H. perforatum* has been observed when tested on human keratinocytes.[90] A review of the chemistry of phenanthroperylene quinones from hypericin reveals photosensory pigments.[91] After oral administration, concentrations of hypericin in human serum and blister fluid have been detected.[92] However, most reports of photosensitivity have been limited to those taking excessive quantities of *H. perforatum*, primarily to treat HIV.[41] For example, IV (eg, 0.5 mg/kg twice weekly) and oral dosing (eg, 0.5 mg/kg/day) of *H. perforatum* caused significant phototoxicity in

30 HIV patients tested, with 16 of 30 discontinuing treatment for this reason.[62]

A number of studies report no serious adverse effects. In a 22-patient study evaluating St. John's wort, 50% reported no side effects. Those reported include jitteriness, insomnia, change in bowel habits, or headache.[93] In a study of 3250 patients taking St. John's wort for 1 month, fewer than 3% suffered from dry mouth, GI distress, or dizziness.[94] In another review of clinical trials, St. John's wort was associated with fewer and milder adverse reactions as compared with any other conventional antidepressant. Adverse effects from *H. perforatum* were "rare and mild." No information on overdose was found.[95] A case report describes acute neuropathy after sun exposure in a patient using St. John's wort.[96] A review on photodermatitis in general is available, discussing mechanisms, clinical features, and treatment options.[97] Various other reports regarding other adverse effect studies concerning St. John's wort are available. A 7-patient evaluation reports St. John's wort to be unlikely to inhibit cytochrome P-450 enzymes 2D6 and 3A4 activity.[98] Reports of mania induction have been associated with St. John's wort.[99,100] Uterotonic actions also have been reported.[101] A letter discussing St. John's wort's use during pregnancy has been published.[102] Due to lack of toxicity data in this area, St. John's wort is best avoided during pregnancy.[63] Potent inhibition of sperm motility was observed from in vitro experimentation of St. John's wort.[103] The volatile oil of St. John's wort is an irritant.[63]

[1] Awang D. *CPJ-RPC*. 1991 Jan:33.

[2] Tyler V. *The New Honest Herbal*. Philadelphia, PA: G.F. Stickley Co., 1987.

[3] Upton R, ed. St. John's wort *Hypericum perforatum*. Austin TX: American Herbal Pharmacopoeia and Therapeutic Compendium, 1997.

[4] Hahn G. *J Naturopathic Med*. 1992;3(1):94–6.

[5] Bombardelli E, et al. *Fitoterapia*. 1995;66(1):43-68.

[6] Gruenwald J. *Nutraceuticals World*. 1999;May/June: 22-25.

[7] Muller W, et al. *J Geriatr Psychiatry Neurol*. 1994;7(suppl. 1):S63–4.

[8] Neary J, et al. *Brain Res*. 1999;816(2):358–63.

[9] Franklin M, et al. *Biol Psychiatry*. 1999;46(4):581–4.

[10] Thiede H, et al. *J Geriatr Psychiatry Neurol*. 1994;7(suppl. 1):S54–6.

[11] Raffa R. *Life Sci*. 1998;62(16):PL265–70.

[12] Gobbi M, et al. *Arch Pharmacol*. 1999;360(3)262–9.

[13] Helgason C, et al. *Immunopharmacology*. 2000;46(3):247–51.

[14] Kleber E, et al. *Arzneimittelforschung*. 1999;49(2):106–9.

[15] Chatterjee S, et al. *Life Sci*. 1998;63(6):499–510.

[16] Chatterjee S, et al. *Pharmacopsychiatry*. 1998;31(suppl):7–15.

[17] Muller W, et al. *Pharmacopsychiatry*. 1998;31(suppl):16–21.

[18] Kaehler S, et al. *Neurosci Lett*. 1999;262(3):199–202.

[19] Bhattacharya S, et al. *Pharmacopsychiatry*. 1998;31(suppl):22–29.

[20] Dimpfel W, et al. *Pharmacopsychiatry*. 1998;31(suppl):30–5.

[21] Chatterjee S, et al. *Life Sci*. 1999;65(22):2395–2405.

[22] Singer A, et al. *J Pharmacol Exp Ther*. 1999;290(3):1363–8.

[23] Laakmann G, et al. *Pharmacopsychiatry*. 1998;31(suppl. 1):54–9.

[24] Okpanyi V, et al. *Arzneimittelforschung*. 1987;37:10.

[25] Muldner V, et al. *Arzneimittelforschung*. 1984;34:918.

[26] Ernst E. *Fortschr Med*. 1995;113(25):354-55.

[27] Mueller W, et al. *Deutsche Apotheker Zeitung*. 1996 Mar 28;136:17-22,24.

[28] DeSmet P, et al. *Br Med J*. 1996 Aug 3;313:241-42.

[29] Harrer G, et al. *Phytomedicine*. 1994;1:3-8.

[30] Linde K, et al. *Br Med J*. 1996;313(7052):253-58.

[31] Witte B, et al. *Fortschritte Der Medizin*. 1995;113(28):404-8.

[32] Heiligenstein E, et al. *J Am Coll Health*. 1998;46(6):271–6.

[33] Cott J, et al. *J Nerv Ment Dis*. 1988;186(8):500–1.

[34] Rey J, et al. *Med J Aust*. 1998;169(11–12):583–6.

[35] Nordfors M, et al. *Lakartidningen*. 1999;96(1–2):12–13.

[36] Clark C. *Nurs Spectr.* (Wash. DC) 1999;9(4):19.

[37] Meier B. *Adv Ther.* 1999;16(3):135–47.

[38] Josey E, et al. *Int J Clin Pharmacol Ther.* 1999;37(3):111–19.

[39] Muller W, et al. *Dtsch Apoth Ztg.* 1999;139(17):1741–6, 1748–50.

[40] Gaster B, et al. *Arch Intern Med.* 2000;160(2):152–6.

[41] Murray M. *Am J Nat Med.* 1997;4(7):14–19.

[42] Miller A. *Altern Med Rev.* 1998;3(1):18–26.

[43] Hippius H. *Curr Med Res Opin.* 1998;14(3):171–84.

[44] Kim H, et al. *J Nerv Ment Dis.* 1999;187(9):532–8.

[45] Kasper S, et al. *Wien Med Wochenschr.* 1999;149(8–10):191–6.

[46] Mulrow C, et al.*Psychopharmacol Bull.* 1998;34(4):409–795.

[47] Stevinson C, et al. *Eur Neuropsychopharmacol.* 1999;9(6):501–5.

[48] Deltito J, et al. *J Affect Disord.* 1998;51(3):345–51.

[49] Bennet D, et al. *Ann Pharmacother.* 1998;32(11):1201–8.

[50] Lenoir S, et al. *Phytomedicine.* 1999;6(3):141–6.

[51] Walter G, et al. *J Child Adolesc Psychopharmacol.* 1999;9(4):307–11.

[52] Chatterjee S, et al. *Pct Int Appl.* 1999.

[53] Ernst E. *Drugs Aging.* 1999;15(6):423–28.

[54] DeVry J, et al. *Eur Neuropsychopharmacol.* 1999;9(6):461–8.

[55] Harrer G, et al. *Arzneimittelforschung.* 1999;49(4):289–96.

[56] Sharpley A, et al. *Psychopharmacology.* 1998;139(3):286–7.

[57] Martinez B, et al. *J Geriatr Psychiatry Neurol.* 1994;7(suppl. 1):S29–33.

[58] Staffeldt B, et al. *J Geriatr Psychiatry Neurol.* 1994 Oct 7;Suppl 1:547-53.

[59] Kerb R, et al. *Antimicrob Agents Chemother.* 1996;40(9):2087-93.

[60] Hebel SK, Burnham TH, eds. *Drug Facts and Comparisons.* St. Louis, MO: Facts and Comparisons, 1998.

[61] *VimRxyn* press release taken from the Internet, dated 10/19/96.

[62] Gulick R, et al. *Ann Intern Med.* 1999;130(6):510–14.

[63] Newall C, et al. *Herbal Medicines.* London, England: Pharmaceutical Press 1996;250-52.

[64] Taylor R, et al. *J Ethnopharmacol.* 1996;52(3):157-63.

[65] Diwu Z. *Photochem Photobiol.* 1995;61(6):529-39.

[66] Barbagallo C, et al. *Fitoterapia.* 1987;58:175.

[67] Ang C, et al. *Antimicrobial activities of St. John's wort extracts.* Book of Abstracts, 217th ACS National Meeting, Anaheim, CA, March 21–25, 1999.

[68] Schempp C, et al. *Lancet.* 1999;353(9170):2129.

[69] Hayakawa A. *Food Style.* 21 1999;3(4):74–77.

[70] Duke J. *Handbook of Medicinal Herbs.* Boca Raton, FL: CRC Press, 1985.

[71] *Business Wire.* April 25, 1997.

[72] Berghofer R, et al. *Planta Med.* 1989;55:91.

[73] *Business Wire.* Oct. 28, 1998.

[74] Grube B, et al.*Adv Ther.* 1999;16(4):117–86.

[75] Evstifeeva T, et al. *Eksperimentalnaia I Klinicheskaia Farmakologiia.* 1996;59(1):51-54.

[76] Shan J, et al. *Pct Int Appl.* 2000.

[77] Klepser T, et al. *Am J Health Syst Pharm.* 1999;56(2):125–38.

[78] Duncan M. *J Ren Nutr.* 1999;9(2):58–62.

[79] Fugh-Berman A. *Lancet.* 2000;355(9198):134–38.

[80] Cupp M. *Am Fam Physician.* 1999;59(5):1239–46.

[81] Tatro D. *Drug Link.* 2000;4(5):34.

[82] Ciordia R. *J Clin Monit Comput.* 1998;14(3):215.

[83] Nebel A, et al. *Ann Pharmacother.* 1999;33(4):502.

[84] Johne A, et al. *Clin Pharm Ther.* 1999;66(4):338–45.

[85] Piscitelli S, et al. *Lancet.* 2000; 355 (9203):547–8.

[86] Ruschitzka F, et al. *Lancet.* 2000;355 (9203):548–9.

[87] Yue Q-Y, et al. *Lancet.* 2000;355:576.

[88] Lantz M, et al. *J Geriatr Psychiatry Neurol.* 1999;12(1):7–10.

[89] Ernst E. *Lancet.* 1999 Dec 11;354:2014–16.

[90] Bernd A, et al. *Photochem Photobiol.* 1999;69(2):218–21.

[91] Falk H. *Angew Chem.* Int. Ed. 1999;38(21):3117–3136.

[92] Schempp C, et al. *Skin Pharmacol Appl Skin Physiol.* 1999;12(5):299–304.

[93] Carey B. *Health.* 1998;Jan/Feb:52–5.

[94] Wagner P, et al. *J Pharm Pract.* 1999;48:615–19.

[95] Stevinson C, et al. *CNS Drugs.* 1999;11(2):125–32.

[96] Bove G. *Lancet.* 1998;352(9134):1121–2.

[97] Bowers A. Phytodermatitis. *Am J Contact Dermat.* 1999;10(2):89–93.

[98] Markowitz J, et al. *Life Sci.* 2000;66(9):PL133-9.

[99] Nierenberg A, et al. *Biol Psychiatry.* 1999;46(12):1707–8.

[100] Moses E, et al. *J Clin Psychopharmacol.* 2000;20(1):115–17.

[101] Shipochliev T. *Vet Med Nauki.* 1981;18(4):94–8.

[102] Grush L, et al. *JAMA.* 1998;28(18):1566.

[103] Ondrizek R, et al. *J Assist Reprod Genet.* 1999;16(2):87–91.

Stevia

SCIENTIFIC NAME(S): *Stevia rebaudiana* Bertoni. Family: Asteraceae

COMMON NAME(S): Stevia, Sweet Leaf of Paraguay, Caa-he-é, Ca-a-yupi, Eira-caa, Capim doce

---

⊱⊰⊱⊰ PATIENT INFORMATION ⊱⊰⊱⊰

Uses: Stevia is used as a sweetening agent. It has also been found to have hypotensive, hypoglycemic, and bactericidal properties.

Side Effects: No major contraindications, warnings, or side effects have been documented.

Dosing: Stevia leaf is used ad lib for sweetening foods.

BOTANY: Stevia is a perennial shrub indigenous to northern South America, but commercially grown in areas such as Central America, Israel, Thailand, and China. The plant can grow to 1 m in height, with 2- to 3-cm long leaves. The leaves are the parts of the plant used.[1]

HISTORY: Stevia has been used to sweeten tea for centuries, dating back to the Guarani Indians of South America. For hundreds of years, native Brazilians and Paraguayans also have employed the leaves of the plant as a sweetening agent. Europeans learned about stevia in the 16th century, whereas North American interest in the plant began in the 20th century when researchers heard of its sweetening properties. Paraguayan botanist Moises Bertoni documented stevia in the early 1900s. Glycosides responsible for the plant's sweeteners were discovered in 1931. Stevia extracts are used today as food additives by the Japanese and Brazilians as a noncaloric sweetener. However, in the US, use is limited to supplement status only.[1,2]

PHARMACOLOGY: Stevia has been used for centuries as a natural sweetener.[1] The plant contains sweet ent-kaurene glycosides,[3] with the most intense sweetness belonging to the *S. rebaudina* species.[4] Stevia has been evaluated for sweetness in animal response testing.[5] In humans, stevia as a sweetening agent works well in weight-loss programs to satisfy "sugar cravings," and it is low in calories. The Japanese are the largest consumers of stevia leaves and use the plant to sweeten foods (as a replacement for aspartame and saccharin) such as soy sauce, confections, and soft drinks.[1]

Stevia may be helpful in treating diabetes. Oral use of stevia extract in combination with chrysanthemum to manage hyperglycemia has been discussed.[6] Aqueous extracts of the plant increased glucose tolerance in 16 healthy volunteers, as well as markedly decreasing plasma glucose levels.[7]

Stevia's effects on blood pressure have been reported. The plant displayed vasodilatory actions in normotensive and hypertensive animals.[8] The plant has cardiotonic actions, which normalize blood pressure and regulate heartbeat.[1]

Stevia extract has exhibited strong bactericidal activity against a wide range of pathogenic bacteria, including certain *E. coli* strains.[9] Steviol, stevia's aglycone, is mutagenic toward salmonella and other bacterial strains, under various conditions and toward certain cell lines.[10-13] Stevia may also be effective against *Candida albicans*.[1] One report addresses stevia's role against dental plaque.[14]

TOXICOLOGY: Stevia has been shown not to be mutagenic or genotoxic.[1] One report indicates that constituents of stevioside and steviol are not mutagenic in vitro.[15] Stevioside was found to be nontoxic in acute toxicity studies in a variety of laboratory animals.[1] Chronic administration of stevia to male rats had no effect in fertility vs. controls.[16] Another report concludes that stevioside in high doses affected neither growth nor reproduction in hamsters of both sexes.[17]

1 Sousa M. *Constituintes Quimicos Ativos De Planta Medicinais Brasileiras*. Fortaleza, Brasil: Laboratorio de Produtos Naturais.

2 Blumenthal M. *Whole Foods*. Feb. 1996.

3 Kinghorn A, et al. *J Nat Prod*. 1984; 47(3):439–44.

4 Soejarto D, et al. *J Nat Prod*. 1982; 45(5):590–99.

5 Jakinovich W, et al. *J Nat Prod*. 1990; 53(1):190–95.

6 White J, et al. *Diabetes Care*. 1994; 17(8):940.

7 Curi R, et al. Effect of Stevia rebaudiana on glucose tolerance in normal adult humans. *Braz J Med Biol Res*. 1986; 19(6):771–74.

8 Melis MS. *Braz J Med Biol Res*. 1996; 29(5):669–75.

9 Tomita T, et al. *Microbiol Immunol*. 1997; 41(12): 1005–9.

10 Pezzuto J, et al. *Proc Natl Acad Sci*. 1985; 82(8):2478–82.

11 Pezzuto J, et al. *Mutat Res*. 1986; 169(3):93–103.

12 Matsui M, et al. *Mutagenesis*. 1996; 11(6):573–79.

13 Klongpanichpak S, et al. *J Med Assoc*. 1997; 80 Suppl 1: S121–28.

14 Pinheiro C, et al. *Rev Odontol Univ Sao Paulo*. 1987; 1(4):9–13.

15 Suttajit M, et al. *Environ Health Perspect*. 1993; 101 Suppl 3:53–56.

16 Oliveira-Filho RM, et al. *Gen Pharmacol*. 1989; 20(2):187–91.

17 Yodyingyuad V, et al. *Hum Reprod*. 1991; 6(1):158–65.

SCIENTIFIC NAME(S): *Melaleuca alternifolia* (Cheel) Family: Myrtaceae

COMMON NAME(S): Tea tree oil

❧❧❧ PATIENT INFORMATION ❧❧❧

Uses: Tea tree oil has been used mainly for its antimicrobial effects. Apply tea tree oil topically; do not ingest orally.

Side Effects: Use of tea tree oil has resulted in allergic contact eczema and dermatitis.

Dosing: TTO has been studied for its topical antifungal activity incorporated in cream formulations of 5% and 10% and as the neat oil. Standardized tea tree oil contains less than 10% cineole and greater than 30% terpinen-4-ol. Dosage should initially start low to avoid irritation caused by cineole. CNS toxicity has been observed at internal doses of 10 to 70 mL.[1-3]

BOTANY: There are many plants known as "tea trees," but *Melaleuca alternifolia* is responsible for the "tea tree oil," which has recently gained popularity. Native to Australia, the tea tree is found in coastal areas. It is an evergreen shrub that can grow to 6 m tall. Its narrow, 4 cm, needle-like leaves release a distinctive aroma when crushed. The fruits grow in clusters, and its white flowers bloom in the summer.[4]

HISTORY: Tea tree oil (TTO) was first used in surgery and dentistry in the mid-1920s. Its healing properties were also used during World War II for skin injuries to those working in munition factories. TTO's popularity has resurfaced within the last few years with help from promotional campaigns. The oil may be present in soaps, shampoos, and lotions.[4]

PHARMACOLOGY: TTO has been used mainly for its antimicrobial effects without irritating sensitive tissues. It has been applied to cuts, stings, acne, and burns. In hospitals, TTO has been used in soap and soaked in blankets to make an antibacterial covering for burn victims. When run through air-conditioning ducts, TTO has been shown to exert bactericidal effects.[4] A considerable amount of literature has become available on this topic.

Disc diffusion and broth microdilution methods have been used to determine antimicrobial effects against 8 TTO constituents. Terpin-4-ol was active against all test organisms including *Candida albicans*, *Escherichia coli*, *Staphylococcus aureus*, and *Pseudomonas aeruginosa*. Other constituents of the oil (such as linalool and α-terpineol) had some antimicrobial activity as well.[5,6] In addition, constituents terpin-4-ol, α-terpineol, and α-pinene were found to possess antimicrobial effects against *Staphylococcus epidermidis* and *Propionibacterium acnes*.[7]

TTO may be useful in removing "transient skin flora while suppressing but maintaining resident flora."[8] TTO was also shown to be an effective topical treatment of monilial and fungal dermatoses and superficial skin infections in 50 subjects for 6 months with minimal or no side effects reported.[9] One report suggests TTO to be useful in treatment of "methicillin-resistant *S. aureus* (MRSA) carriage." In this evaluation, all 66 isolates of *S. aureus* were susceptible to the essential oil (64 isolates being MRSA, 33 being mupirocin-resistant).[10]

TTO's activity against anaerobic oral bacteria has been surveyed.[11] One case report exists, discussing antibacterial efficacy of TTO in a 40-year-old woman with anaerobic vaginosis.[12]

In a randomized, double-blind study comparing the efficacy of 10% (w/w) TTO cream with 1% tolnaftate (and placebo creams) against tinea pedis (athlete's foot), TTO was found to be as effective as tolnaftate in reducing symptoms but no more effective than placebo in achieving a mycological cure.[13] In a report on onychomycosis (nail fungus), TTO (100%) vs clotrimazole solution (1%) application yielded similar results in treatment. Both therapies had high recurrence rates.[14]

TTO can be added to baths or vaporizers to help treat respiratory disorders. Related oils have been used for nasal antiseptic purposes, pulmonary anti-inflammatory use, and coughs.[1,2,4] TTO is also used in perfumery and aromatherapy.[5]

TOXICOLOGY: Allergic contact eczema was found to be caused primarily by the α-limonene constituent (in TTO) in 7 patients tested. In this same report, alpha-terpinene and aromadendrene additionally caused dermatitis in 5 of the patients.[15] Eucalyptol was found to be the contact allergan in a Dutch report.[16] Contact allergy caused by TTO may be related to cross-sensitization to colophony.[17] A case report describes a petechial body rash and marked neutrophil leukocytosis in a 60-year-old man who ingested about ½ teaspoonful of the oil (for common cold symptoms). He recovered 1 week later.[18]

Another case report describes ataxia and drowsiness as a result of oral TTO ingestion (less than 10 mL) by a 17-month-old male. He was treated with activated charcoal, which was only partially successful, but after a short time appeared normal and was discharged 7 hours after ingestion.[19]

[1] Tong M, et al. *Australas J Dermatol.* 1992;33(3):145-49.

[2] Buck D, et al. *J F Pract.* 1994;38(6):601-5.

[3] Syed TA, et al. *Trop Med Int Health.* 1999;4:284-287.

[4] Low T, et al. (contributing editors). *Reader's Digest (Aust) Magic and Medicines of Plants.* Surry Hills, NSW, 2010 Australia: PTY Limited 1994;349.

[5] Bruneton J. *Medicinal Plants.* Seacus, NY: Lavoisier Publ. Inc., 1995;461.

[6] Osol, et al, eds. *The Dispensatory of the United States of America.* Philadelphia, PA: JB Lippincott, 1960;1750.

[7] Carson C, et al. *J Appl Bacteriol.* 1995;78(3):264-69.

[8] Carson C, et al. *Microbios.* 1995;82(332):181-85.

[9] Raman A, et al. *Letters in Applied Microbiology.* 1995;21(4):242-45.

[10] Hammer K, et al. *Am J Infect Control.* 1996;24(3):186-89.

[11] Shemesh A, et al. *Aust J Pharm.* 1991 Sep;72:802-3.

[12] Carson C, et al. *J Antimicrob Chemother.* 1995;35(3):421-24.

[13] Shapiro S, et al. *Oral Microbiology and Immunology.* 1994;9(4):202-8.

[14] Blackwell A. *Lancet.* 1991 Feb 2;337:300.

[15] Knight T, et al. *J Am Acad Dermatol.* 1994;30(3):423-27.

[16] Van der Valk P, et al. *Ned Tijdschr Geneeskd.* 1994;138(16):823-25.

[17] Selvaag E, et al. *Contact Dermatitis.* 1994;31(2):124-25.

[18] Elliott C. *Med J Aust.* 1993 Dec 6;159:830-31.

[19] Del Beccaro M. *Vet Hum Toxicol.* 1995;37(6):557-58.

SCIENTIFIC NAME(S): *Terminalia arjuna, Terminalia bellirica (T. belerica), Terminalia chebula* Family: Combretaceae[1,2,3,4,5]

COMMON NAME(S): Arjuna, Axjun, Argun (*T. arjuna*); Behada, Bahera (Bahira), Balera (*T. belerica*); Hara, Harada, Hirala, Myrobalan, Haritaki (*T. chebula*); Bala harade (*T. chebula* black variety).

❧❧❧ PATIENT INFORMATION ❧❧❧

Uses: *T. arjuna's* traditional use as a cardiotonic has been confirmed by modern research. It also has been used as an aphrodisiac, diuretic, and for earaches.[1,2] It may play a role as an anti-atherogenic,[6] and has reduced cholesterol. *T. belerica* has been used in treating liver disorders[1] and as a primary treatment for digestive and respiratory (eg, cough, sore throat) problems.[2] Other uses include the following: as an astringent, laxative,[2,7] lotion for sore eyes,[2] and retroviral reverse transcriptase inhibitory activity in murine leukemia enzymes.[8] *T. chebula* is used in Indian medicine to treat digestive problems. Other uses include as a mouthwash/gargle, astringent, and douche for vaginitis.[2] *T. chebula* and *T. belerica* have demonstrated antimicrobial properties.[9,10] Certain *Terminalia* species demonstrate antifungal[11] and antiviral[12-15] activities.

Side Effects: Few toxicity reports exist; do not use during pregnancy.

Dosing: Daily doses of 0.5 to 1.5 g of powdered *Terminalia* bark have been studied for their clinical effects on heart failure and serum cholesterol levels. A 10% solution also has been used as a mouthwash.[16-18]

BOTANY: The *Terminalia* species are evergreen trees. *T. arjuna* reaches about 30 m, has light-yellow flowers and cone-shaped leaves. *T. belerica* has clustered oval leaves and greenish, foul-smelling flowers with brown, hairy fruit about the size of walnuts. *T. chebula* grows about 21 m in height with white flowers and small, ribbed fruits.[2]

T. arjuna is used for its bark. In other *Terminalia* species, the fruit is the plant part used.[1] For example, in India, 100,000 metric tons of *T. chebula* fruit was produced in 1 year.[19]

A traditional Ayurvedic herbal combination dating back 5000 years is a mixture of 3 herbs, 2 of which are terminalia species: *T. belerica* (for health-harmonizing qualities), *T. chebula* (to normalize body balance), and *Emblica officinalis*.[3]

HISTORY: Arjuna bark has been used in Indian medicine for at least 3000 years as a remedy for heart ailments. *T. chebula* also has been used by this culture as a digestive aid.[2] This species, referred to as "King of Medicine" by Tibetans, is often depicted in the extended palm of Buddha. The *E. officinalis/T. chebula/T. belerica* herbal combination product is said to have been formulated by Ayurvedic physicians thousands of years ago.[3]

PHARMACOLOGY: Some similarity in pharmacologic actions exist among the 3 species. *T. arjuna's* traditional use as a cardiotonic has been confirmed by modern research. Although some results of these studies (performed since the 1930s) appear conflicting, (eg, increases and decreases in heart rate or blood pressure), the herb seems to work best when blood supply to the heart is compromised as in ischemic heart disease or angina.[2] Ayurvedic medicine employs *T. arjuna* to restore balance of the "3 humors."[3] *T. arjuna* also has been used as an aphrodisiac, diuretic, and for earaches.[1,2] This species has reduced cholesterol levels, as well.[2] Studies done on *T. arjuna* combinations find the herb to be the most potent hypolipidemic agent compared with *T. belerica* and *T. chebula*. *T. arjuna* may also play a role as an anti-atherogenic.[6]

T. belerica has been studied for its effects on similar disease states. *T. belerica's* role in treating liver disorders is apparent.[1] Constituent gallic acid displays significant hepatoprotective effects. Marked reversal of most altered parameters was shown including lipid peroxidation, drug metabolizing enzymes, and others.[20] *T. belerica* also has been used as primary treatment for digestive and respiratory (eg, cough, sore throat) problems.[2] Other uses include the following: as an astrigent, laxative,[2,7] lotion for sore eyes,[2] and retroviral reverse transcriptase inhibitory activity in murine leukemia enzymes.[8]

T. chebula is used in Indian medicine to treat digestive problems. It improves bowel regularity, thus making it possibly useful as a laxative and to treat diarrhea and dysentery.[1,2] Other uses include as a mouthwash/gargle, astringent, and douche for vaginitis.[2]

T. chebula and *T. belerica* have demonstrated antimicrobial properties.[9,10] *T. chebula* also has been evaluated for activity aganist methicillin-resistant *Staphylococcus aureus*.[21]

Certain *Terminalia* species demonstrate antifungal[11] and antiviral[12-15] activities, as well.

TOXICOLOGY: Few reports were found from recent literature searches regarding *Terminalia* species and toxicity. One source warns against taking *T. belerica* and *T. chebula* during pregnancy.[2]

[1] Evans W. *Trease and Evans' Pharmacognosy*, 14th ed. WB Saunders Co. Ltd, 1996;493.

[2] Chevallier A. *Encyclopedia of Medicinal Plants*. New York, NY: DK Publishing, 1996;141,273.

[3] Khorana M, et al. *Indian J Pharm.* 1959;21:331.

[4] Rukmini C, et al. *J Am Oil Chem Soc.* 1986;63(3):360-63.

[5] Thakur C, et al. *Int J Cardiol.* 1988;21(2):167-75.

[6] Shaila H, et al. *Int J Cardiol.* 1998;67(2):119-24.

[7] Dhar H, et al. *Indian J Med Res.* 1969;57(1):103-05.

[8] Suthienkul O, et al. *Southeast Asian J Trop Med Public Health.* 1993;24(4):751-55.

[9] Ahmad I, et al. *J Ethnopharmacol.* 1998;62(2):183-93.

[10] Phadke S, et al. *Indian J Med Sci.* 1989;43(5):113-17.

[11] Dutta B, et al. *Mycoses.* 1998;41(11-12):535-36.

[12] Shiraki K, et al. *Nippon Rinsho.* 1998;56(1):156-60.

[13] Yukawa T, et al. *Antiviral Res.* 1996;32(2):63-70.

[14] Kurokawa M, et al. *Antiviral Res.* 1995;27(1-2):19-37.

[15] el-Mekkawy S, et al. *Chem Pharm Bull.* 1995;43(4):641-48.

[16] Gupta R, et al. *J Assoc Physicians India.* 2001;49:231-235.

[17] Bharani A, et al. *Int J Cardiol.* 1995;49:191-199.

[18] Jagtap AG, et alG. *J Ethnopharmacol.* 1999;68:299-306.

[19] Bruneton J. *Pharmacognosy, Phytochemistry, Medicinal Plants*. Paris, France: Lavoisier Publishing, 1995;333.

[20] Anand K, et al. *Pharmacol Res.* 1997;36(4):315-21.

[21] Sato Y, et al. *Biol Pharm Bull.* 1997;20(4):401-04.

Turmeric

SCIENTIFIC NAME(S): *Curcuma longa* L. Synonymous with *C. domestica* Vahl. Family: Zingiberaceae

COMMON NAME(S): Turmeric, curcuma, Indian saffron

❧❧❧ PATIENT INFORMATION ❧❧❧

Uses: Turmeric is used as a spice. Recent investigations indicate that the strong antioxidant effects of several components of turmeric result in an inhibiton of carcinogenesis and may play a role in limiting the development of cancers.

Side Effects: There are no known side effects.

Dosing: Powdered turmeric root has been used as a stimulant and carminative at doses of 0.5 to 3 g/day. Higher doses of 6 g/day were investigated for protective effects against ulcer.[1]

BOTANY: Turmeric is a perennial member of the ginger family characterized by a thick rhizome. The plant grows to a height of about 0.9 to 1.5 m and has large oblong leaves. It bears funnel-shaped yellow flowers.[2] The plant is cultivated widely throughout Asia, India, China, and tropical countries. The primary (bulb) and secondary (lateral) rhizomes are collected, cleaned, boiled, and dried; and lateral rhizomes contain more yellow coloring material than the bulb.[3] The dried rhizome forms the basis for the culinary spice.

HISTORY: Turmeric has a warm, bitter taste and is a primary component of curry powders and some mustards. The powder and its oleoresins are used extensively as food flavorings in the culinary industry. The spice has a long history of use in Asian medicine. In Chinese medicine, it has been used to treat problems as diverse as flatulence and hemorrhage. It also has been used topically as a poultice, as an analgesic, and to treat ringworms.[4] The spice has been used for the management of jaundice and hepatitis.[3] The oil is sometimes used as a perfume component.

PHARMACOLOGY: Several soluble fractions of turmeric, including curcumin, have been reported to have antioxidant properties. Turmeric inhibits the degradation of polyunsaturated fatty acids.[5] The curcumins inhibit cancer at initiation, promotion, and progression stages of development.[6]

In smokers, turmeric given at a daily dose of 1.5 g for 30 days significantly reduced the urinary excretion of mutagens compared with controls; turmeric had no effect on hepatic enzyme levels or lipid profiles suggesting that the spice may be an effective antimutagen useful in chemoprevention.[7]

Ukonan-A, a polysaccharide with phagocytosis-activating activity has been isolated from *C. longa*,[8] and ukonan-D has demonstrated strong reticuloendothelial system-potentiating activity.[9] Aqueous extract of *C. longa* has been shown to have cytoprotective effects that inhibit chemically induced carcinogenesis, forming a basis for the traditional use of turmeric as an anticancer treatment.[10]

A combination of turmeric and neem (*Azadirachta indica*) applied topically has been shown to effectively eradicate scabies in 97% of 814 people treated within 3 to 15 days.[11] Other pharmacologic properties of turmeric include choleretic, hypotensive, antibacterial, and insecticidal activity.

The choleretic (bile-stimulating) activity of curcumin has been recognized for almost 40 years, and these compounds have been shown to possess strong antihepatotoxic properties.[12]

TOXICOLOGY: No reports of toxicity have been reported following the ingestion of turmeric. No change in weight was observed following chronic treatment, although changes in heart and lung weights were observed; a decrease in white and red blood cell levels were observed. Although a gain in weight of sexual organs and an increase in sperm motility was observed, no spermatotoxic effects were found.[13]

[1] Dobelis IN, ed. *Magic and Medicine of Plants.* Pleasantville, NY: Reader's Digest Association, Inc., 1986.

[2] Evans WC. *Trease and Evans' Pharmacognosy,* 13th ed. London, England: Balliere Tindall, 1989.

[3] Dau NV, et al. *Phytomed.* 1998;5:29-34.

[4] Leung AY. *Encyclopedia of Common Natural Ingredients Used in Food, Drugs and Cosmetics.* New York, NY: John Wiley and Sons, 1980.

[5] Reddy AC, et al. *Mol Cell Biochem.* 1992;111:117.

[6] Nagabhushan M, et al. *J Am Coll Nutr.* 1992;11:192.

[7] Polasa K, et al. *Mutagenesis.* 1992;7:107.

[8] Gonda R, et al. *Chem Pharm Bull.* 1992;40:990.

[9] Ibid. 1992;40:185.

[10] Azuine MA, et al. *J Cancer Res Clin Oncol.* 1992;118:447.

[11] Charles V, et al. *Trop Geogr Med.* 1992;44:178.

[12] Kiso Y, et al. *Phytochemistry.* 1983;49:185.

[13] Qureshi S, et al. *Planta Med.* 1992;58:124.

Ubiquinone

SCIENTIFIC NAME(S): Coenzyme Q-10, ubidecarenone, mitoquinone

COMMON NAME(S): Adelir, heartcin, inokiton, neuquinone, taidecanone, udekinon, ubiquinone

---

✺✺✺ PATIENT INFORMATION ✺✺✺

Uses: Ubiquinone may have applications in treating ischemic heart disease, congestive heart failure (CHF), toxin-induced cardiopathy and hypertension, and protects ischemic myocardium during surgery.

Side effects: Rare side effects include epigastric discomfort, loss of appetite, nausea, and diarrhea. Use is not recommended in pregnancy and lactation and in people with demonstrated hypersensitivity.

Dosing: Ubiquinone has been studied in clinical trials at doses of 90 to 200 mg/day for heart failure, cirrhosis, and antioxidant properties.[1-8]

HISTORY: The first ubiquinone was isolated in 1957. Since that time, ubiquinones have been extensively studied in Japan, Russia, and Europe. Research in the US began more recently. Lay press accounts claim that roughly 12 million Japanese use ubiquinones for the management of cardiovascular diseases, supplying the demand for more than 250 commercially available preparations. Ubiquinone is touted as an effective treatment of CHF, cardiac arrhythmias, hypertension, and in the reduction of hypoxic injury to the myocardium. Other health claims include the increase of exercise tolerance, stimulation of the immune system, and slowing the aging process. Clinical uses include the treatment of diabetes, obesity, and periodontal disease. Ubiquinone is not approved for therapeutic use in the US, but it is available as a food supplement.[9]

PHARMACOLOGY: Biomedical evidence provides the rationale for the use of ubiquinone in cardiovascular diseases. Endogenous forms function as essential cofactors in several metabolic pathways, especially in oxidative respiration. Supraphysiologic doses of ubiquinone may benefit tissues that have been rendered ischemic and then reperfused. Ubiquinone appears to function in such tissues as a free-radical scavenger, membrane stabilizer, or both.[10] Ubiquinone as a mobile component in mitochondrial membrane and its role in electron transfer has been reported.[11] It may have applications in treating ischemic heart disease, CHF, toxin-induced cardiopathy, and possibly hypertension. It protects ischemic myocardium during surgery.[10]

Ubiquinone's role in cardiac treatment using human subjects is promising. In geriatric patients, ubiquinone treatment improved both symptoms and clinical conditions of all 34 patients with CHF.[12] It also was effective for symptomatic mitral valve prolapse and improved stress-induced cardiac dysfunction in 400 pediatric patients.[13] Activity tolerance improvements were observed in a double-blind study of 19 patients with chronic myocardial disease given oral ubiquinone-10.[14] In advanced heart failure, 12 patients given 100 mg daily of the drug showed marked clinical improvement.[15] Immune system effects were enhanced in myocardial failure in another report, when ubiquinone was used in conjunction with other drugs.[16] Aiding defective myocardial supply, ubiquinone's role in oxidative phosphorylation offers positive results in adjunctive treatment, clinical outcomes, symptoms, and quality of life in these cardiac patients.[17]

Ubiquinone's actions on lipids also have been reported. The mechanism may be membrane phospholipid protection against phospholipase attack.[18] In its reduced form, ubiquinone's presence in all cellular membrane, blood serum, and serum lipoproteins, allows protection from lipid peroxidation.[19] Its ability to remain stable in hypercholesterolemia patients has been studied.[20,21] Ubiquinol can also sustain vitamin E's antioxidant effects by regenerating the vitamin from its oxidized form.[19,22]

One report describes ubiquinone and its role in human nutrition.[23] A case report

uses ubiquinone to treat drug-induced rhabdomyolysis and hepatotoxicity.[24]

INTERACTIONS: There exists the potential for herb-drug interactions to occur between ubiquinone and warfarin. Avoid concurrent use.[25]

TOXICOLOGY: No serious side effects have been associated with the use of ubiquinone. Use of the substance is contraindicated in people with demonstrated hypersensitivity. Use during pregnancy or lactation is not recommended because studies have not demonstrated the safety of ubiquinone for fetuses and infants. Rare side effects have included epigastric discomfort, loss of appetite, nausea and diarrhea.[8]

[1] Khatta M, et al. *Ann Intern Med.* 2000;132:636-640.

[2] Munkholm H, et al. *Biofactors.* 1999;9:285-289.

[3] Eriksson JG, et al. *Biofactors.* 1999;9:315-318.

[4] Barbieri B, et al. *Biofactors.* 1999;9:351-357.

[5] Henriksen JE, et al. *Diabet Med.* 1999;16:312-318.

[6] Raitakari OT, et al. *Free Radic Biol Med.* 2000;28:1100-1105.

[7] Kaikkonen J, et al. *Free Radic Res.* 2000;33:329-340.

[8] Watson JP, et al. *J Gastroenterol Hepatol.* 1999;14:1034-1040.

[9] Lay press accounts and promotional brochures.

[10] Greenberg SM, et al. *Med Clin North Am.* 1987;72:243.

[11] Lenaz G, et al. *Drugs Exp Clin Res.* 1985;11(8):547-56.

[12] Cascone A, et al. *Boll Chim Farm.* 1985;124(May):435-525.

[13] Oda T. *Drugs Exp Clin Res.* 1985;11(8):557-76.

[14] Langsjoen P, et al. *Drugs Exp Clin Res.* 1985;11(8):577-9.

[15] Mortensen S, et al. *Drugs Exp Clin Res.* 1985;11(8):581-3.

[16] Folkers K, et al. *Drugs Exp Clin Res.* 1985;11(8):539-45.

[17] Mortensen S. *Clin Investigator.* 1993;71(8 Suppl):S116-23.

[18] Sugiyama S, et al. *Arzneimittelforschung.* 1985;35(1):23-5.

[19] Ernster L, et al. *Biochem Biophys Acta.* 1995;1271(1):195-204.

[20] Mabuchi H, et al. *N Engl J Med.* 1981;305(Aug 27):478-82.

[21] Laaksonen R, et al. *Clin Pharmacol Ther.* 1995;57(Jan):62-6.

[22] Ernster L, et al. *Clin Investigator.* 1993;71(8 Suppl):S60-5.

[23] Hotzel D. *Dtsch Apothek Zeit.* 1995;135(Jul 6):27-8, 31-2, 35-6.

[24] Lees R, et al. *N Engl J Med.* 1995;333(Sept 7):664-5.

[25] Spigset O. *Lancet.* 1994;344;1372.

SCIENTIFIC NAME(S): *Valeriana officinalis* L. Family: Valerianaceae. A number of other species have been used medicinally, including *V. wallichi* DC, *V. sambucifolia* Mik., and the related *Centranthus ruber* L.

COMMON NAME(S): Valerian, baldrian, radix valerianae, Indian valerian (*V. wallichii*), red valerian (*C. ruber*)

❧❧❧ PATIENT INFORMATION ❧❧❧

Uses: Valerian has been used for the treatment of restlessness and sleep disorders. Valerian is classified as generally recognized as safe (GRAS) in the US for food use. Extracts and the root oil are used as flavoring in foods and beverages.

Side Effects: Studies have generally found valerian to have fewer side effects than other positive control drugs.

Dosing: Valerian root (fresh or dried) has been used at doses of 2 to 3 g given 1 to 3 times/day for nervousness or as an antispasmodic, and at bedtime for insomnia. Several types of extracts have been tested; an aqueous extract has shown activity in sleep studies at doses of 270 to 900 mg, while an ethanolic extract has been recommended at 600 mg for sleep. Combinations with extracts of hops (eg, *ReDormin, Ze 91019*) or with lemon balm (*EuVegal Forte*) are quite common as sleep aids and the valerian extract dose in combinations is 320 to 500 mg. Lipophilic extracts such as *Baldrian-Dispert* have fallen out of favor because of toxicity concerns and the failure to identify active principles in them.[1-9]

BOTANY: Members of the genus *Valeriana* are herbaceous perennials widely distributed in the temperate regions of North America, Europe, and Asia. Of the 200 known species, the Eurasian *V. officinalis* is the species most often cultivated for medicinal use. The dried rhizome contains a volatile oil with a distinctive, unpleasant odor.[10] The fresh drug has no appreciable smell, but drying liberates the odiferous constituent isovaleric acid.[1]

HISTORY: Despite its odor, valerian was considered a perfume in 16th century Europe. The tincture has been used for its sedative properties for centuries; it is still widely used in France, Germany, and Switzerland as a sleep aid. About 50 tons of valerian are sold each year in France.[1]

PHARMACOLOGY: While there is substantial debate over the constituents responsible for valerian's sedative activity, it is undeniable that valerian preparations have sedative effects. Human studies have documented valerian's effectiveness as a sleep aid.

Aqueous and hydroalcoholic extracts of valerian induced release of [3H]GABA from synaptosomal preparations, which was interpreted as an effect on the GABA transporter. Thus GABA may be responsible for some of the peripheral effects of valerian, while glutamine, another free amino acid in the extract, can cross the blood-brain barrier and be metabolized to GABA in situ, producing central sedation.[11]

Valerenic acid has been found to inhibit GABA transaminase, the principle enzyme that catabolizes GABA. GABA-T inhibition increases the inhibitory effect of GABA in the CNS, and contributes to valerian's sedative properties.[12]

Clinical trials: There is abundant evidence that valerian is effective as a sleep aid and as a mild antianxiety agent, although the effect appears to be weaker in healthy subjects than in poor sleepers. An aqueous extract of the root (400 mg extract) improved sleep quality in a number of subjective parameters in 128 healthy volunteers using a crossover design.[1] Elderly patients with nervous disorders responded positively to a commercial valerian preparation in a placebo-controlled study, as measured by subjective and objective parameters.[13] Sleep latency was decreased in a group of 8 poor sleepers given an aqueous extract of valerian in a double-blind, placebo-controlled study.[2] A sleep laboratory study found minor sedative effects in healthy volunteers.[3] An uncontrolled multicenter study of more than 11,000 patients suffering from sleep-related disorders found subjective improvements in 94% of those treated.[4] Another multicenter trial of the same preparation in a younger study population found progressive symptomatic improvement over 10 days of treatment.[14] Valerian was found to increase slow-wave sleep in a pilot study of poor sleepers.[15] In contrast to previous studies that demonstrated a prompt decrease in symptoms, one study found that 2 to 4 weeks was required to see improvement in 121 patients with serious insomnia.[16] These studies have been reviewed.[17]

Combination studies: Valerian is combined with other herbs such as hops, St. John's wort, or balm in commercial products. A combination of hyperion and valerian was evaluated for antidepressant activity in a double-blind study of 93 patients treated for 6 weeks. All psychometric scales showed statisti-

cally significant improvement.[18] A second study of the same combination in the treatment of anxiety reached similar positive conclusions.[19] A combination of valerian and *Hibiscus syriacus* (rose of sharron) was active in 130 depressed patients over 6 weeks.[20] A valerian combination preparation containing valerenic acid sesquiterpenes, but not valepotriates, improved sleep quality in a small crossover study of poor sleepers.[5] Valerian and *Melissa officinalis* (balm) were effective in combination in a study (20 patients) of poor sleepers.[21] The same combination was found to be tolerated in healthy volunteers and increased the quality of sleep.[6] A complex product made up of 6 herbs (*Crataegus*, *Ballota*, *Passiflora*, *Valeriana*, *Cola*, and *Paullinia*) treated generalized anxiety, producing progressive decreases in the Hamilton Anxiety Scale that were greater than with placebo.[22]

TOXICOLOGY: Concern was raised over the discovery that valepotriates are mutagenic in the Ames assay; their poor bioavailability makes them a dubious source of toxicity for patients.[23]

Clinical studies have generally found valerian to have fewer side effects than positive control drugs such as diazepam, producing little hangover effect when used as a sleep aid. An intentional overdose has been reported in which 20 times the recommended dose was ingested; the patient experienced mild symptoms that resolved within 24 hours.[24] A case of withdrawal after chronic use of valerian has been reported; however, the complex nature of the patient's medical history provides weak support for valerian's role.[25]

[1] Leathwood P, et al. *Pharmacol Biochem Behav.* 1982;17(1):65-71.

[2] Leathwood P, et al. *Planta Med.* 1985;Apr(2):144-48.

[3] Balderer G, et al. *Psychopharmacology (Berl).* 1985;87(4):406-09.

[4] Schmidt-Vogt J. *Therapiewoche.* 1986;36:663-67.

[5] Lindahl O, et al. *Pharmacol Biochem Behav.* 1989;32(4):1065-66.

[6] Cerny A, et al. *Fitoterapia.* 1999;70:221-28.

[7] Kohnen R, Oswald WD. *Pharmacopsychiatry.* 1988;21:447-448.

[8] Dressing H, et al. *Psychpharmakotherapie.* 1996;3:123-130.

[9] Fussel A, et al. *Eur J Med Res.* 2000;5:385-390.

[10] Houghton P. *J Pharm Pharmacol.* 1999;51(5):505-12.

[11] Santos M, et al. *Planta Med.* 1994;60(5):475-76.

[12] Riedel E, et al. *Planta Med.* 1982;46:219-20.

[13] Kamm-Kohl A, et al. *Med Welt.* 1984;35:1450.

[14] Seifert T. *Therapeutikon.* 1988;2:94-98.

[15] Schulz H, et al. *Pharmacopsychiatry.* 1994;27(4):147-51.

[16] Vorbach E, et al. *Psychopharmakotherapie.* 1996;3109.

[17] Schulz V, et al. *Phytomedicine.* 1997;4(4):379-87.

[18] Steger W. *Therapeutisches Erfahrungen.* 1985;61:914-18.

[19] Panijel M. Therapy of symptoms of anxiety. *Therapiewoche* . 1985;414659.

[20] Kniebel R, et al. *Therapeutisches Erfahrungen.* 1988;64:689-96.

[21] DreBing H, et al. *Therapiewoche.* 1992;42:726-36.

[22] Bourin M, et al. *Fundam Clin Pharmacol.* 1997;11:127-32.

[23] von der Hude W, et al. *Mutat Res.* 1986;169:23-27.

[24] Willey L, et al. *Vet Hum Toxicol.* 1995;37(4):364.

[25] Garges H, et al. *JAMA.* 1998;280(18):1566-67.

SCIENTIFIC NAME(S): *Dioscorea villosa* L. Dioscoreaceae (Yams)

COMMON NAME(S): Wild yam root, colic root, yuma, devil's bones, rheumatism root, China root

---

❧❧❧ PATIENT INFORMATION ❧❧❧

Uses: *Dioscorea* has been promoted for the treatment of menstrual dysfunction, nausea in pregnancy, urinary tract infections, rheumatoid arthritis, cholera, nervous excitement, and gas expulsion.

Side Effects: In large doses, *D. villosa* root may cause nausea, vomiting, and diarrhea.

Dosing: Wild yam root was used traditionally as a diaphoretic and expectorant at doses of 0.4 to 4 g/day, although there are no recent clinical studies to substantiate this dosage.[1]

BOTANY: *D. villosa* is a twining vine native to the central southeastern US and found less frequently in the Appalachian region. It is a dioecious plant with inconspicuous white to greenish yellow female flowers and smooth heart-shaped leaves. A Chinese species, *Dioscorea opposita* Thunb., is also occasionally found in herbal commerce. There are more than 500 species of *Dioscorea* worldwide.

HISTORY: Wild yam was popularized by the Eclectic medical movement in the 19th century for its supposed antispasmodic properties and prescribed for biliary colic and spasm of the bowel. More recently, it has been promoted for the relief of nausea in pregnancy, and for amenorrhoea and dysmenorrhoea.[1] Wild yam use for urinary tract infections, rheumatoid arthritis, cholera, nervous excitement, and gas expulsion have been reported.

PHARMACOLOGY: The root of *D. villosa* is reported to be diaphoretic and expectorant in a dose of 4 g.[2] Much of the current herbal use of wild yam is predicated on the misconception that the diosgenin contained in the product can be converted by the human body into steroid hormones, particularly progesterone, through the intermediate dehydroepiandrosterone (DHEA). This notion appears to be based on diosgenin's use as a synthetic precursor of cortisone[3] and of the steroids found in birth control pills. There is no scientific evidence to support the notion that diosgenin or dioscin can be converted by the body into human hormones. In a pilot study of women using wild yam products (*D. villosa*), it was found that progesterone synthesis appeared to be suppressed compared with controls.[4] No direct effect of wild yam extract on the estrogen or progesterone receptors was found.

Work with ginseng saponins has shown that metabolism by specific microbes in the gut can substantially enhance uptake of the metabolites into the body.[5,6] Thus, one may postulate a similar mechanism of uptake with other, otherwise poorly absorbed plant saponins such as dioscin. Research needs to be done to understand the pharmacodynamics of saponin-containing plants in humans.

Topical formulations of *Dioscorea* are also poorly understood, though it is unlikely that they can serve as "progesterone replacement" vehicles. The sale of supplemental DHEA as an "anti-aging" product has carried over to *Dioscorea* by analogy. In fact, several products containing *Dioscorea* and DHEA are available.

TOXICOLOGY: In large doses, *D. villosa* root may cause nausea, vomiting, and diarrhea.

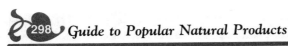

[1] Brinker F. *J Naturopathic Med.* 1996;7:11.
[2] Claus E. *Textbook of Pharmacognosy*, 5th ed. Philadelphia, PA: Lea & Febiger, 1956:151-52.
[3] Correll D, et al. *Econ Bot.* 1955;9:307.
[4] Zava D, et al. *Proc Soc Exp Biol Med.* 1998;217:369.
[5] Akao T, et al. *Biol Pharm Bull.* 1998;21:245.
[6] Hasegawa H, et al. *Planta Med.* 1996;62:453.

SCIENTIFIC NAME(S): *Salix alba* L., *Salix purpurea* L., *Salix fragilis* L., and other species. Family: Salicaceae (willow family)

COMMON NAME(S): Willow, weidenrinde, white willow (*S. alba*), purple osier willow/basket willow (*S. purpurea*), crack willow (*S. fragilis*)

༭༭༭ PATIENT INFORMATION ༭༭༭

Uses: Willow bark can be an effective analgesic if the content of salicylates is adequate.

Side Effects: Adverse effects are those of salicylates in general. Use with caution in patients with peptic ulcers and other medical conditions in which aspirin is contraindicated.

Dosing: Willow bark has been used for analgesia at daily doses of 1 to 3 g of bark, corresponding to 60 to 120 mg of salicin. A clinical study of low back pain used willow bark at a daily dose of 120 to 240 mg salicin.[1]

BOTANY: Willows are small trees or shrubs, many of which grow in moist places or along riverbanks in temperate and cold climates. Most of the several hundred species are dioecious, with male and female catkins (flowers) on separate plants. Largely insect pollinated, different species of willow hybridize freely. Medicinal willow bark is collected in the early spring from young branches (2 to 3 years of age) of the species listed above. Other species of *Salix* have similar chemistry and pharmacology.

HISTORY: For centuries, the bark of European willows has been used to treat fevers, headache and other pain, and arthritis. North American willows also have been used in folk medicine. Most of the European medicinal willows have been introduced to the Americas and have escaped cultivation. In the late 19th century, salicylic acid was widely used in place of willow bark, and its derivative aspirin was discovered to be less irritating to the mouth and stomach.[2,3]

PHARMACOLOGY: The ester glycosides salicortin, tremulacin, and fragilin can be considered to be prodrugs of salicylic acid, that deliver this compound into the systemic circulation without irritating the GI tract.[4] The pharmacokinetics of salicylic acid delivered from willow bark have been studied, and the plasma half-life is determined as approximately 2.5 hours.[5] The mechanism of action of salicylic acid is inhibition of cyclooxygenase enzymes, which are involved in prostaglandin synthesis. The anti-inflammatory efficacy of tremulacin (a derivative of salicin) has recently been studied.[6] A clinical trial of a willow bark preparation found mild efficacy in arthritis.[7]

TOXICOLOGY: There are no reports of adverse effects because of the use of willow bark; although, additive effects with synthetic salicylates must be considered. Use with caution in patients with peptic ulcers and other medical conditions in which aspirin is contraindicated.

[1] Chrubasik S, et al. *Am J Med.* 2000;109:9-14.
[2] Weissmann G. *Sci Am.* 1991;264(1):84-90.
[3] Jourdier S. *Chem Ber.* 1999;35:33.
[4] Kaul R, et al. *Deutsche Apoth Ztg.* 1999;139:3439.
[5] Pentz R. *Deutsche Apoth Ztg.* 1989;92.
[6] Cheng G, et al. *Phytomed.* 1994;1:209.
[7] Mills S, et al. *Br J Rheumatol.* 1996;35(9):874-78.

Witch Hazel

SCIENTIFIC NAME(S): *Hamamelis virginiana* L. Family: Hamamelidaceae

COMMON NAME(S): Witch hazel, hamamelis, snapping hazel, winter bloom, spotted alder, tobacco wood, hamamelis water

---

♠♣♥♦ PATIENT INFORMATION ♠♣♥♦

Uses: Witch hazel has astringent and hemostatic properties, making it useful as a skin astringent to promote healing in hemorrhoid treatment, diarrhea, dysentery, and colitis, as well as other skin inflammations such as eczema. It also can be gargled to treat mucous membrane inflammations of the mouth, throat, and gums. Witch hazel has been used to treat damaged veins, bruises, and sprains; it rapidly stops bleeding, making it useful as an enema.

Side Effects: Internal use is not recommended. Doses of 1 g of witch hazel will cause nausea, vomiting, or constipation, possibly leading to impactions. Hepatic damage may occur if the tannins are absorbed to an appreciable extent.

Dosing: Witch hazel leaves or bark have been used traditionally at daily oral doses of 2 to 3 g. Suppositories containing witch hazel contain from 0.1 to 1 g/dose.[1,2]

BOTANY: Witch hazel grows as a deciduous bush, often reaching about 6 m in height. The plant is found throughout most of North America. Its broad, toothed leaves are ovate, and the golden yellow flowers bloom in the fall. Brown fruit capsules appear after the flowers, then when ripe, eject their 2 seeds away from the tree. The dried leaves, bark, and twigs are used medicinally.[3,4]

HISTORY: Witch hazel is a widely known plant with a long history of use in the Americas. One source lists more than 30 traditional uses for witch hazel including the treatment of hemorrhoids, burns, cancers, tuberculosis, colds, and fever. Preparations have been used topically for symptomatic treatment of itching and other skin inflammations and in ophthalmic preparations for ocular irritations.[5]

The plant is used in a variety of forms including the crude leaf and bark, fluid extracts, a poultice, and most commonly as witch hazel water. The latter, also known as hamamelis water or distilled witch hazel extract, is obtained from the recently cut and partially dormant twigs of the plant. This plant material is soaked in warm water followed by distillation and the addition of alcohol to the distillate. Witch hazel water is the most commonly found commercial preparation, usually kept in most homes as a topical cooling agent or astringent.[4,5]

Traditionally, witch hazel was known to native North American people as a treatment for tumors and eye inflammations. Its internal use was for hemorrhaging. Eighteenth century European settlers came to value the plant for its astringency, and it is still used today for this and other purposes.[4]

PHARMACOLOGY: Witch hazel leaves, bark, and its extracts have been reported to have astringent and hemostatic properties. These effects have been ascribed to the presence of a relatively high concentration of tannins in the leaf, bark, and extract. Tannins are protein precipitants in appropriate concentrations.[6]

Witch hazel water is devoid of tannins but still retains its astringency, suggesting that other constituents may possess astringent qualities.[4]

The mechanism of witch hazel astringency involves the tightening of skin proteins, which come together to form a protective covering that promotes skin healing.[4] This quality is desirable in treatment of hemorrhoids (including preventive measures for recurring hemorroids).[7] A preparation of tea has been used in cases of diarrhea, dysentery, and colitis.[3-5,8]

Skin problems are also treated with witch hazel. Its drying and astringent effects help treat skin inflammations such as eczema. Witch hazel's action on skin lesions also protects against infection.[4] Skin lotions may also contain witch hazel for these purposes.[3] Inflammation of mucous membranes including mouth, throat, and gums may also be treated with witch hazel in the form of a gargle.[3]

Witch hazel is also used to treat damaged veins. Its ability to tighten distended veins and restore vessel tone is employed in varicose vein treatment and is also valuable for bruises and sprains.[3,4] This hemostatic property of witch hazel is said to stop bleeding instantly and, if used as an enema, offers a rapid cure for inwardly bleeding piles.[5]

TOXICOLOGY: Although the volatile oil contains the carcinogen safrole, this is found in much smaller quantities than in plants such as sassafras.[5] Although extracts of witch hazel are available commercially, it is not recommended that these extracts be taken internally because the toxicity of the tannins has not been well defined.[8] Although tannins are not usually absorbed following oral administration, doses of 1 g of witch hazel will cause nausea, vomiting, or constipation, possibly leading to impactions; hepatic damage may occur if the tannins are absorbed to an appreciable extent.[3,9] Witch hazel water is not intended for internal use. Teas can be brewed from leaves and twigs available commercially in some health-food stores, but their safety is undefined.

At least one report is available discussing contact allergy to witch hazel.[10]

[1] Claus E, ed. *Pharmacognosy*. 3rd ed. Philadelphia, PA: Lea & Febiger; 1956.

[2] Blumenthal M, Brinckmann J, Goldberg A, eds. *Herbal Medicine: Expanded Commission E Monographs*. Newton, MA: Integrative Medicine Communications; 2000.

[3] Bisset N. *Herbal Drugs and Phytopharmaceuticals*. Stuttgart, Germany: CRC Press, 1994.

[4] Chevallier A. *Encyclopedia of Medicinal Plants*. New York, NY: DK Publishing Inc., 1996.

[5] Duke JA. *Handbook of Medicinal Herbs*, Boca Raton, FL: CRC Press, 1985.

[6] Bate-Smith EC. *Phytochemistry*. 1973;12:907.

[7] Weiner B, et al. *Nat Assoc Retail Drug J*. 1983 Apr;105:45-49.

[8] Newall C, et al. *Herbal Medicine*. London, England: Pharmaceutical Press, 1996.

[9] Spoerke DG. *Herbal Medications*. Santa Barbara, CA: Woodbridge Press, 1980.

[10] Granlund H. *Contact Dermatitis*. 1994;31(3):195.

SCIENTIFIC NAME(S): *Withania somnifera* (L.) Dunal, also *W. coagulans* Dunal Family: Solanaceae (nightshade family)

COMMON NAME(S): Withania, Ashwagandha, Aswaganda, winter cherry, Indian ginseng, Ajagandha, Kanaje Hindi, Samm Al Ferakh, Asgand (Hindi), Amukkirag (Tamil), Amangura (Kannada), Asvagandha (Bengali), Ashvagandha (Sanskrit), Asundha (Gujarati), Kuthmithi, clustered wintercherry

---

♣♣♣♣ PATIENT INFORMATION ♣♣♣♣

Uses: Withania has adaptogenic, immunomodulatory, and anti-inflammatory effects in animals; it also has been studied in animals as a cytotoxic agent and has different CNS applications.

Side Effects: Acute toxicity of *W. somnifera* is modest. A 180-day study involving rats found unfavorable increases in catecholamine content of the heart and decreases in the adrenal glands.

Dosing: Despite a large volume of basic scientific studies on the plant, there is minimal evidence for a proper dose of this herb. A single study in which *W. somnifera* was the principal component of a polyherbal mixture administered 450 mg of root powder 4 times/day for arthritis.[1]

BOTANY: *W. somnifera* is an erect, grayish, slightly hairy evergreen shrub with fairly long tuberous roots. It is widely cultivated in India and throughout the Middle East, and is found in eastern Africa. The flowers are small and greenish, single or in small clusters in the leaf axils. The fruit is smooth, round, fleshy, and has many seeds, orange-red when ripe, enclosed in a membranous covering.

HISTORY: The root of *W. somnifera* is used to make the Ayurvedic sedative and diuretic "Ashwagandha," which is also considered an adaptogen. Other parts of the plant (eg, seeds, leaves) are used to relieve pain, kill lice, and make soap. The fresh berries have been used as an emetic.

PHARMACOLOGY: The majority of studies of *W. somnifera* pharmacology have not related bioactivity to specific chemical constitutents present. Given the noted variation in withanolides, it is obvious that this has limited reproducibility of results.

Adaptogenic effects: Pretreatment with the alcoholic extract of defatted seeds increased swimming endurance in mice, and significantly reduced cold-, stress-, restraint-, and aspirin-induced ulcers in rats.[2] A combination of withaferin A and two sterol glucosides from roots of *W. somnifera* showed antistress activity in a panel of tests.[3] Aqueous suspensions from the roots of Ashwagandha and ginseng were compared in a mouse swimming model and for anabolic activity (weight gain) in rats and both were found to possess oral activity when animals were treated for 7 days.[4] Ashwagandha extract given orally to rabbits and mice prevented stress-induced increases in lipid peroxidation.[5] Stress-induced increases in plasma corticosterone, phagocytic index, and avidity index were blocked by administration of *W. somnifera* to rats, while swimming time was increased.[6] Another study in rats and frogs found the extract to be adaptogenic when given as a pretreatment for up to 3 months, as measured by swimming tests, glycogen content of various tissues, coagulation time, and catecholamine content, among others.[7] The effect of *W. somnifera* extract on thyroid hormone levels[8] and corticosterone levels[9] in animals has been studied. A review of adaptogenic effects of *W. somnifera* and other Ayurvedic adaptogens has been published.[10]

Immunomodulatory and anti-inflammatory effects: *W. somnifera* extracts given interphalangeal suppressed rat paw edema induced by carrageenan,[11] as well as in a granuloma pouch assay.[12] Orally administered proprietary extracts of *W. somnifera* were found to have modest activity in an active paw anaphylaxis model and to suppress cyclophosphamide-induced delayed-type hypersensitivity.[13] Withanolides inhibit murine spleen cell proliferation,[14] and an extract of *W. somnifera* reversed ochratoxin's suppressive effect on murine macrophage chemotaxis.[15] Withanolide glycosides activated murine macrophages, phagocytosis, and increased lysosomal enzymatic activity secreted by the macrophages, while also displaying anti-stress activity and positive effects on learning and memory in rats.[16] Alpha-2 macroglobulin synthesis stimulated by inflammation was reduced by *W. somnifera* extract.[17] Similarly, the extract prevented myelosuppression caused by cyclophosphamide, azathioprine, or prednisolone in mice.[18]

The stimulation of macrophages was invoked to explain activity versus experimental aspergillosis in mice.[19] Similar activity in other experimental infections was observed in rats.[20]

Cancer: Withaferin A was first isolated as a cytotoxic agent,[21] and a considerable amount of investigation followed. The compound produced mitotic arrest in Ehrlich ascites carcinoma cells in vitro[22] while in vivo effects were mediated by macrophage activation.[16,23] Further investigations on peripheral blood lymphocytes determined that withaferin A destroyed spindle microtubules of cells in metaphase.[24] Mouse sarcoma cells showed similar effects, with additional effects on nuclear membranes of cells.[25] A structure-activity comparison of withaferin A analogues in P388 cells attributed reaction of its lactone and epoxide moieties with cysteine as important to its cytotoxicity.[26] Withaferin was synergistic with radiation treatment in a mouse Ehrlich ascites carcinoma model.[27] Recently, several withanolides were identified as inducers of differentiation of myeloid leukemia cells.[28]

CNS: Withania extract protected against pentylenetetrazol-induced seizures in a mouse anticonvulsant model when administered over a 9-week period.[29] The same research group found the extract active in a rat status epilepticus model.[30] A further study of the extract found that it inhibited the development of tolerance to morphine in mice, while suppressing withdrawal symptoms precipitated by naloxone.[31] A withanolide-containing fraction reversed morphine-induced reduction in intestinal motility and confirmed the previous finding of inhibition of development of tolerance to morphine.[32] A depressant effect on the CNS was indicated by potentiation of pentobarbital effects on the righting reflex in mice.[33] Effects on learning and memory attributed to the plant in Ayurvedic medicine were supported by an experiment in which ibotenic acid-induced lesions in intact rat brain which led to cognitive deficit, as measured by performance in a learning task, were found to be reversed by treatment with a withanolide mixture.[34]

Miscellaneous: *W. somnifera* seed extract was found to protect against carbon tetrachloride-induced liver damage in rats.[35] The leaf extract also showed a modest protective effect in a subacute model of liver damage, and an anti-inflammatory effect.[36] Damage to the bladder by cyclophosphamide was ameliorated by *W. somnifera* extract given IP,[37] as was leukopenia induced by cyclophosphamide.[38] The extract decreased arterial and diastolic blood pressure in normotensive dogs, while preventing the hypotensive effect of acetylcholine and increasing the hypertensive effects of adrenaline.[39]

TOXICOLOGY: Acute toxicity of *W. somnifera* is modest. In mice an LD-50 was determined to be 1750 mg/kg PO[2] in one study and 1260 mg/kg by the intraperitoneal route.[40] Subacute IP toxicity studies at 100 mg/kg/day for 30 days led to decreased spleen, thymus, and adrenal weights, but no mortality or hematological changes.[41] A longer-term study (180 days) in rats at a dose of 100 mg/kg PO found no lethality but unfavorable increases in catecholamine content of the heart and decreases in the adrenal glands.[7]

[1] Kulkarni RR, et al. *J Ethnopharmacol.* 1991;33:91-95.

[2] Singh N, et al. *Int J Crude Drug Res.* 1982;20:29.

[3] Bhattacharya S, et al. *Phytother Res.* 1987;1:32.

[4] Grandhi A, et al. *J Ethnopharmacol.* 1994;44:131.

[5] Dhuley J. *J Ethnopharmacol.* 1998;60:173.

[6] Archana R, et al. *J Ethnopharmacol.* 1999;64:91.

[7] Dhuley J. *J Ethnopharmacol.* 2000;70:57.

[8] Panda S, et al. *J Ethnopharmacol.* 1999;67:233.

[9] Singh A, et al. *Phytother Res.* 2000;14:122.

[10] Rege N, et al. *Phytother Res.* 1999;13:275.

[11] al Hindawi M, et al. *J Ethnopharmacol.* 1989;26:163.

[12] al Hindawi M, et al. *J Ethnopharmacol.* 1992;37:113.

[13] Agarwal R, et al. *J Ethnopharmacol.* 1999;67:27.

[14] Bähr V, et al. *Planta Med.* 1982;44:32.

[15] Dhuley J. *J Ethnopharmacol.* 1997;58:15.

[16] Ghosal S, et al. *Phytother Res.* 1989;3:201.

[17] Anbalagan K, et al. *Int J Crude Drug Res.* 1985;23:177.

[18] Ziauddin M, et al. *J Ethnopharmacol.* 1996;50:69.

[19] Dhuley J. *Immunopharmacol Immunotoxicol.* 1998;20:191.

[20] Thatte U, et al. *Phytother Res.* 1989;3:43.

[21] Kupchan S, et al. *J Am Chem Soc.* 1965;37:5805.

[22] Shohat B, et al. *Int J Cancer.* 1970;5:244.

[23] Shohat B, et al. *Int J Cancer.* 1971;8:487.

[24] Shohat B, et al. *Cancer Lett.* 1976;2:63.

[25] Shohat B, et al. *Cancer Lett.* 1976;2:71.

[26] Fuska J, et al. *Neoplasma.* 1984;31:31.

[27] Devi P, et al. *Cancer Lett.* 1995;95:189.

[28] Kuroyanagi M, et al. *Chem Pharm Bull.* 1999;47:1646.

[29] Kulkarni S, et al. *Phytother Res.* 1996;10:447.

[30] Kulkarni S, et al. *Phytother Res.* 1998;12:451.

[31] Kulkarni S, et al. *J Ethnopharmacol.* 1997;57:213.

[32] Ramarao P, et al. *Phytother Res.* 1995;9:66.

[33] Ahumada F, et al. *Phytother Res.* 1991;5:29.

[34] Bhattacharya S, et al. *Phytother Res.* 1995;9:110.

[35] Singh N, et al. *Quart J Crude Drug Res.* 1978;16:8.

[36] Sudhir S, et al. *Planta Med.* 1986;36:61.

[37] Davis L, et al. *Cancer Lett.* 2000;148:9.

[38] Davis L, et al. *J Ethnopharmacol.* 1998;62:209.

[39] Ahumada F, et al. *Phytother Res.* 1991;5:111.

[40] Sharada A, et al. *Int J Pharmacognosy.* 1993;31:205.

[41] Singh S, et al. *Withania somnifera: The Indian ginseng ashwagandha.* New Dehli: Vedams Books Intl., 1998.

SCIENTIFIC NAME(S): *Achillea millefolium* L.; Family: Compositae

COMMON NAME(S): Yarrow, thousand-leaf, mil foil, green arrow, wound wort, nosebleed plant

---

⚡⚡⚡ PATIENT INFORMATION ⚡⚡⚡

Uses: Yarrow has been used to induce sweating and to stop wound bleeding. It can also reduce heavy menstrual bleeding and pain. It has been used to relieve gastrointestinal (GI) ailments, for cerebral and coronary thromboses, to lower high blood pressure, to improve circulation, and to tone varicose veins. It has antimicrobial actions, is a natural source for food flavoring, and is used in alcoholic beverages and bitters.

Side Effects: Contact dermatitis is the most commonly reported side effect. It is generally not considered toxic.

Dosing: A typical dose of yarrow herb is 4.5 g/day for inflammatory conditions. However, there are no modern clinical studies to validate this dose.

BOTANY: The name yarrow applies to any of roughly 80 species of daisy plants native to the north temperate zone. *A. millefolium* L. has finely divided leaves and whitish, pink, or reddish flowers. It can grow up to 0.9 m in height. This hardy perennial weed blooms from June to November. Golden yarrow is *Eriophyllum confertiflorum*.[1,2]

HISTORY: Yarrow is native to Europe and Asia and has been naturalized in North America. Its use in food and medicine dates back to the Trojan War, around 1200 B.C.[3] In classical times, yarrow was referred to as "herba militaris" because it stopped wound bleeding caused by war.[2] Yarrow leaves have been used for tea, and young leaves and flowers have been used in salads. Infusions of yarrow have served as cosmetic cleansers and medicines. Sneezewort leaves (*A. ptarmica*) have been used in sneezing powder, while those of *A. millefolium* have been used for snuff.[1] Yarrow has been used therapeutically as a strengthening bitter tonic and astringent. Chewing fresh leaves has been used to relieve toothaches.[3,4] Yarrow oil has been used in shampoos for a topical healing effect.

PHARMACOLOGY: Yarrow acts as a sudorific to induce sweating. It is also classified as a wound-healing herb because it stops wound bleeding.[4] It has been used for this purpose for centuries and is a component in some healing ointments, lotions, and percolates or extracts.[2,5] Its healing and regenerating effects have been reported when used as a constituent in medicated baths to remove perspiration and to remedy inflammation of skin and mucous membranes.[5,6,7] One study reports wound-healing properties of yarrow oil in napalm burns.[8]

Chamazulene, a constituent in yarrow essential oil, has anti-inflammatory and antiallergenic properties.[9]

The yarrow component achilleine arrests internal and external bleeding.[2]

Yarrow helps regulate the menstrual cycle and reduces heavy bleeding and pain.[2,9] It has been used as an herbal remedy for cerebral and coronary thromboses.[9] Yarrow has also been used to lower high blood pressure, improve circulation, and tone varicose veins.[2,3]

Antispasmodic activity of yarrow has also been documented, probably caused by the plant's flavonoid fractions[2,9] or azulene.[9] Yarrow has relieved GI ailments such as diarrhea, flatulence, and cramping.[5] Yarrow's antimicrobial actions also have been documented. In vitro fungistatic effect from the oil has been proven.[10] The oil has also exhibited marked activity against *S. aureus* and *C. albicans*.[11] Another report discusses antistaphylococcal activity from yarrow grass extract.[12] Antibacterial actions have also been demonstrated against *B. subtillus, E. coli, Shigella sonnei*, and *flexneri*.[9] Other actions of yarrow include growth inhibiting effects on seed germination caused by constituents phenylcarbonic acids, coumarins, herniarin, and umbelliferone,[13] marked hypoglycemic and glycogen-sparing properties.[14] Yarrow is a natural source for

food flavoring and is used in alcoholic beverages and bitters.[9] Thujone-free yarrow extract is generally recognized as safe (GRAS) for use in beverages.

TOXICOLOGY: Contact dermatitis is the most commonly reported adverse reaction from yarrow. Guaianolide peroxides from yarrow have caused this reaction,[15] as have α-peroxyachifolid,[16] 10 sesquiterpene lactones, and 3 polyines.[17] Terpinen-4-ol, a yarrow oil component, has irritant properties and may contribute to its diuretic actions.[9] Thujone, a known toxin and minor component in the oil, is in too low a concentration to cause any health risk.[9] Yarrow is not generally considered toxic.[3,9]

[1] Seymour ELD. *The Garden Encyclopedia.* Wise, 1936.

[2] Chevallier A. *Encyclopedia of Medicinal Plants.* New York, NY: DK Publishing, 1996;54.

[3] Duke J. *CRC Handbook of Medicinal Herbs.* Boca Raton, FL: CRC Press Inc., 1989;9-10.

[4] Loewenfeld C, et al. *The Complete Book of Herbs and Spices.* London, England: David E Charles, 1979.

[5] Bisset N. *Herbal Drugs and Phytopharmaceuticals.* Stuttgart, Germany: CRC Press Inc., 1994;342-44.

[6] Gafitanu E, et al. *Revista Medico-Chirurgicala A Societatii de Medici Si Naturalisti Din Iasi.* 1988;92(1):121-22.

[7] Taran D, et al. *Voenno-Meditsinskii Zhurnal.* 1989;(8):50-52.

[8] Popovici A, et al. *Rev Med.* 1970;16(3-4):384-89.

[9] Newall C, et al. *Herbal Medicines.* London, England: Pharmaceutical Press, 1996;271-73.

[10] Kedzia B, et al. *Herba Polonica.* 1990;36(3):117-25.

[11] Molochko V, et al. *Vestnik Dermatologii I Venerologii.* 1990;(8):54-56.

[12] Detter A. *Pharmazeutische Zeitung.* 1981 Jun 4;126:1140-42.

[13] Molokovskii D, et al. *Problemy Endokrinologii.* 1989;35(6):82-87.

[14] Paulsen E, et al. *Contact Dermatitis.* 1993;29(1):6-10.

[15] Chandler R, et al. *J Pharm Sci.* 1982 Jun 71:690-93.

[16] Tozyo T, et al. *Chem Pharm Bull.* 1994;42(5):1096-1100.

[17] Rucker G, et al. *Pharmazie.* 1994;49(2-3):167-69.

Appendix

Appendix

With the exception of a few herbal products (eg, grapefruit juice), most documentation regarding potential interactions between natural products and drugs in humans is based on case reports and often lacks relevant information. Evaluating these reports is difficult because of medications the patient may be receiving concurrently or because of the presence of comorbidity. In addition, the lack of herbal product standardization, purity, and potency, as well as multiple ingredients in products, product adulteration, misidentification, and batch-to-batch variations in crop conditions and yield complicate the assessment of drug interactions with herbs. The absorption, metabolism, distribution, and elimination characteristics and physiologic effects of most herbal products are poorly understood. Until this information is available, many herb-drug interactions remain speculative and one cannot predict the clinical outcome of potential interactions. Take special care when considering the use of natural products in patients taking drugs with a narrow therapeutic index. Ask patients experiencing adverse reactions if they are using herbal products, especially if the reaction cannot be attributed to another cause.

Because herb-drug interactions are sporadically reported and epidemiologically derived, practitioners should report any potential interactions to the Food and Drug Administration through its MedWatch program by phone at 1-800-FDA-1088 or via the Internet at http://www.accessdata.fda.gov/scripts/medwatch/.

Evidence-Based Herb-Drug Interactions		
Herbal product	Drug or drug class	Potential interaction
Artemether	Grapefruit	*Documentation*: Noncontrolled trial.[1]
		Effect: Grapefruit juice may increase the bioavailability of artemether.
		Management: No special precautions are necessary.
Ascorbic Acid (Vitamin C)	Propranolol	*Documentation*: Noncontrolled trial.[2]
		Effect: The pharmacologic effects of propranolol may be decreased.
		Management: No special precautions are necessary with usual doses of ascorbic acid. Advise patients taking propranolol to avoid excessive amounts of ascorbic acid (more than 500 mg/day).
Avocado	Warfarin	*Documentation*: Case reports.[3]
		Effect: Decreased anticoagulant effect of warfarin.
		Management: Because warfarin has a narrow therapeutic index, avoid concurrent ingestion of avocado.
Betel Nut	Procyclidine	*Documentation*: Case reports.[4]
		Effects: The risk of occurrence of extrapyramidal symptoms may be increased.
		Management: Avoid concurrent use.
Bitter Melon		See Karela.
Boldo	Warfarin	*Documentation*: Case report.[5]
		Effect: Enhanced anticoagulant effect of warfarin, increasing the risk of bleeding.
		Management: Because warfarin has a narrow therapeutic index, avoid concurrent use.

Evidence-Based Herb-Drug Interactions		
Herbal product	Drug or drug class	Potential interaction
Broccoli	Warfarin	*Documentation*: Controlled trial and case reports.[6,7]
		Effect: The anticoagulant effect of warfarin may be antagonized.
		Management: Because warfarin has a narrow therapeutic index, patients receiving warfarin should avoid ingestion of large daily amounts of broccoli.
Caffeine	Clozapine	*Documentation*: Controlled trial and case reports.[8-11]
		Effect: Elevated clozapine plasma levels, which may increase the risk of side effects.
		Management: Substantial fluctuations in caffeine intake may affect the response to clozapine. Adverse responses are most likely in patients drinking more than 4 cups of caffeinated coffee daily or who ingest large quantities of caffeine (ie, more than 400 mg/day) from other sources.
	Lithium	*Documentation*: Noncontrolled trial and case reports.[12,13]
		Effect: Decreased lithium serum levels, which may decrease the therapeutic effect.
		Management: Inform patients who ingest large amounts of caffeine (ie, at least 4 cups of coffee daily) to inform their physician or pharmacist before eliminating caffeine and to avoid large fluctuations in their caffeine intake.
	Theophylline	*Documentation*: Open-label study in healthy volunteers.[14]
		Effect: Elevated plasma theophylline levels, increasing the risk of toxicity.
		Management: Advise patients to avoid drastic fluctuations in their daily caffeine intake.
Capsaicin	ACE Inhibitors (eg, captopril)	*Documentation*: Controlled study (capsaicin inhalation) and case report (capsaicin topical).[15,16]
		Effect: Increased risk of cough.
		Management: Avoid concomitant use.
Coenzyme Q10		See Ubiquinone.
Cucurbita	Warfarin	*Documentation*: Case reports.[17]
		Effect: Increased anticoagulant effect of warfarin.
		Management: No special precautions are necessary.
Danshen	Digoxin	*Documentation*: Controlled trial.[18]
		Effect: Digoxin plasma levels measured by the fluorescence polarization immunoassay may be falsely elevated and levels measured by the microparticle enzyme immunoassay may be falsely decreased.
		Management: No special precautions are warranted. Use the ultrafiltration technique to measure digoxin plasma levels. Monitor free digoxin levels.
	Warfarin	*Documentation*: Case reports.[19-21]
		Effect: Increased anticoagulant effect of warfarin.
		Management: Because warfarin has a narrow therapeutic index, avoid concurrent use.
Dong Quai	Warfarin	*Documentation*: Case report.[22]
		Effect: Increased anticoagulant effect of warfarin.
		Management: Because warfarin has a narrow therapeutic index, avoid concurrent use.

Evidence-Based Herb-Drug Interactions		
Herbal product	Drug or drug class	Potential interaction
Eleutherococcus (Siberian Ginseng)	Digoxin	*Documentation*: Case report.[23]
		Effect: Falsely elevated digoxin serum assay or increased digoxin plasma levels.
		Management: Because digoxin has a narrow therapeutic index, avoid concurrent use.
Fenugreek	Warfarin	*Documentation*: Case report.[5]
		Effect: The anticoagulant effect of warfarin may be enhanced, increasing the risk of bleeding.
		Management: Because warfarin has a narrow therapeutic index, avoid concurrent use.
Fiddleheads	Warfarin	*Documentation*: Case report.[24]
		Effect: The anticoagulant effect of warfarin may be antagonized.
		Management: Because warfarin has a narrow therapeutic index, question patients about their food and beverage consumption. Avoid ingestion of large daily amounts of fiddleheads.
Garlic	Saquinavir	*Documentation*: Controlled trial.[25]
		Effect: Reduced saquinavir plasma levels, decreasing the pharmacologic effects.
		Management: Avoid concurrent use.
	Warfarin	*Documentation*: Based on inhibition of platelet aggregation in individuals ingesting garlic.[26-32]
		Effect: The risk of bleeding may be increased.
		Management: No special precautions are necessary.
Ginger	Warfarin	*Documentation*: Based on inhibition of platelet aggregation in individuals ingesting ginger.[33-36]
		Effect: The risk of bleeding may be increased.
		Management: No special precautions are necessary.
Ginkgo biloba	Aspirin	*Documentation*: Case report.[37,38]
		Effect: Increased risk of bleeding.
		Management: Avoid concurrent use.
	Nifedipine	*Documentation*: Controlled trial.[39]
		Effect: Elevated nifedipine plasma levels, which may increase the pharmacologic and adverse effects.
		Management: Avoid concurrent use.
	Trazodone	*Documentation*: Case report.[40]
		Effect: Increased risk of sedation.
		Management: Avoid concurrent use.
	Warfarin	*Documentation*: Case reports.[41-43]
		Effect: Increased risk of bleeding.
		Management: Because warfarin has a narrow therapeutic index, avoid concurrent use.

Evidence-Based Herb-Drug Interactions		
Herbal product	Drug or drug class	Potential interaction
Ginseng	Furosemide	*Documentation*: Case report.[44]
		Effect: Decrease in diuretic effect of furosemide.
		Management: Avoid concurrent use.
	Nifedipine	*Documentation*: Controlled trial.[39]
		Effect: Elevated nifedipine plasma levels, which may increase the pharmacologic and adverse effects.
		Management: Avoid concurrent use.
	Phenelzine	*Documentation*: Case reports.[45,46]
		Effect: Manic-like symptoms, headache, and tremulousness have been reported.
		Management: Avoid concurrent use.
	Warfarin	*Documentation*: Case report.[47]
		Effect: Anticoagulant effect of warfarin may be decreased.
		Management: Because warfarin has a narrow therapeutic index, avoid concurrent use.
Ginseng, Siberian		See Eleutherococcus.
Glycyrrhizin		See Licorice.
Grapefruit Juice	Amlodipine	*Documentation*: Controlled trials.[48,49]
		Effect: Elevated amlodipine serum levels, increasing the pharmacologic and adverse effects.
		Management: Avoid simultaneous administration. However, patients who routinely drink grapefruit juice may have been stabilized on a higher than usual dose and should not abruptly stop drinking grapefruit juice.
	Amprenavir	*Documentation*: Controlled trial.[50]
		Effect: Amprenavir peak levels may be slightly decreased.
		Management: No special precautions are necessary.
	Benzodiazepines (ie, midazolam, triazolam)	*Documentation*: Controlled trials and product information.[51-57]
		Effect: Pharmacologic effects may be increased and onset delayed.
		Management: Avoid coadministration. Take with a liquid other than grapefruit juice.
	Buspirone	*Documentation*: Controlled trial.[58]
		Effect: Elevated plasma levels of buspirone, increasing the pharmacologic and adverse effects.
		Management: Avoid concomitant use. Take with a liquid other than grapefruit juice.
	Carbamazepine	*Documentation*: Controlled trial.[59]
		Effect: Carbamazepine plasma levels may be elevated, increasing the pharmacologic and adverse effects.
		Management: Avoid concomitant ingestion. Take with a liquid other than grapefruit juice.
	Cisapride (available from the manufacturer on a limited-access protocol)	*Documentation*: Controlled trials.[60-62]
		Effect: Elevated cisapride plasma levels with increased risk of adverse effects, including life-threatening cardiac arrhythmias (eg, torsades de pointes).
		Management: Cisapride is contraindicated in patients receiving grapefruit juice.

Evidence-Based Herb-Drug Interactions		
Herbal product	Drug or drug class	Potential interaction
Grapefruit Juice (cont.)	Clomipramine	*Documentation*: Case reports.[63]
		Effect: Elevated plasma levels of clomipramine and reduced levels of the desmethylclomipramine, which may improve outcome in treatment of obsessive-compulsive disorders.
		Management: Avoid concurrent use unless coadministration of clomipramine and grapefruit juice is being used to improve symptom control of obsessive-compulsive disorder.
	Cyclosporine	*Documentation*: Controlled trials, noncontrolled trials, case reports, and product information.[64-76]
		Effect: Trough cyclosporine whole blood concentrations may be elevated, increasing the risk of toxicity.
		Management: Because cyclosporine has a narrow therapeutic index, avoid concurrent use.
	Digoxin	*Documentation*: Controlled trial.[77]
		Effect: Digoxin plasma levels may be slightly elevated.
		Management: No special precautions are warranted.
	Erythromycin	*Documentation*: Controlled trial.[78]
		Effect: Erythromycin plasma levels may be elevated, increasing the risk of side effects.
		Management: Avoid taking erythromycin with grapefruit products. Take erythromycin with a liquid other than grapefruit juice.
	Estrone	*Documentation*: Controlled trial.[79]
		Effect: Estrone serum levels may be increased.
		Management: The effect of grapefruit or grapefruit juice ingestion on estrone is unlikely to result in a clinically important interaction.
	Ethinyl Estradiol	*Documentation*: Controlled trial.[80]
		Effect: Ethinyl estradiol serum levels may be increased.
		Management: Advise patients to avoid grapefruit and grapefruit juice while taking ethinyl estradiol.
	HMG-CoA Reductase Inhibitors (ie, atorvastatin, lovastatin, simvastatin)	*Documentation*: Controlled trials.[81-85]
		Effect: The AUC and elimination half-life of atorvastatin may be increased. Lovastatin and simvastatin plasma levels may be elevated, increasing the risk of side effects (eg, rhabdomyolysis).
		Management: Take with a liquid other than grapefruit juice.
	Indinavir	*Documentation*: Controlled trial and product information.[86,87]
		Effect: Taking indinavir with grapefruit juice may delay the time to reach indinavir peak plasma concentrations.
		Management: Because indinavir is a substrate for CYP3A4 and grapefruit inhibits CYP3A4, patients taking indinavir should avoid chronic ingestion of grapefruit products.
	Itraconazole	*Documentation*: Controlled trials.[88,89] Data are conflicting.
		Effect: Plasma levels and therapeutic effects of itraconazole may be decreased.
		Management: Avoid coadministration. Take with a liquid other than grapefruit juice.

Evidence-Based Herb-Drug Interactions		
Herbal product	Drug or drug class	Potential interaction
Grapefruit Juice (cont.)	Losartan	*Documentation*: Controlled trial.[90]
		Effect: The rate and magnitude of losartan metabolism to its major active metabolite may be decreased.
		Management: Advise patients to take losartan with a liquid other than grapefruit juice.
	Nicardipine	*Documentation*: Controlled trial.[91]
		Effect: Nicardipine plasma levels may be elevated, increasing the pharmacologic and adverse effects.
		Management: Avoid grapefruit products and take nicardipine with a liquid other than grapefruit juice.
	Nisoldipine	*Documentation*: Controlled trials.[92-94]
		Effect: Elevated plasma levels of nisoldipine, increasing the pharmacologic and adverse effects.
		Management: Avoid coadministration. Take with a liquid other than grapefruit juice.
	Praziquantel	*Documentation*: Controlled trial.[95]
		Effect: Elevated praziquantel plasma levels, increasing the pharmacologic and adverse effects.
		Management: Avoid taking praziquantel with grapefruit products. Take praziquantel with a liquid other than grapefruit juice.
	Quinidine	*Documentation*: Controlled trials.[53,96,97]
		Effect: The onset of action of quinidine may be delayed.
		Management: Avoid coadministration. Take with a liquid other than grapefruit juice.
	Saquinavir	*Documentation*: Controlled trials and product information.[98-100]
		Effect: Elevated plasma levels of saquinavir, increasing the pharmacologic and adverse effects.
		Management: Avoid coadministration. Take with a liquid other than grapefruit juice.
	Scopolamine	*Documentation*: Controlled trial.[101]
		Effect: Scopolamine absorption may be delayed and bioavailability may be increased.
		Management: No special precautions are needed.
	Sildenafil	*Documentation*: Controlled trial and case report.[102,103]
		Effect: Sildenafil plasma levels may be increased and absorption delayed.
		Management: A clinically important interaction is unlikely; however, it would be prudent to take sildenafil with a liquid other than grapefruit juice.
	Verapamil	*Documentation*: Controlled trial.[104]
		Effect: Verapamil plasma concentrations may be elevated, increasing the pharmacologic and adverse effects.
		Management: Avoid grapefruit products. Take with a liquid other than grapefruit juice.

Evidence-Based Herb-Drug Interactions		
Herbal product	Drug or drug class	Potential interaction
Green Tea	Warfarin	*Documentation*: Case report.[105]
		Effect: The anticoagulant effect of warfarin may be antagonized.
		Management: Because warfarin has a narrow therapeutic index, question patients about food and beverage consumption. Avoid ingestion of large amounts (more than 4 cups/day) of green tea.
Guar Gum	Metformin	*Documentation*: Controlled trials.[106,107]
		Effect: Metformin serum levels may be reduced, decreasing the hypoglycemic effect.
		Management: No special precautions are necessary.
Ispaghula	Lithium	*Documentation*: Case report.[108]
		Effect: Possible decrease in lithium absorption, reducing the pharmacologic effect.
		Management: Avoid concomitant use.
Karela	Chlorpropamide	*Documentation*: Case report.[109]
		Effect: A greater than expected hypoglycemic response may occur.
		Management: Avoid concurrent use of karela and chlorpropamide.
Kava	Alprazolam	*Documentation*: Case report.[110]
		Effect: CNS side effects may be increased.
		Management: It would be prudent to avoid concurrent use.
Khat	Penicillins (ie, amoxicillin, ampicillin)	*Documentation*: Noncontrolled trial.[111]
		Effect: Antimicrobial effectiveness may be reduced.
		Management: Avoid khat chewing or take the penicillin 2 hours after khat chewing.
Licorice (Glycyrrhizin)	Prednisolone	*Documentation*: Controlled trials.[117-119]
		Effect: Prednisolone plasma levels may be elevated, increasing the pharmacologic and adverse effects.
		Management: Avoid excessive ingestion of licorice-containing products while taking prednisolone.
Lime Juice	Felodipine	*Documentation*: Controlled trial.[120]
		Effect: Elevated felodipine serum levels, increasing the pharmacologic and adverse efffects.
		Management: Until more clinical data are available, it would be prudent to avoid lime juice while taking felodipine.
Lycium barbarum L.	Warfarin	*Documentation*: Case report.[121]
		Effect: The anticoagulant effect of warfarin may be increased.
		Management: Because warfarin has a narrow therapeutic index, avoid concurrent use.
Mango	Warfarin	*Documentation*: Noncontrolled trial.[122]
		Effect: Increased anticoagulant effect of warfarin.
		Management: Because warfarin has a narrow therapeutic index, avoid concurrent use.

Evidence-Based Herb-Drug Interactions		
Herbal product	Drug or drug class	Potential interaction
Melatonin	Fluvoxamine	*Documentation*: Noncontrolled trials.[123-125]
		Effect: Elevated plasma levels of melatonin, increasing the effects (eg, drowsiness).
		Management: No special precautions are necessary.
	Nifedipine	*Documentation*: Controlled trial.[126]
		Effect: Interference with antihypertensive effect, which may increase blood pressure.
		Management: Avoid concurrent use. If melatonin use cannot be avoided, it may be necessary to adjust the nifedipine dose when starting or stopping melatonin.
Milk Thistle	Indinavir	*Documentation*: Controlled trial.[127]
		Effect: Pharmacologic effects of indinavir may be decreased.
		Management: A clinically important interaction is unlikely; however, be prepared to make appropriate changes in dosage if there is evidence of a decrease in virologic effect.
Oat Bran	Lovastatin	*Documentation*: Noncontrolled trial.[128]
		Effect: The pharmacologic effect of lovastatin may be decreased.
		Management: Do not take oat bran and lovastatin at the same time. If both must be taken, separate oat bran ingestion and lovastatin administration by as much time as possible.
Orange Juice	Fexofenadine	*Documentation*: Controlled trial.[129]
		Effect: Fexofenadine plasma levels may be decreased, reducing the clinical effect.
		Management: A higher dose of fexofenadine may be required when taken with orange juice. Take with a liquid other than orange juice.
	Itraconazole	*Documentation*: Controlled trial.[89]
		Effect: Plasma levels and therapeutic effects of itraconazole may be reduced.
		Management: Avoid coadminstration. Take with a liquid other than orange juice.
Orange Juice (calcium fortified)	Ciprofloxacin	*Documentation*: Controlled trial.[130]
		Effects: Ciprofloxacin plasma levels may be reduced, decreasing the clinical effect.
		Management: Avoid concurrent use.
Pectin	Lovastatin	*Documentation*: Noncontrolled trial.[128]
		Effect: Decreased pharmacologic effect of lovastatin.
		Management: Avoid concurrent use. If concomitant use cannot be avoided, separate pectin ingestion and lovastatin administration by as much time as possible.
Peppermint Oil	Felodipine	*Documentation*: Controlled trial.[131]
		Effect: Elevated felodipine serum levels, increasing the pharmacologic and adverse effects.
		Management: Avoid concurrent use.
	Simvastatin	*Documentation*: Controlled trial.[131]
		Effect: Elevated simvastatin serum levels, increasing the pharmacologic and adverse effects.
		Management: Avoid concurrent use.

Evidence-Based Herb-Drug Interactions		
Herbal product	Drug or drug class	Potential interaction
Plantain (Psyllium)	Lithium	*Documentation*: Case report.[108]
		Effect: Lithium plasma levels may be reduced, decreasing the pharmacologic efficacy.
		Management: Avoid coadministration.
Psyllium		See Plantain.
Quinine	Amantadine	*Documentation*: Controlled trials.[132,133]
		Effect: Elevated amantadine levels in men but not women, increasing the risk of toxicity in men.
		Management: Although the effect of drinking quinine beverages on amantadine levels has not been assessed, it would be prudent to limit quinine ingestion during amantadine administration.
	Carbamazepine	*Documentation*: Controlled trials.[133,134]
		Effect: Elevated carbamazepine plasma levels, increasing the pharmacologic and adverse effects.
		Management: Although the effect of quinine in tonic beverages has not been assessed, it would be prudent to limit quinine ingestion during carbamazepine administration.
	Digoxin	*Documentation*: Controlled studies using prescription doses of quinine (ie, at least 200 mg).[133-139]
		Effect: Elevated digoxin levels, increasing the risk of digoxin toxicity. However, studies have not reported digoxin toxicity.
		Management: If used concurrently, it may be necessary to decrease the dose of digoxin. Closely monitor the patient and digoxin serum levels. However, the effect of quinine in tonic beverages has not been assessed. Until studied, it would be prudent to limit quinine ingestion during digoxin administration.
	Phenobarbital	*Documentation*: Controlled trials.[133,134]
		Effect: Elevated phenobarbital plasma levels, increasing the pharmacologic and adverse effects.
		Management: Although the effect of drinking quinine beverages has not been assessed, it would be prudent to limit quinine ingestion during phenobarbital administration.
	Warfarin	*Documentation*: Case reports of excessive hypoprothrombinemia and bleeding during concurrent use.[140,141]
		Effect: Increased anticoagulant activity, increasing the risk of bleeding.
		Management: Closely monitor anticoagulant parameters and adjust the warfarin dose as needed.
Saw Palmetto	Warfarin	*Documentation*: Case reports.[17]
		Effect: The anticoagulant effect of warfarin may be increased.
		Management: No special precautions are necessary.
Seaweed	Warfarin	*Documentation*: Case report.[142]
		Effect: The anticoagulant effect of warfarin may be antagonized.
		Management: Because warfarin has a narrow therapeutic index, advise patients receiving warfarin to avoid ingestion of large amounts of vitamin K-containing seaweed.

Evidence-Based Herb-Drug Interactions		
Herbal product	Drug or drug class	Potential interaction
Spinach	Warfarin	*Documentation*: Controlled trials.[6,7]
		Effect: The anticoagulant effect of warfarin may be antagonized.
		Management: Because warfarin has a narrow therapeutic index, advise patients receiving warfarin to avoid ingestion of large daily amounts of spinach.
St. John's Wort (See Appendix: "Potential Drug Interactions with St. John's Wort" for additional interactions.)	Amitriptyline	*Documentation*: Noncontrolled trial.[143]
		Effect: Amitriptyline plasma levels may be reduced, decreasing the pharmacologic effects.
		Management: If use of St. John's wort cannot be avoided, assess the patient's clinical response to amitriptyline when St. John's wort is started or stopped. Adjust the amitriptyline dose as needed.
	Contraceptives, Oral	*Documentation*: Case report.[144]
		Effect: The efficacy of oral contraceptives may be reduced.
		Management: Inform women of increased risk of oral contraceptive failure with concomitant use of St. John's wort. If use of St. John's wort cannot be avoided, consider an alternative nonhormonal contraceptive or an additional method of contraception.
	Cyclosporine	*Documentation*: Case reports.[145-150]
		Effect: Cyclosporine levels may be reduced, resulting in organ transplant rejection.
		Management: Because cyclosporine has a narrow therapeutic index, avoid St. John's wort.
	Digoxin	*Documentation*: Controlled trial and noncontrolled trial.[151,152]
		Effect: Decreased digoxin plasma levels and clinical efficacy.
		Management: If use of St. John's wort cannot be avoided, the patient's response to digoxin should be assessed when St. John's wort is started or stopped. Monitoring digoxin plasma levels may be useful.
	Fexofenadine	*Documentation*: Noncontrolled trials.[153,154]
		Effect: Fexofenadine plasma levels may be reduced, decreasing the pharmacologic effect. Increased fexofenadine concentrations have been reported after a single dose of St. John's wort.
		Management: If use of St. John's wort cannot be avoided, assess the patient's clinical response to fexofenadine when St. John's wort is started or stopped. Adjust the fexofenadine dose as needed.
	Indinavir	*Documentation*: Noncontrolled trial and product information.[155,156]
		Effect: Indinavir plasma levels may be reduced, decreasing the clinical efficacy.
		Management: Avoid coadministration.
	Midazolam	*Documentation*: Controlled trial and noncontrolled trial.[153,157]
		Effect: Midazolam plasma levels may be reduced, decreasing the pharmacologic effect.
		Management: If use of St. John's wort cannot be avoided, assess the patient's clinical response to midazolam when St. John's wort is started or stopped. Adjust the midazolam dose as needed.

Evidence-Based Herb-Drug Interactions

Evidence-Based Herb-Drug Interactions		
Herbal product	Drug or drug class	Potential interaction
St. John's wort (cont.)	Nefazodone	*Documentation*: Case report.[158]
		Effect: A "serotonin syndrome" (eg, CNS irritability, shivering, myoclonus, altered consciousness) may occur.
		Management: Avoid concurrent use. Patients taking nefazodone should inform their physician or pharmacist before taking St. John's wort.
	Nevirapine	*Documentation*: Case reports.[159]
		Effect: Nevirapine plasma levels may be reduced, decreasing the clinical efficacy.
		Management: Avoid coadministration of nevirapine and St. John's wort.
	Nifedipine	*Documentation*: Controlled trial.[39]
		Effect: Nifedipine plasma levels may be reduced, decreasing the pharmacologic effects.
		Management: If use of St. John's wort cannot be avoided, assess the patient's clinical response to nifedipine when St. John's wort is started or stopped. Adjust the nifedipine dose or discontinue St. John's wort if needed.
	Nortriptyline	*Documentation*: Noncontrolled trial.[143]
		Effect: Nortriptyline plasma levels may be reduced, decreasing the pharmacologic effects.
		Management: If use of St. John's wort cannot be avoided, assess the patient's clinical response to nortriptyline when St. John's wort is started or stopped. Adjust the nortriptyline dose as needed.
	Paroxetine	*Documentation*: Case report.[160]
		Effect: Increased sedative-hypnotic effects.
		Management: Avoid concurrent use. When starting paroxetine in patients receiving St. John's wort, discontinue St. John's wort at least 2 weeks prior to starting paroxetine. Patients taking paroxetine should inform their physician or pharmacist before taking St. John's wort.
	Propofol	*Documentation*: Case report.[161]
		Effect: Delayed emergence from general anesthesia.
		Management: Discontinue St. John's wort at least 5 days prior to surgery.
	Sertraline	*Documentation*: Case reports.[158]
		Effect: A "serotonin syndrome" (eg, CNS irritability, shivering, myoclonus, altered consciousness) may occur.
		Management: Avoid concurrent use. Patients taking sertraline should inform their physician or pharmacist before taking St. John's wort.
	Sevoflurane	*Documentation*: Case report.[161]
		Effect: Delayed emergence from general anesthesia.
		Management: Discontinue St. John's wort at least 5 days prior to surgery.
	Simvastatin	*Documentation*: Controlled trial.[162]
		Effect: Cholesterol-lowering effect of simvastatin may be reduced.
		Management: Avoid concurrent use.

Evidence-Based Herb-Drug Interactions		
Herbal product	Drug or drug class	Potential interaction
St. John's wort (cont.)	Theophylline	*Documentation*: Case report.[163]
		Effect: Decreased theophylline plasma levels.
		Management: If use of St. John's wort cannot be avoided, assess the patient's response to theophylline when starting or stopping St. John's wort. Closely monitor theophylline plasma levels and adjust the dose as needed.
	Warfarin	*Documentation*: Controlled trial and case reports.[144,164]
		Effect: Anticoagulant effect of warfarin may be decreased.
		Management: Because warfarin has a narrow therapeutic index, avoid concurrent use of St. John's wort. If concomitant use cannot be avoided, closely monitor coagulation parameters when starting or stopping St. John's wort and adjust the warfarin dose as needed.
L-Tryptophan	Fluoxetine	*Documentation*: Noncontrolled study.[112]
		Effect: Symptoms related to central and peripheral toxicity may occur.
		Management: Avoid concurrent use. The FDA requested a nationwide recall of all nonprescription supplements containing L-tryptophan as the major component because of a possible link with eosinophilia myalgia.
	MAO Inhibitors (ie, isocarboxazid, phenelzine, tranylcypromine)	*Documentation*: Case reports.[113-116]
		Effect: Possible additive effect, leading to serotonin syndrome (eg, CNS irritability, motor weakness, shivering, altered consciousness).
		Management: Concomitant use of MAO inhibitors and L-tryptophan is contraindicated. The FDA requested a nationwide recall of all nonprescription supplements containing L-tryptophan as the major component because of a possible link with eosinophilia myalgia.
Tyramine-Containing Foods	MAO Inhibitors (ie, isocarboxazid, phenelzine, tranylcypromine)	*Documentation*: Controlled trial, noncontrolled trial, case reports, and product information.[165-188]
		Effect: Marked elevation in blood pressure, hypertensive crisis, hemorrhagic stroke, and death may occur.
		Management: Advise patients taking isocarboxazid not to eat foods high in tyramine or other pressor amine content during and for at least 2 weeks after isocarboxazid therapy is discontinued.
Ubiquinone (Co-enzyme Q10)	Warfarin	*Documentation*: Case reports.[189]
		Effect: Anticoagulant effect of warfarin may be decreased.
		Management: Because warfarin has a narrow therapeutic index, avoid concurrent use.
Vitamin E-Containing Herbs (eg, sunflower seeds)	Warfarin	*Documentation*: Case reports and controlled study.[12,190-192]
		Effect: Increased risk of bleeding caused by vitamin E interference with vitamin K-dependent clotting factors.
		Management: Minimize variable consumption of foods or nutritional supplements containing vitamin E. Monitor coagulation parameters during coadministration of warfarin and vitamin E supplements.

Evidence-Based Herb-Drug Interactions		
Herbal product	Drug or drug class	Potential interaction
Vitamin K-Containing Herbs (eg, alfalfa)	Warfarin	*Documentation*: Resistance to warfarin has been associated with vitamin K content of foods and nutritional supplements.[193-196]
		Effect: Decreased anticoagulant activity.
		Management: Minimize variable consumption of foods or nutritional supplements containing vitamin K.
Watercress	Chlorzoxazone	*Documentation*: Controlled trial.[197]
		Effect: Elevated chlorzoxazone plasma levels, increasing the therapeutic and adverse effects.
		Management: Advise patients taking chlorzoxazone to avoid watercress and that concurrent use could lead to increased chlorzoxazone side effects (eg, CNS depression).
Yohimbe	Tricyclic Antidepressants (eg, clomipramine)	*Documentation*: Controlled study in depressed patients.[198]
		Effect: May cause hypertension in patients receiving tricyclic antidepressants.
		Management: Avoid concomitant use.

1 van Agtmael MA, Gupta V, van der Graaf CA, van Boxtel CJ. The effect of grapefruit juice on the time-dependent decline of artemether plasma levels in healthy subjects. *Clin Pharmacol Ther.* 1999;66:408-414.

2 Gonzalez JP, Valdivieso A, Calvo R, et al. Influence of vitamin C on the absorption and first pass metabolism of propranolol. *Eur J Clin Pharmacol.* 1995;48:295-297.

3 Blickstein D, Shaklai M, Inbal A. Warfarin antagonism by avocado. *Lancet.* 1991;337:914-915.

4 Deahl M. Betel nut-induced extrapyramidal syndrome: an unusual drug interaction. *Mov Disord.* 1989;4:330-332.

5 Lambert JP, Cormier A. Potential interaction between warfarin and boldo-fenugreek. *Pharmacotherapy.* 2001;21:509-512.

6 Kempin SJ. Warfarin resistance caused by broccoli. *N Engl J Med.* 1983;308:1229-1230.

7 Karlson B, Leijd B, Hellstrom K. On the influence of vitamin K-rich vegetables and wine on the effectiveness of warfarin treatment. *Acta Med Scand.* 1986;220:347-350.

8 Carrillo JA, Jerling M, Bertilsson L. Comments to "interaction between caffeine and clozapine." *J Clin Psychopharmacol.* 1995;15:376-377.

9 Hägg S, Spigset O, Mjorndal T, Dahlqvist R. Effect of caffeine on clozapine pharmacokinetics in healthy volunteers. *Br J Clin Pharmacol.* 2000;49:59-63.

10 Vainer JL, Chouinard G. Interaction between caffeine and clozapine. *J Clin Psychopharmacol.* 1994;14:284-285.

11 Odom-White A, de Leon J. Clozapine levels and caffeine. *J Clin Psychiatry.* 1996;57:175-176.

12 Mester R, Toren P, Mizrachi I, Wolmer L, Karni N, Weizman A. Caffeine withdrawal increases lithium blood levels. *Biol Psychiatry.* 1995;37:348-350.

13 Jefferson JW. Lithium tremor and caffeine intake: two cases of drinking less and shaking more. *J Clin Psychiatry.* 1988;49:72-73.

14 Sato J, Nakata H, Owada E, Kikuta T, Umetsu M, Ito K. Influence of usual intake of dietary caffeine on single-dose kinetics of theophylline in healthy human subjects. *Eur J Clin Pharmacol.* 1993;44:295.

15 Morice AH, Lowry R, Brown MJ, Higenbottam T. Angiotensin-converting enzyme and the cough reflex. *Lancet.* 1987;2:1116.

16 Hakas JF Jr. Topical capsaicin induces cough in patient receiving ACE inhibitor. *Ann Allergy.* 1990;65:322-323.

17 Yue QY, Jansson K. Herbal drug *Curbicin* and anticoagulant effect with and without warfarin: possibly related to the vitamin E component. *J Am Geriatr Soc.* 2001;49:838.

18 Wahed A, Dasgupta A. Positive and negative in vitro interference of Chinese medicine dan shen in serum digoxin measurement. Elimination of interference by monitoring free digoxin concentration. *Am J Clin Pathol.* 2001;116:403-408.

19 Tam LS, Chan TY, Leung WK, Critchley JA. Warfarin interactions with Chinese traditional medicines: danshen and methyl salicylate medicated oil. *Aust N Z J Med.* 1995;25:258.

20 Yu CM, Chan JC, Sanderson JE. Chinese herbs and warfarin potentiation by "danshen." *J Intern Med.* 1997;241:337-339.

21 Izzat MB, Yim AP, El-Zufari MH. A taste of Chinese medicine! *Ann Thorac Surg.* 1998;66:941-942.

[22] Page RL 2nd, Lawrence JD. Potentiation of warfarin by dong quai. *Pharmacotherapy.* 1999;19:870-876.

[23] McRae S. Elevated serum digoxin levels in a patient taking digoxin and Siberian ginseng. *CMAJ.* 1996;155:293-295.

[24] Bartle WR, Ferland G. Fiddleheads and the international normalized ratio. *N Engl J Med.* 1998;338:1550.

[25] Piscitelli SC, Burstein AH, Welden N, Gallicano KD, Falloon J. The effect of garlic supplements on the pharmacokinetics of saquinavir. *Clin Infect Dis.* 2002;34:234-238.

[26] Morris J, Burke V, Mori TA, Vandongen R, Beilin LJ. Effects of garlic extract on platelet aggregation: a randomized placebo-controlled double-blind study. *Clin Exp Pharmacol Physiol.* 1995;22:414-417.

[27] Rose KD, Croissant PD, Parliament CF, Levin MB. Spontaneous spinal epidural hematoma with associated platelet dysfunction from excessive garlic ingestion: a case report. *Neurosurgery.* 1990;26:880-882.

[28] Burnham BE. Garlic as a possible risk for postoperative bleeding. *Plast Reconstr Surg.* 1995;95:213.

[29] Bordia A. Effect of garlic on human platelet aggregation in vitro. *Atherosclerosis.* 1978;30:355-360.

[30] Anon. The effect of essential oil of garlic on hyperlipemia and platelet aggregation—an analysis of 308 cases. *J Tradit Chin Med.* 1986;6:117-120.

[31] German K, Kumar U, Blackford HN. Garlic and the risk of TURP bleeding. *Br J Urol.* 1995;76:518.

[32] Samson RR. Effect of dietary garlic and temporal drift on platelet aggregation. *Atherosclerosis.* 1982;44:119-120.

[33] Lumb AB. Effect of dried ginger on human platelet function. *Thromb Haemost.* 1994;71:110-111.

[34] Srivastava KC. Effect of onion and ginger consumption on platelet thromboxane production in humans. *Prostaglandins Leukot Essent Fatty Acids.* 1989;35:183-185.

[35] Dorso CR, Levin RI, Eldor A, Jaffe EA, Weksler BB. Chinese food and platelets. *N Engl J Med.* 1980;303:756-757.

[36] Verma SK, Singh J, Khamesra R, Bordia A. Effect of ginger on platelet aggregation in man. *Indian J Med Res.* 1993;98:240-242.

[37] Chung KF, Dent G, McCusker M, Guinot P, Page CP, Barnes PJ. Effect of ginkgolide mixture (BN 52063) in antagonising skin and platelet responses to platelet activating factor in man. *Lancet.* 1987;1:248-250.

[38] Rosenblatt M, Mindel J. Spontaneous hyphema associated with ingestion of *Ginkgo biloba* extract. *N Engl J Med.* 1997;336:1108.

[39] Smith M, et al. An open trial of nifedipine-herb interactions: nifedipine with St. John's wort, ginseng, or *Ginkgo biloba. Clin Pharmacol Ther.* 2001;69:P86.

[40] Galluzzi S, et al. Coma in a patient with Alzheimer's disease taking low dose trazodone and *Ginkgo biloba. J Neurol Neurosurg Psychiatry.* 2000;68:679-680.

[41] Matthews MK Jr. Association of *Ginkgo biloba* with intracerebral hemorrhage. *Neurology.* 1998;50:1933-1934.

[42] Rowin J, Lewis SL. Spontaneous bilateral subdural hematomas associated with chronic *Ginkgo biloba* ingestion. *Neurology.* 1996;46:1775-1776.

[43] Gilbert GJ. *Gingkgo biloba. Neurology.* 1997;48:1137.

[44] Becker BN, Greene J, Evanson J, Chidsey G, Stone WJ. Ginseng-induced diuretic resistance. *JAMA.* 1996;276:606-607.

[45] Shader RI, Greenblatt DJ. Phenelzine and the dream machine—ramblings and reflections. *J Clin Psychopharmacol.* 1985;5:65.

[46] Jones BD, Runikis AM. Interaction of ginseng with phenelzine. *J Clin Psychopharmacol.* 1987;7:201-202.

[47] Janetzky K, Morreale AP. Probable interaction between warfarin and ginseng. *Am J Health Syst Pharm.* 1997;54:692-693.

[48] Josefsson M, Zackrisson AL, Ahlner J. Effect of grapefruit juice on the pharmacokinetics of amlodipine in healthy volunteers. *Eur J Clin Pharmacol.* 1996;51:189-193.

[49] Vincent J, Harris SI, Foulds G, Dogolo LC, Willavize S, Friedman HL. Lack of effect of grapefruit juice on the pharmacokinetics and pharmacodynamics of amlodipine. *Br J Clin Pharmacol.* 2000;50:455-463.

[50] Demarles D, Gillotin C, Bonaventure-Paci S, Vincent I, Fosse S, Taburet AM. Single-dose pharmacokinetics of amprenavir coadministration with grapefruit juice. *Antimicrob Agents Chemother.* 2002;46:1589-1590.

[51] Kupferschmidt HHT, Ha HR, Ziegler WH, Meier PJ, Krahenbuhl S. Interaction between grapefruit juice and midazolam in humans. *Clin Pharmacol Ther.* 1995;58:20-28.

[52] Vanakoski J, Mattila MJ, Seppala T. Grapefruit juice does not enhance the effects of midazolam and triazolam in man. *Eur J Clin Pharmacol.* 1996;50:501-508.

[53] Ha HR, Chen J, Leuenberger PM, Freiburghaus AU, Follath F. In vitro inhibition of midazolam and quinidine metabolism by flavonoids. *Eur J Clin Pharmacol.* 1995;48:367-371.

[54] Yasui N, Kondo T, Furukori H, et al. Effects of repeated ingestion of grapefruit juice on the single and multiple oral-dose pharmacokinetics and pharmacodynamics of alprazolam. *Psychopharmacology.* 2000;150:185-190.

[55] Product information. Triazolam (*Halcion*). Pharmacia & Upjohn Company. May 1999.

[56] Hukkinen SK, Varhe A, Olkkola KT, Neuvonen PJ. Plasma concentrations of triazolam are increased by concomitant ingestion of grapefruit juice. *Clin Pharmacol Ther.* 1995;58:127-131.

[57] Lilja JJ, Kivisto KT, Backman JT, Neuvonen PJ. Effect of grapefruit juice dose on grapefruit juice-triazolam interaction; repeated consumption prolongs triazolam half-life. *Eur J Clin Pharmacol.* 2000;56:411-415.

[58] Lilja JJ, Kivisto KT, Backman JT, Lamberg TS, Neuvonen PJ. Grapefruit juice substantially increases plasma concentrations of buspirone. *Clin Pharmacol Ther.* 1998;64:655-660.

[59] Garg SK, Kumar N, Bhargava VK, Prabhakar SK. Effect of grapefruit juice on carbamazepine bioavailability in patients with epilepsy. *Clin Pharmacol Ther.* 1998;64:286-288.

[60] Gross AS, Goh YD, Addison RS, Shenfield GM. Influence of grapefruit juice on cisapride pharmacokinetics. *Clin Pharmacol Ther.* 1999;65:395-401.

[61] Kivistö KT, Lilja JJ, Backman JT, Neuvonen PJ. Repeated consumption of grapefruit juice considerably increases plasma concentrations of cisapride. *Clin Pharmacol Ther.* 1999;66:448-453.

[62] Offman EM, Freeman DJ, Dresser GK, Munoz C, Bend JR, Bailey DG. Red wine-cisapride interaction: comparisons with grapefruit juice. *Clin Pharmacol Ther.* 2001;70:17-23.

[63] Oesterheld J, Kallepalli BR. Grapefruit juice and clomipramine: shifting metabolitic ratios. *J Clin Psychopharmacol.* 1997;17:62-63.

[64] Lee M, Min DI, Ku YM, Flanigan M. Effect of grapefruit juice on pharmacokinetics of microemulsion cyclosporine in African American subjects compared with Caucasian subjects: does ethnic difference matter? *J Clin Pharmacol.* 2001;41:317-323.

[65] Ducharme MP, et al. Trough concentrations of cyclosporine in blood following administration with grapefruit juice. *Br J Clin Pharmacol.* 1993;36:457-459.

[66] Herlitz H, Edgar B, Hedner T, Lidman K, Karlberg I. Grapefruit juice: a possible source of variability in blood concentration of cyclosporine A. *Nephrol Dial Transplant.* 1993;8:375.

[67] Yee GC, Stanley DL, Pessa LJ, et al. Effect of grapefruit juice on blood cyclosporin concentration. *Lancet.* 1995;345:955-956.

[68] Hollander AA, van Rooij J, Lentjes GW, et al. The effect of grapefruit juice on cyclosporine and prednisone metabolism in transplant patients. *Clin Pharmacol Ther.* 1995;57:318-324.

[69] Ducharme MP, Warbasse LH, Edwards DJ. Disposition of intravenous and oral cyclosporine after administration with grapefruit juice. *Clin Pharmacol Ther.* 1995;57:485-491.

[70] Proppe DG, Hoch OD, McLean AJ, Visser KE. Influence of chronic ingestion of grapefruit juice on steady-state blood concentrations of cyclosporine A in renal transplant patients with stable graft function. *Br J Clin Pharmacol.* 1995;39:337.

[71] Min DI, Ku YM, Perry PJ, et al. Effect of grapefruit juice on cyclosporine pharmacokinetics in renal transplant patients. *Transplantation.* 1996;62:123-125.

[72] Ioannides-Demos LL, Christophidis N, Ryan P, Angelis P, Liolios L, McLean AJ. Dosing implications of a clinical interaction between grapefruit juice and cyclosporine and metabolite concentrations in patients with autoimmune diseases. *J Rheumatol.* 1997;24:49-54.

[73] Edwards DJ, Fitzsimmons ME, Schuetz EG, et al. 6',7'-Dihydroxybergamottin in grapefruit juice and Seville orange juice: effects on cyclosporine disposition, enterocyte CYP3A4, and P-glycoprotein. *Clin Pharmacol Ther.* 1999;65:237-244.

[74] Emilia G, Longo GE, Bertesi M, Gandini G, Ferrara L, Valenti C. Clinical interaction between grapefruit juice and cyclosporine: is there any interest for the hematologists? *Blood.* 1998;91:362-363.

[75] Ku YM, Min DI, Flanigan M. Effect of grapefruit juice on the pharmacokinetics of microemulsion cyclosporine and its metabolite in healthy volunteers: does the formulation difference matter? *J Clin Pharmacol.* 1998;38:959-965.

[76] Product information. Cyclosporine (*Neoral*). Novartis Pharmaceutical Corporation. 1999.

[77] Becquemont L, Verstuyft C, Kerb R, et al. Effect of grapefruit juice on digoxin pharmacokinetics in humans. *Clin Pharmacol Ther.* 2001;70:311-316.

[78] Kanazawa S, Ohkubo T, Sugawara K. The effect of grapefruit juice on the pharmacokinetics of erythromycin. *Eur J Clin Pharmacol.* 2001;56:799-803.

[79] Schubert W, Cullberg G, Edgar B, Hedner T. Inhibition of 17 β-estradiol metabolism by grapefruit juice in ovariectomized women. *Maturitas.* 1994;20:155-163.

[80] Weber A, Jager R, Borner A, et al. Can grapefruit juice influence ethinylestradiol bioavailability? *Contraception.* 1996;53:41.

[81] Lilja JJ, Kivisto KT, Neuvonen PJ. Grapefruit juice increases serum concentrations of atorvastatin and has no effect on pravastatin. *Clin Pharmacol Ther.* 1999;66:118-127.

[82] Kantola T, Kivisto KT, Neuvonen PJ. Grapefruit juice greatly increases serum concentrations of lovastatin and lovastatin acid. *Clin Pharmacol Ther.* 1998;63:397-402.

[83] Rogers JD, Zhao J, Liu L, et al. Grapefruit juice has minimal effects on plasma concentrations of lovastatin-derived 3-hydroxy-3-methylglutaryl

coenzyme A reductase inhibitors. *Clin Pharmacol Ther.* 1999;66:358-366.

[84] Lilja JJ, Kivisto KT, Neuvonen PJ. Grapefruit juice-simvastatin interaction: effect on serum concentrations of simvastatin, simvastatin acid, and HMG-CoA reductase inhibitors. *Clin Pharmacol Ther.* 1998;64:477-483.

[85] Lilja JJ, Kivisto KT, Neuvonen PJ. Duration of effect of grapefruit juice on the pharmacokinetics of the CYP3A4 substrate simvastatin. *Clin Pharmacol Ther.* 2000;68:384-390.

[86] Shelton MJ, Wynn HE, Hewitt RG, Di-Francesco R. Effects of grapefruit juice on pharmacokinetic exposure to indinavir in HIV-positive subjects. *J Clin Pharmacol.* 2001;41:435-442.

[87] Product information. Indinavir (*Crixivan*). Merck & Co., Inc. February 2001.

[88] Penzak SR, Gubbins PO, Gurley BJ, Wang PL, Saccente M. Grapefruit juice decreases the systemic availability of itraconazole capsules in healthy volunteers. *Ther Drug Monit.* 1999;21:304-309.

[89] Kawakami M, Suzuki K, Ishizuka T, Hidaka T, Matsuki Y, Nakamura H. Effect of grapefruit juice on pharmacokinetics of itraconazole in healthy subjects. *Int J Clin Pharmacol Ther.* 1998;36:306-308.

[90] Zaidenstein R, Soback S, Gips M, et al. Effect of grapefruit juice on the pharmacokinetics of losartan and its active metabolite E3174 in healthy volunteers. *Ther Drug Monit.* 2001;23:369-373.

[91] Uno T, Ohkubo T, Sugawara K, Higashiyama A, Motomura S, Ishizaki T. Effects of grapefruit juice on the stereoselective disposition of nicardipine in humans: evidence for dominant presystemic elimination at the gut site. *Eur J Clin Pharmacol.* 2000;56:643-649.

[92] Takanaga H, Ohnishi A, Murakami H, et al. Relationship between time after intake of grapefruit juice and the effect on pharmacokinetics and pharmacodynamics of nisoldipine in healthy subjects. *Clin Pharmacol Ther.* 2000;67:201-214.

[93] Bailey DG, Arnold JM, Strong HA, Munoz C, Spence JD. Effect of grapefruit juice and naringin on nisoldipine pharmacokinetics. *Clin Pharmacol Ther.* 1993;54:589-594.

[94] Azuma J, et al. Effects of grapefruit juice on the pharmacokinetics of the calcium channel blockers nifedipine and nisoldipine. *Curr Ther Res.* 1998.59:619-634.

[95] Castro N, Jung H, Medina R, Gonzalez-Esquivel D, Lopez M, Sotelo J. Interaction between grapefruit juice and praziquantel in humans. *Antimicrob Agents Chemother.* 2002;46:1614-1616.

[96] Min DI, Ku YM, Geraets DR, Lee H. Effect of grapefruit juice on the pharmacokinetics and pharmacodynamics of quinidine in healthy volunteers. *J Clin Pharmacol* 1996;36:469-476.

[97] Ho PC, Chalcroft SC, Coville PF, Wanwimolruk S. Grapefruit juice has no effect on quinine pharmacokinetics. *Eur J Clin Pharmacol.* 1999;55:393-398.

[98] Eagling VA, Profit L, Back DJ. Inhibition of the CYP3A4-mediated metabolism and P-glycoprotein-mediated transport of the HIV-1 protease inhibitor saquinavir by grapefruit juice components. *Br J Clin Pharmacol.* 1999;48:543-552.

[99] Kupferschmidt HH, Fattinger KE, Ha HR, Follath F, Krahenbuhl S. Grapefruit juice enhances the bioavailability of the HIV protease inhibitor saquinavir in man. *Br J Clin Pharmacol.* 1998;45:355-359.

[100] Product information. Saquinavir (*Fortovase*). Roche Laboratories Inc. October 2000.

[101] Ebert U, Oertel R, Kirch W. Influence of grapefruit juice on scopolamine pharmacokinetics and pharmacodynamics in healthy male and female subjects. *Int J Clin Pharmacol Ther.* 2000;38:523-531.

[102] Lee M, Min DI. Determination of sildenafil citrate in plasma by high-performance liquid chromatography and a case for potential interaction of grapefruit juice with sildenafil citrate. *Ther Drug Monit.* 2001;23:21-26.

[103] Jetter A, Kinzig-Schippers M, Walchner-Bonjean M, et al. Effects of grapefruit juice on the pharmacokinetics of sildenafil. *Clin Pharmacol Ther.* 2002;71:21-29.

[104] Ho PC, Ghose K, Saville D, Wanwimolruk S. Effect of grapefruit juice on pharmacokinetics and pharmacodynamics of verapamil enantiomers in healthy volunteers. *Eur J Clin Pharmacol.* 2000;56:693-698.

[105] Taylor JR, Wilt VM. Probable antagonism of warfarin by green tea. *Ann Pharmacother.* 1999;33:426-428.

[106] DerMarderosian A, Beutler JA, eds. Guar Gum. *The Review of Natural Products.* St. Louis, Mo: Facts and Comparisons; 2002.

[107] Gin H, Orgerie MB, Aubertin J. The influence of Guar gum on absorption of metformin from the gut in healthy volunteers. *Horm Metab Res.* 1989;21:81-83.

[108] Perlman B. Interaction between lithium salts and ispaghula husk. *Lancet.* 1990;335:416.

[109] Aslam M, Stockley IH. Interaction between curry ingredient (karela) and drug (chlorpropamide). *Lancet.* 1979;1:607.

[110] Almeida JC, Grimsley EW. Coma from the health food store: interaction between kava and alprazolam. *Ann Intern Med.* 1996;125:940-941.

111 Attef OA, Ali AA, Ali HM. Effect of khat chewing on the bioavailability of ampicillin and amoxycillin. *J Antimicrob Chemother.* 1997;39:523-525.

112 Steiner W, Fontaine R. Toxic reaction following the combined administration of fluoxetine and L-tryptophan: five case reports. *Biol Psychiatry.* 1986;21:1067-1071.

113 Thomas JM, Rubin EH. Case report of a toxic reaction from a combination of tryptophan and phenelzine. *Am J Psychiatry.* 1984;141:281.

114 Kline SS, Mauro LS, Scala-Barnett DM, Zick D. Serotonin syndrome versus neuroleptic malignant syndrome as a cause of death. *Clin Pharm* 1989;8:510.

115 Alvine G, Black DW, Tsuang D. Case of delirium secondary to phenelzine/L-tryptophan combination. *J Clin Psychiatry.* 1990;51:311.

116 *FDA Drug Bull* 1990;20:2.

117 Chen MF, Shimada F, Kato H, Yano S, Kanaoka M. Effect of oral administration of glycyrrhizin on the pharmacokinetics of prednisolone. *Endocrinol Jpn.* 1991;38:167-174.

118 Chen MF, Shimada F, Kato H, Yano S, Kanaoka M. Effect of glycyrrhizin on the pharmacokinetics of prednisolone hemisuccinate. *Endocrinol Jpn.* 1990;37:331-341.

119 Homma M, Oka K, Ikeshima K, et al. Different effects of traditional Chinese medicines containing similar herbal constituents on prednisolone pharmacokinetics. *J Pharm Pharmacol.* 1995;47:687-692.

120 Bailey DG, Dresser G, Bend J. Lime juice/red wine-felodipine interaction: comparison with grapefruit juice. *Clin Pharmacol Ther.* 2002;71:P62.

121 Lam AY, Elmer GW, Mohutsky MA. Possible interaction between warfarin and *Lycium barbarum L. Ann Pharmacother.* 2001;35:1199-1201.

122 Monterrey-Rodriguez J. Interaction between warfarin and mango fruit. *Ann Pharmacother.* 2002;36:940-941.

123 Härtter S, Wang X, Weigmann H, et al. Differential effects of fluvoxamine and other antidepressants on the biotransformation of melatonin. *J Clin Psychopharmacol.* 2001;21:167-174.

124 Facciolá G, Hidestrand M, von Bahr C, Tybring G. Cytochrome P450 isoforms involved in melatonin metabolism in human liver microsomes. *Eur J Clin Pharmacol.* 2001;56:881-888.

125 Härtter S, Grozinger M, Weigmann H, Roschke J, Hiemke C. Increased bioavailability of oral melatonin after fluvoxamine coadministration. *Clin Pharmacol Ther.* 2000;67:1-6.

126 Lusardi P, Piazza E, Fogari R. Cardiovascular effects of melatonin in hypertensive patients well controlled by nifedipine: a 24-hour study. *Br J Clin Pharmacol.* 2000;49:423-427.

127 Piscitelli SC, Formentini E, Burstein AH, Alfaro R, Jagannatha S, Falloon J. Effect of milk thistle on pharmacokinetics of indinavir in healthy volunteers. *Pharmacotherapy.* 2002;22:551-556.

128 Richter WO, Jacob BG, Schwandt P. Interaction between fibre and lovastatin. *Lancet.* 1991;338:706.

129 Dresser GK, Bailey DG, Leake BF, et al. Fruit juices inhibit organic anion transporting polypeptide-mediated drug uptake to decrease the oral bioavailability of fexofenadine. *Clin Pharmacol Ther.* 2002;71:11-20.

130 Neuhofel AL, Wilton JH, Victory JM, Hejmanowsk LG, Amsden GW. Lack of bioequivalence of ciprofloxacin when administered with calcium-fortified orange juice: a new twist on an old interaction. *J Clin Pharmacol.* 2002;42:461-466.

131 Dresser GK, Wacher V, Ramtoola Z, Cumming K, Bailey D. Peppermint oil increases the oral bioavailability of felodipine and simvastatin. *Clin Pharmacol Ther.* 2002;71:P67.

132 Gaudry SE, Sitar DS, Smyth DD, McKenzie JK, Aoki FY. Gender and age as factors in the inhibition of renal clearance of amantadine by quinine and quinidine. *Clin Pharmacol Ther.* 1993;54:23-27.

133 Evaluation of certain food additives and contaminants: forty-first report of the joint FAO/WHO expert committee on food additives. *WHO Tech Rep Ser.* 1993;837:13.

134 Amabeoku GJ, Chikuni O, Akino C, Mutetwa S. Pharmacokinetic interaction of single doses of quinine and carbamazepine, phenobarbitone and phenytoin in healthy volunteers. *East Afr Med J.* 1993;70:90-93.

135 Wandell M, Powell JR, Hager WD, et al. Effect of quinine on digoxin kinetics. *Clin Pharmacol Ther.* 1980;28:425.

136 Aronson JK, Carver JG. Interaction of digoxin with quinine. *Lancet.* 1981;1:1418.

137 Pedersen KE, Lysgaard Madsen J, Klitgaard NA, Kjaer K, Hvidt S. Effect of quinine on plasma digoxin concentration and renal digoxin clearance. *Acta Med Scand.* 1985;218:229.

138 Hedman A, Angelin B, Arvidsson A, Dahlqvist R, Nilsson B. Interactions in the renal and biliary elimination of digoxin: stereoselective difference between quinine and quinidine. *Clin Pharmacol Ther.* 1990;47:20.

139 Hedman A. Inhibition by basic drugs of digoxin secretion into human bile. *Eur J Clin Pharmacol.* 1992;42:457.

140 Pirk LA, et al. Hypoprothrombinemic action of quinine sulfate. *JAMA.* 1945;128:1093-1095.

141 Jarnum S. Cinchophen and acetylsalicylic acid in anticoagulant treatment. *Scand J Clin Lab Invest.* 1954;6:91-93.

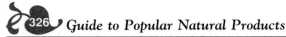

142 Bartle WR, Madorin P, Ferland G. Seaweed, vitamin K, and warfarin. *Am J Health Syst Pharm*. 2001;58:2300.

143 Johne A, Schmider J, Brockmoller J, et al. Decreased plasma levels of amitriptyline and its metabolites on comedication with an extract from St. John's wort (*Hypericum perforatum*). *J Clin Psychopharmacol*. 2001;2:46-54.

144 Yue QY, Bergquist C, Gerden B. Safety of St. John's wort (*Hypericum perforatum*). *Lancet*. 2000;355:576-577.

145 Ahmed SM, Banner NR, Dubrey SW. Low cyclosporin-A level due to Saint-John's-wort in heart transplant patients. *J Heart Lung Transplant*. 2001;20:795.

146 Ruschitzka F, Meier PJ, Turina M, Luscher TF, Noll G. Acute heart transplant rejection due to Saint John's wort. *Lancet*. 2000;355:548-549.

147 Breidenbach TH, Hoffmann MW, Becker T, Schlitt H, Klempnauer J. Drug interaction of St. John's wort with cyclosporin. *Lancet*. 2000;355:1912.

148 Mai I, Kruger H, Budde K, et al. Hazardous pharmacokinetic interaction of Saint John's wort (*Hypericum perforatum*) with the immunosuppressant cyclosporin. *Int J Clin Pharmacol Ther*. 2000;38:500-502.

149 Barone GW, Gurley BJ, Ketel BL, Abul-Ezz SR. Herbal supplements: a potential for drug interaction in transplant recipients. *Transplantation*. 2001;71:239-241.

150 Karliova M, Treichel U, Malago M, Frilling A, Gerken G, Broelsch CE. Interaction of *Hypericum perforatum* (St. John's wort) with cyclosporin A metabolism in a patient after liver transplantation. *J Hepatol*. 2000;33:853-855.

151 Dürr D, Steiger B, Kullack-Ublick GA, et al. St. John's wort induces intestinal P-glycoprotein/MDRI and intestinal and hepatic CYP3A4. *Clin Pharmacol Ther*. 2000;68:598-604.

152 Johne A, Brockmoller J, Bauer S, Maurer A, Langheinrich M, Roots I. Pharmacokinetic interaction of digoxin with an herbal extract from St. John's wort (*Hypericum perforatum*). *Clin Pharmacol Ther*. 1999;66:338-345.

153 Dresser GK, et al. St John's wort induces intestinal and hepatic CYP3A4 and P-glycoprotein in healthy volunteers. *Clin Pharmacol Ther*. 2001;69:P23.

154 Hamman MA, et al. Effect of acute and chronic St. John's wort (SJW) administration on fexofenadine (FEX) disposition. *Clin Pharmacol Ther*. 2001;69:P53.

155 Product information. Indinavir (*Crixivan*). Merck & Co., Inc. 2001.

156 Piscitelli SC, Burstein AH, Chaitt D, Alfaro RM, Falloon J. Indinavir concentrations and St. John's wort. *Lancet*. 2000;355:547-548.

157 Wang Z, Gorski JC, Hamman MA, Huang SM, Lesko LJ, Hall SD. The effects of St. John's wort (*Hypericum perforatum*) on human cytochrome P450 activity. *Clin Pharmacol Ther*. 2001;70:317-326.

158 Lantz MS, Buchalter E, Giambanco V. St. John's wort and antidepressant drug interactions in the elderly. *J Geriatr Psychiatry Neurol*. 1999;12:7-10.

159 de Maat MM, Hoetelmans RM, Math t RA, et al. Drug interaction between St. John's wort and nevirapine. *AIDS*. 2001;15:420-421.

160 Gordon JB. SSRIs and St. John's wort: possible toxicity? *Am Fam Physician*. 1998;57:950.

161 Crowe S, McKeating K. Delayed emergence and St. John's wort. *Anesthesiology*. 2002;96:1025-1027.

162 Sugimoto K, Ohmori M, Tsuroka S, et al. Different effects of St. John's wort on the pharmacokinetics of simvastatin and pravastatin. *Clin Pharmacol Ther*. 2001;70:518-524.

163 Nebel A, Schneider BJ, Baker RK, Kroll DJ. Potential metabolic interaction between St. John's wort and theophylline. *Ann Pharmacother*. 1999;33:502.

164 Maurer A, et al. Interaction of St. John's wort extract with phenprocoumon. *Eur J Clin Pharmacol*. 1999;55:A22.

165 Generali JA, Hogan LC, McFarlane M, Schwab S, Hartman CR. Hypertensive crisis resulting from avocados and a MAO inhibitor. *Drug Intell Clin Pharm*. 1981;15:904-906.

166 Foster AR, et al. Tranylcypromine and cheese. *Lancet*. 1963;2:587.

167 Cuthill JM, et al. Death associated with tranylcypromine and cheese. *Lancet*. 1964;1:1076-1077.

168 Horwitz D, et al. Monoamine oxidase inhibitors, tyramine, and cheese. *JAMA*. 1964;188:1108-1110.

169 Hedberg DL, Gordon MW, Glueck BC Jr. Six cases of hypertensive crisis in patients on tranylcypromine after eating chicken livers. *Am J Psychiatry*. 1966;122:933-937.

170 Wing YK, Chen CN. Tyramine content in Chinese food. *J Clin Psychopharmacol*. 1997;17:227.

171 Blackwell B. Effects of yeast extract after monoamine-oxidase inhibition. *Lancet*. 1965;1:940-943.

172 Nuessle WF, et al. Pickled herring and tranylcypromine reaction. *JAMA*. 1965;192:726-727.

173 Walker SE, Shulman KI, Tailor SA, Gardner D. Tyramine content of previously restricted foods in monoamine oxidase inhibitor diets. *J Clin Psychopharmacol*. 1996;16:383-388.

174 Shulman KI, Walker SE, MacKenzie S, Knowles S. Dietary restriction, tyramine, and the use of monoamine oxidase inhibitors. *J Clin Psychopharmacol*. 1989;9:397-402.

175 Tailor SA, Shulman KI, Walker SE, Moss J, Gardner D. Hypertensive episode associated with phenelzine and tap beer—a reanalysis of the role of pressor amines in beer. *J Clin Psychopharmacol.* 1994;14:5-14.

176 Mesmer RE. Don't mix miso with MAOIs. *JAMA.* 1987;258:3515.

177 Gardner DM, Shulman KI, Walker SE, Tailor SA. The making of a user friendly MAOI diet. *J Clin Psychiatry.* 1996;57:99-104.

178 Blackwell B, Marley E, Price J, Taylor D. Hypertensive interactions between monoamine oxidase inhibitors and foodstuffs. *Br J Psychiatry.* 1967;113:349-365.

179 Marley E, Blackwell B. Interactions of monoamine oxidase inhibitors, amines, and foodstuffs. *Adv Pharmacol Chemother.* 1970;9:185-239.

180 Walker JL, Davidson J, Zung WW. Patient compliance with MAO inhibitor therapy. *J Clin Psychiatry.* 1984;45:78-80.

181 Davidson J, Zung WW, Walker JI. Practical aspects of MAO inhibitor therapy. *J Clin Psychiatry.* 1984;45:81-84.

182 *Med Lett Drugs Ther.* 1980;22:58-60.

183 Maxwell MB. Reexamining the dietary restrictions with procarbazine (an MAOI). *Cancer Nurs.* 1980;3:451-457.

184 Pettinger WA, Oates JA. Supersensitivity to tyramine during monoamine oxidase inhibition in man: mechanism at the level of the adrenergic neuron. *Clin Pharmacol Ther.* 1968;9:341-344.

185 Blackwell B. Hypertensive crisis due to monoamine oxidase inhibitors. *Lancet.* 1963;2:849-851.

186 Product information. Tranylcypromine (*Parnate*). GlaxoSmithKline. 1994.

187 Livingston MG. Interactions with selective MAOIs. *Lancet.* 1995;345:533-534.

188 Dollow S. Selective MAOIs. *Lancet.* 1995;345:1055-1056.

189 Spigset O. Reduced effect of warfarin caused by ubidecarenone. *Lancet.* 1994;344:1372-1373.

190 Corrigan JJ Jr, Marcus FI. Coagulopathy associated with vitamin E ingestion. *JAMA.* 1974;230:1300-1301.

191 Schrogie JJ. Coagulopathy and fat-soluble vitamins. *JAMA.* 1975;232:19.

192 Kim JM, White RH. Effect of vitamin E on the anticoagulant response to warfarin. *Am J Cardiol.* 1996;77:545-546.

193 O'Reilly RA, Rytand DA. "Resistance" to warfarin due to unrecognized vitamin K supplementation. *N Engl J Med.* 1980;303:160-161.

194 Walker FB. Myocardial infarction after diet-induced warfarin resistance. *Arch Intern Med.* 1984;144:2089-2090.

195 Chow WH, Chow TC, Tse TM, Tai YT, Lee WT. Anticoagulation instability with life-threatening complication after dietary modification. *Postgrad Med J.* 1990;66:855-857.

196 Pedersen FM, Hamberg O, Hess K, Ovesen L. The effect of dietary vitamin K on warfarin-induced anticoagulation. *J Intern Med.* 1991;229:517-520.

197 Leclercq I, Desager JP, Horsmans Y. Inhibition of chlorzoxazone metabolism, a clinical probe for CYP2E1, by a single ingestion of watercress. *Clin Pharmacol Ther.* 1998;64:144-149.

198 Lacomblez L, Bensimon G, Isnard F, Diquet B, Lecrubier Y, Puech AJ. Effect of yohimbine on blood pressure in patients with depression and orthostatic hypotension induced by clomipramine. *Clin Pharmacol Ther.* 1989;45:241-251.

St. John's wort (*Hypericum perforatum*) is a natural product that is used in various herbal preparations, primarily for the treatment of anxiety and depression. Among other components, St. John's wort consists of flavonoids, glycosides, phenols, and tannins; however, the anthraquinone derivative hypericin, which is considered to have antidepressant activity, may be the best known component. While St. John's wort has been considered to be safe, several potentially serious drug interactions have been identified. Because of increasing and widespread use of St. John's wort, health care providers should be aware of potential drug interactions with this product, encourage patients to discuss their use of herbal products with their health care providers, and standardization of products is desirable.[1]

The precise mechanisms of many drug interactions with St. John's wort are not known. It has been suggested that St. John's wort induces CYP1A2, CYP2C9, and CYP3A4 hepatic metabolism. In addition, it is suspected that St. John's wort induces P-glycoprotein transporter, interfering with drug absorption.[2] Although these mechanisms are not mutually exclusive, it is important to determine the mechanisms of reported interactions in order to anticipate other drugs that may interact with St. John's wort. Numerous drugs are potential substrates for enzymes, depending on the CYP isozymes that may be induced (see Table 1). Many drugs are potential substrates for the P-glycoprotein transporter (see Table 2). P-glycoprotein is found in high amounts in normal tissues, including the large and small intestines, kidneys (eg, proximal tubules), liver (eg, biliary hepatocytes), brain, testes, adrenal gland, and pregnant uterus.[3-5]

Although the exact function of P-glycoprotein is not known, it does protect humans and other organisms against toxic compounds by acting as a transporter to excrete these substances into the intestinal lumen, bile, and urine.[3-5] Thus, if a drug is a substrate of P-glycoprotein in the renal tubules, active secretion into the urine could result, whereas, if a drug is a substrate of P-glycoprotein in the GI tract, uptake from the intestine will be incomplete (ie, decreasing drug levels).[3-5] Inhibition of P-glycoprotein in the proximal tubules by a substance (eg, drug, natural product) may reduce the elimination of another compound or drug, resulting in increased levels of that substance.

Without standardization of herbal products, it is difficult to determine the amount of the ingredient (eg, hypericin) an individual may be ingesting, which may confound the prediction of possible drug interactions. It is unlikely that clinically important interactions will occur with St. John's wort and many of the drugs listed in Tables 1 and 2. Naturopathic physicians, herbalists, and those taking St. John's wort are not seeing or reporting many difficulties. However, until more information is available, it would be prudent to use caution when patients taking these agents are starting or stopping St. John's wort. When possible, consider avoiding use of St. John's wort in patients taking drugs listed in Tables 1 and 2, especially when the drug has a narrow therapeutic index (eg, cyclosporine, digoxin, theophylline, tolbutamide, warfarin).

Table 1. Cytochrome P450[3-28]		
Substrates of CYP1A2		
Acetaminophen	Naproxen	Theophylline (major)
Caffeine	Ofloxacin	TCAs (demethylation)
Clozapine (major)	Olanzapine	Amitriptyline
Cyclobenzaprine	Ondansetron	Clomipramine
Diazepam*	Phenacetin	Desipramine
Fluvoxamine	Propafenone	Imipramine
Haloperidol	Propranolol	Nortriptyline
Isotretinoin	Riluzole	Verapamil
Lomefloxacin	Ritonavir	R-warfarin
Melatonin (major)	Ropivacaine (major)	Zileuton
Methadone	Tacrine	Zolpidem
Mexiletine (minor)	Tamoxifen	
Mirtazapine	Testosterone	
Substrates of CYP2C9		
Barbiturates	Ibuprofen	Sertraline
Hexobarbital	Indomethacin	Sildenafil
Mephobarbital	Losartan	Suprofen*
Carvedilol	Mefenamic acid	Terbinafine
Celecoxib	Melatonin (minor)	Tetrahydrocannabinol
Cilostazol	Mephenytoin	Tolbutamide
Dapsone	Mirtazapine	Torsemide
Diclofenac	Montelukast	TCAs
Dronabinol	Naproxen	Amitriptyline
Fluoxetine	Nateglinide	Imipramine
Flurbiprofen	Phenytoin	S-warfarin
Fluvastatin	Piroxicam	Zafirlukast
Glimepiride	Ritonavir	Zileuton

Continued on following page ...

Table 1. Cytochrome P450[3-28] (*Cont.*)		
Substrates of CYP3A4		
Acetaminophen	Ethosuximide	Paclitaxel (minor)
Alfentanil	Etoposide	Pimozide
Alprazolam	Exemestane	Progesterone
Amiodarone	Felodipine	Propafenone
Amlodipine	Fentanyl	Quinidine
Astemizole	Finasteride	Quinine
Atorvastatin	Flutamide	Ritonavir
Benzphetamine	Granisetron	Ropivacaine (minor)
Bromocriptine	Glyburide	Salmeterol
Busulfan	Halofantrine	Saquinavir
Cerivastatin	Hydrocortisone	Sertraline
Chlorpromazine	Ifosfamide	Sildenafil
Cilostazol	Indinavir	Simvastatin
Cisapride	Isradipine	Sufentanil
Citalopram	Itraconazole*	Tacrolimus
Clarithromycin	Ketoconazole	Tamoxifen
Clindamycin	Lansoprazole	Teniposide
Clonazepam	Lidocaine	Terfenadine
Clozapine	Loratadine	Testosterone
Cocaine	Losartan	Theophylline (minor)
Codeine	Lovastatin	Tiagabine
Colchicine	Methadone	Tolterodine
Cyclobenzaprine	Mibefradil	Tretinoin
Cyclophospha-mide	Miconazole	Triazolam
Cyclosporine	Midazolam	TCAs (demethylation)
Dapsone	Mifepristone	Amitriptyline
Delavirdine	Mirtazapine	Clomipramine
Dexamethasone	Montelukast	Imipramine
Dextromethorphan	Navelbine	Troglitazone
Diazepam	Nateglinide	Troleandomycin
Digitoxin	Nefazodone	Venlafaxine
Diltiazem	Nelfinavir	Verapamil
Disopyramide	Neviramine	Vinblastine
Docetaxel	Nicardipine	Vincristine
Dolasetron	Nifedipine	R-warfarin*
Donepezil	Nimodipine	Yohimbine
Doxorubicin	Nisoldipine	Zileuton
Dronabinol	Nitrendipine	Zolpidem (major)
Erythromycin	Omeprazole	
Ethinyl estradiol	Ondansetron	

* Effect uncertain or minimal.

Table 2. Substrates for P-glycoprotein[3-5,21,29-43]		
Amiodarone	Hydrocortisone	Quinidine
Chlorpromazine	Indinavir	Reserpine
Clarithromycin	Itraconazole	Ritonavir
Cyclosporine	Ketoconazole	Saquinavir
Dactinomycin	Lidocaine	Sirolimus
Daunorubicin	Loperamide	Tacrolimus
Dexamethasone	Lovastatin	Tamoxifen
Digoxin	Mifepristone (RU486)	Teniposide
Diltiazem	Mitoxantrone	Testosterone
Doxorubicin	Nelfinavir	Trifluoperazine
Erythromycin	Nicardipine	Triflupromazine
Estradiol	Nifedipine	Verapamil
Etoposide	Ondansetron	Vinblastine
Fexofenadine	Paclitaxel	Vincristine
Fluphenazine	Progesterone	
	Promethazine	

1 Ernst E. Second thoughts about safety of St. John's wort. *Lancet*. 1999;354:2014-2016.

2 Dürr D, et al. St John's wort induces intestinal P-glycoprotein/MDR1 and intestinal and hepatic CYP3A4. *Clin Pharmacol Ther*. 2000;68:598-604.

3 Yu DK. The contribution of P-glycoprotein to pharmacokinetics drug-drug interactions. *J Clin Pharmacol*. 1999;39:1203-1211.

4 Verschraagen M, et al. P-glycoprotein system as a determinant of drug interactions: the case of digoxin-verapamil. *Pharmacol Res*. 1999;40:301-306.

5 Tanigawara Y. Role of P-glycoprotein in drug disposition. *Ther Drug Monit*. 2000;22:137-140.

6 Guengerich FP. Cytochrome P-450 3A4: regulation and role in drug metabolism. *Annu Rev Pharmacol Toxicol*. 1999;39:1-17.

7 Tatro D. Cytochrome P450 enzyme drug interactions. *DFC News*. 1995;14:59-60.

8 Mullen W, et al. Pharmaceuticals and the cytochrome P450 isoenzymes: A tool for decision making. *Pharm Prac News*. 1998;25:20-24.

9 Miners JO, et al. Cytochrome P4502C9: an enzyme of major importance in human drug metabolism. *Br J Clin Pharmacol*. 1998;45:525-538.

10 Gantmacher J, et al. Interaction between warfarin and oral terbinafine. Manufacturer does not agree that interaction was with terbinafine. *BMJ*. 1998;317:205.

11 Michalets EL. Clinically significant cytochrome P-450 drug interactions—author's reply. *Pharmacotherapy*. 1998;18:892-893.

12 Nakajima M, et al. Involvement of CYP 1A2 in mexiletine metabolism. *Br J Clin Pharmacol*. 1998;46:55-62.

13 Jefferson J. Drug interactions-friend or foe? *J Clin Psychiatry*. 1998;59(suppl 4):37-47.

14 Michalets EL. Update: Clinically significant cytochrome P-450 drug interactions. *Pharmacotherapy*. 1998;18:84-112.

15 Nemeroff C, et al. Newer antidepressants and the cytochrome P450 system. *Am J Psychiatry*. 1996;153:311-320.

16 Bertz R, et al. Use of in vitro and in vivo data to estimate the likelihood of metabolic pharmacokinetic interactions. *Clin Pharmacokinet*. 1997;32:210-258.

17 Goldberg RJ. The P-450 system. Definition and relevance to the use of antidepressants in medical practice. *Arch Fam Med*. 1996;5:406-412.

18 Spatzenegger M, et al. Clinical importance of hepatic cytochrome P450 in drug metabolism. *Drug Metab Rev*. 1995;27:397-417.

19 Halliday R, et al. An investigation of the interaction between halofantrine, CYP2D6 and CYP3A4: Studies with human liver microsomes and heterologous enzyme expression systems. *Br J Clin Pharmacol*. 1995;40:369-378.

20 Kroemer H, et al. Stereoselectivity in drug metabolism and action: Effects of enzyme inhibition and induction. *Ther Drug Monit*. 1996;18:388-392.

21 Abernethy D, et al. Molecular basis of cardiovascular drug metabolism: Implications for predicting clinically important drug interactions. *Circulation*. 2000;101:1749-1753.

[22] Ko JW, et al. In vitro inhibition of the cytochrome P450 (CYP450) system by the antiplatelet drug Ticlopidine: potent effect on CYP2C19 and CYP2D6. *Br J Clin Pharmacol.* 2000;49:343-351.

[23] Cupp MJ, et al. Cytochrome P450: new nomenclature and clinical implications. *Am Fam Physician.* 1998;57:107-116.

[24] Caraco Y. Genetic determinants of drug responsiveness and drug interactions. *Ther Drug Monit.* 1998;20:517-524.

[25] Arlander E, et al. Metabolism of ropivacaine in humans is mediated by CYP1A2 and to a minor extent by CYP3A4: an interaction study with fluvoxamine and ketoconazole as in vivo inhibitors. *Clin Pharmacol Ther.* 1998;64:484-491.

[26] Abdel-Rahman SM, et al. Investigation of terbinafine as a CYP2D6 inhibitor in vivo. *Clin Pharmacol Ther.* 1999;65:465-472.

[27] Tanaka M, et al. Stereoselective pharmacokinetics of Pantoprazole, a proton pump inhibitor, in extensive and poor metabolizers of S-mephenytoin. *Clin Pharmacol Ther.* 2001;69:108-113.

[28] Hyland R, et al. Identification of the cytochrome P450 enzymes involved in the N-demethylation of sildenafil. *Br J Clin Pharmacol.* 2001;51:239-248.

[29] Matheny CJ, et al. Pharmacokinetic and pharmacodynamic implications of P-glycoprotein modulation. *Pharmacotherapy.* 2001;21:778-796.

[30] von Moltke LL, et al. Drug transporters revisited. *J Clin Psychopharmacol.* 2001;21:1-3.

[31] Sadeque AJM, et al. Increased drug delivery to the brain by P-glycoprotein inhibition. *Clin Pharmacol Ther.* 2000;68:231-237.

[32] Fromm MF, et al. Inhibition of P-glycoprotein-mediated drug transport: a unifying mechanism to explain the interaction between digoxin and quinidine. *Circulation.* 1999;99:552-557.

[33] von Moltke LL, et al. Drug transporters in psychopharmacology—are they important? *J Clin Psychopharmacol.* 2000;20:291-294.

[34] Zhang Y, et al. The gut as a barrier to drug absorption: combined role of cytochrome P450 3A and P-glycoprotein. *Clin Pharmacokinet.* 2001;40:159-168.

[35] Fromm MF. P-glycoprotein: a defense mechanism limiting oral bioavailability and CNS accumulation of drugs. *Int J Clin Pharmacol Ther.* 2000;38:69-74.

[36] Greiner B, et al. The role of intestinal P-glycoprotein in the interaction of digoxin and rifampin. *J Clin Invest.* 1999;104:147-153.

[37] Hamman MA, et al. The effect of rifampin administration on the disposition of fexofenadine. *Clin Pharmacol Ther.* 2001;69:114-121.

[38] Kim RB, et al. Interrelationship between substrates and inhibitors of human CYP3A and P-glycoprotein. *Pharm Res.* 1999;16:408-414.

[39] Masuda S, et al. Effect of intestinal P-glycoprotein on daily tacrolimus trough level in a living-donor small bowel recipient. *Clin Pharmacol Ther.* 2000;68:98-103.

[40] Huisman MT, et al. Significance of P-glycoprotein for the pharmacology and clinical use of HIV protease inhibitors. *AIDS.* 2000;14:237-242.

[41] Woodland C, et al. A model for the prediction of digoxin-drug interactions at the renal tubular cell level. *Ther Drug Monit.* 1998;20:134-138.

[42] Levêque D, et al. P-glycoprotein and pharmacokinetics. *Anticancer Res.* 1995;15:331-336.

[43] Clayette P, et al. Significance of P-glycoprotein for the pharmacology and clinical use of HIV protease inhibitors. *AIDS.* 2000;14:235-236.

PHARMACOLOGY: Diuretics remain among the most frequently prescribed drugs in the United States. In addition to the widespread use of prescription diuretics, OTC and natural diuretics continue to play an important role in the self-treatment of menstrual distress, edema, and hypertension.

Numerous OTC menstrual distress preparations contain xanthine alkaloids such as caffeine and theobromine, which are most often derived from inexpensive natural sources. Of these compounds, only caffeine has been found to be both safe and effective for use as an OTC diuretic. In its review of these products, the FDA Advisory Review Panel on Menstrual Drug Products concluded that the frequently used dandelion root (*Taraxacum officinale* Wiggers), a preparation once thought to have strong diuretic properties, is safe but ineffective in the treatment of dysmenorrhea. Nor is there evidence that dandelion is an effective diuretic.

Teas and extracts of buchu (*Barosma betulina*) and quack grass (*Agropyron* spp.) are popular, but their diuretic activity is probably no greater than that of the xanthine alkaloids in coffee or ordinary tea. Significant toxicity from buchu and quack grass have not been reported.[1]

Diuretic teas that should be avoided include juniper berries (*Juniperus communis*), which contain a locally irritating volatile oil capable of causing renal damage, and shave grass or horsetail (*Equisetum* spp.) a weakly diuretic plant that contains several toxic compounds including aconitic acid, equisitine (a neurotoxin), and nicotine.[2] In grazing animals, the ingestion of horsetail has caused excitement, convulsions, and death. Thiamine deficiency has been reported in sheep after the experimental administration of shave grass.

Other teas, such as ephedra (ma huang), contain the mildly diuretic stimulant ephedrine. These teas should be used with caution by hypertensive patients.

All plants and herbal extracts included in OTC products for use as diuretics are not toxic; however, the majority are either clinically ineffective or no more effective than caffeine. The following table lists plants that have been reported to possess diuretic activity. This list has been compiled from old materia medica, herbals, and when documentation is available, the scientific literature. There is generally little scientific evidence to justify the use of most of these plants as diuretics. Some are toxic even in very low doses. The fact that some have been used for centuries in herbal medicine does not necessarily attest to their effectiveness; rather it suggests that such plants have a relatively broad margin of safety and their use does not usually result in toxicity.

Herbal Diuretics[1]		
Scientific name	*Common name*	*Part used*
Abutilon indicum	—	Bark
Acalypha evrardii	—	Flower, leaf
Acanthus spinosus	—	Entire plant
Acorus calamus[2]	**Calamus**	**Rhizome**
Adonis vernalis	Pheasant's eye herb	Above ground
Agave americana	Agave	Roots
Agrimonia eupatoria	**Agrimony**	**Entire plant**

Herbal Diuretics[1]		
Scientific name	*Common name*	*Part used*
Agropyron	**Couch grass**	**Rhizomes, roots, stems**
Alchemilla arvensis	**Lady's mantle**	**Entire plant**
Alisma plantago	—	Entire plant
Allium cepa	Onion	Bulb
Ammi visnaga	—	**Fruit**
Anemone spp.[2]	Windflower	Entire plant
Apium graveolens[2]	**Celery**	**Stalk, oil**
Apocynum cannabinum[2]	—	Entire plant
Arctostaphylos uva-ursi[2]	**Uva ursi**	**Leaves**
Arctium lappa	**Burdock**	**Root**
Asparagus officinale	**Asparagus**	**Roots**
Bacopa monnieri	—	Entire plant
Barosma spp.	**Buchu**	**Leaves**
Begonia cucullata	Begonia	Entire plant
Betula alba[2]	Betula	Leaves, twigs
Blumea lacera	—	Entire plant
Boerhaavia diffusa	—	Entire plant
Borago officinalis	**Borage**	**Leaves, tops**
Buddleja americana	—	Bark, leaf, root
Callistris arborea	—	Gum
Calystegia soldanella	—	Entire plant
Camellia sinensis	Common tea	Leaves
Capsella bursa-pastoris	Shepherd's purse	Above ground
Carex arenaria	—	Entire plant
Chamaelirium luteum	—	Root
Chelidomium majus	Celandine	Root, leaves, latex
Chicorium intybus	**Chicory**	**Root**
Chimaphilia umbellata	Pipsissewa	Above ground
Claytonia sibirica	—	Entire plant
Clematis spp[2]	—	**Entire plant**
Coffea arabica	Coffee	Fruit

Herbal Diuretics[1]		
Scientific name	*Common name*	*Part used*
Collinsonia canadensis	Stoneroot	Root
Convallaria majalis[2]	Lily of the valley	Flowering tops
Costus spicatus	—	Sap
Curanga fel-terrae	—	Leaf
Cynanchium vincetoxicum	—	Entire plant
Cytisus scoparius[2]	**Broom**	**Flowering tops**
Daucus carota	**Carrot**	**Root**
Digitalis purpurea[2]	**Foxglove**	**Leaves**
Drosera rotundifolia	Drosera	Entire plant
Ephedra spp.	**Ephedra**	**Stems**
Equisetum spp.	**Horsetail**	**Above ground**
Eryngium yuccifolium	—	Entire plant
Fumaria officinalis	**Fumitory**	**Flowering tops**
Gaillardia pinnatifida	—	Entire plant
Galega officinalis	Goat's rue	All but root
Galium aparine	Cleavers	Above ground
Glycyrrhiza glabra	**Licorice**	**Rhizome, root**
Helianthus annus	Sunflower	Seeds
Hemidesmus indicus	—	Entire plant
Herniaria glabra	Rupturewort	Above ground
Hibiscus spp.	**Hibiscus**	**Flowers**
Hydrangea arborescens[2]	Hydrangea	Roots
Hypericum perforatum	**St. John's Wort**	**Entire plant**
Hypochoeris scarzonerae	—	Entire plant
Ilex paraguayensis[2]	**Maté**	**Leaves**
Iris florentina	Orris	Peeled rhizome
Juniperus communis[2]	**Juniper**	**Berries**

Herbal Diuretics[1]		
Scientific name	*Common name*	*Part used*
Laportea meyeniana	—	Leaf, root
Levisticum officinale	**Lovage**	**Roots**
Paullinia cupana	**Guarana**	**Seeds**
Petroselinum crispum[2]	**Parsley**	**Leaves, seeds**
Peumus boldus	**Boldo**	**Leaves**
Pinus silvestris	Pine	Cones
Psoralae corylifolia	—	Seeds
Rafnia perfoliata	—	Leaf
Rehmannia lutea	—	Entire plant
Sambucus nigra	**Elderberry**	**Flowers**
Santalum album	**Sandalwood**	**Oil**
Sassafras albidum	**Sassafras**	**Root**
Senecionis herba	Senecio herb	Above ground
Serenoa repens	**Saw palmetto**	**Ripe fruits**
Smilax spp.	Sarsaparilla	Roots
Solanum dulca-mara[2]	**Bittersweet**	**Twigs, branches**
Spiranthes diuretica	—	Entire plant
Tagetes multifida	—	Entire plant
Taraxacum offici-nale	**Dandelion**	**Leaves**
Theobroma cacao	**Cocoa**	**Seeds**
Trianthema portula-castrum	—	Leaves
Tribulus terrestris	—	Fruit
Urginea maritima[2]	**Squill**	**Bulb**
Urtica dioica[2]	**Nettle**	**Leaves**
Viola odorata	Violet	Leaves, flowers
Withania somnifera[2]	**Withania**	**Root**

[1] Plants in **bold** are described in their own monograph in this system.
[2] Noted as toxic in reference; all others should not be considered safe for general use in the absence of valid safety.

❀❀❀

[1] *Med Let.* 1979;21:29.

[2] DerMarderosian AH. *Am Druggist.* 1980 Aug:35.

Photographs

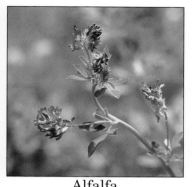

Alfalfa

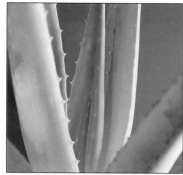

Aloe Vera

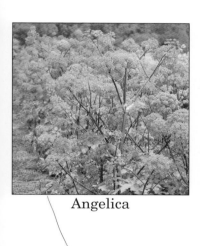

Angelica

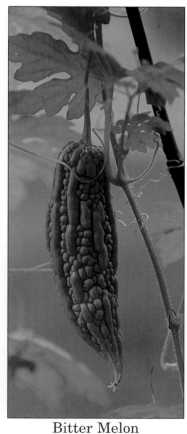

Bitter Melon

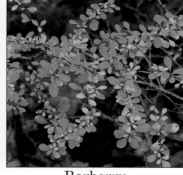

Barberry

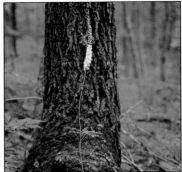

Black Cohosh (flower)

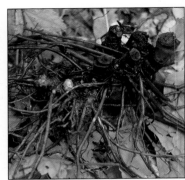

Black Cohosh (root & leaf)

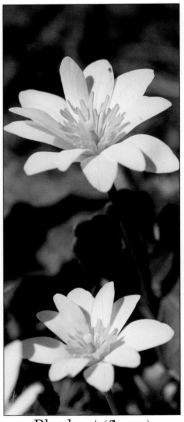

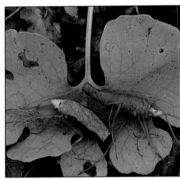

Blood Root (root & leaf)

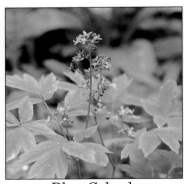

Bloodroot (flower)

Blue Cohosh

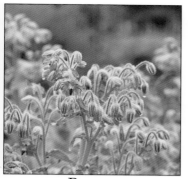

Borage

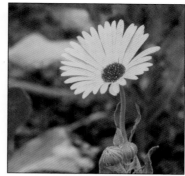

Calendula

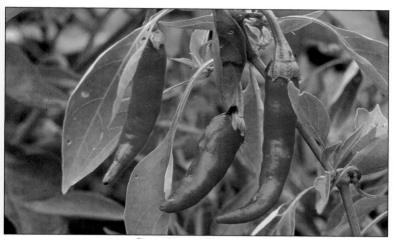

Capsicum Peppers

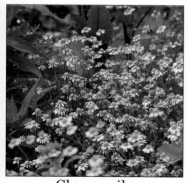

Chamomile

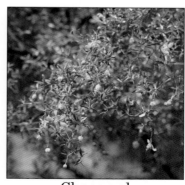

Chaparral

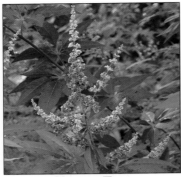

Chaste Tree

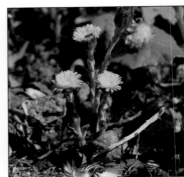

Coltsfoot

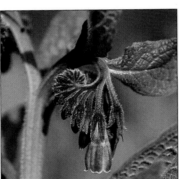

Comfrey

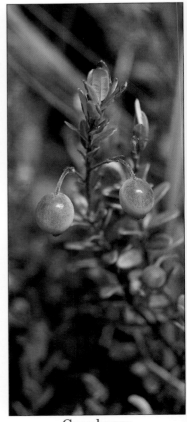

Cranberry

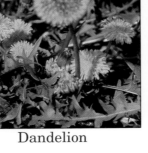

Dandelion

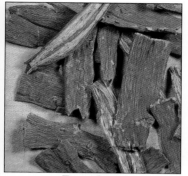

Danshen

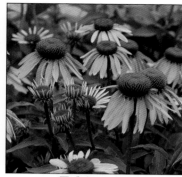

Echinacea

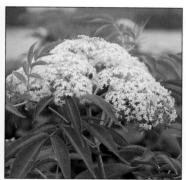

Elderberry

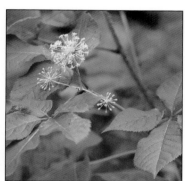

Eleutherococcus

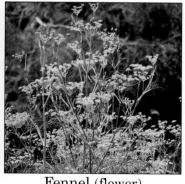

Fennel (flower)

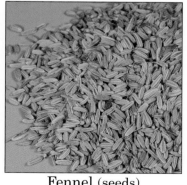

Fennel (seeds)

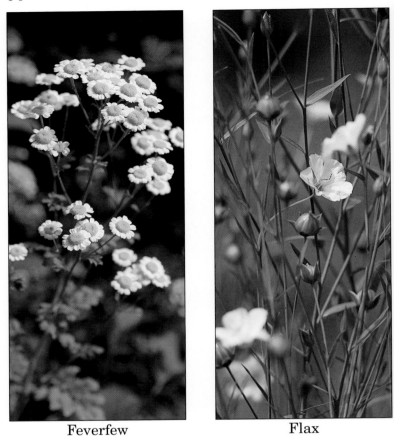

Feverfew

Flax

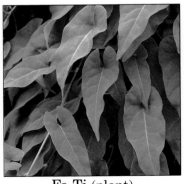

Fo-Ti (plant)

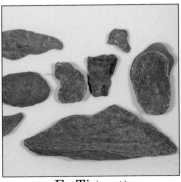

Fo-Ti (root)

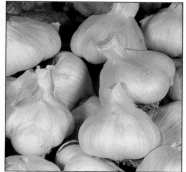

Garlic (bulb)

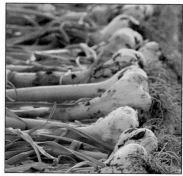

Garlic (bulb & root)

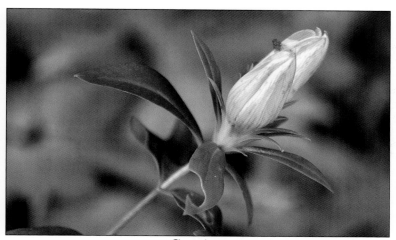

Gentian

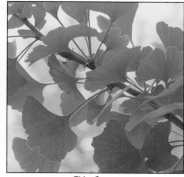

Ginkgo

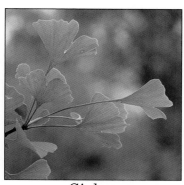

Ginkgo

I-8

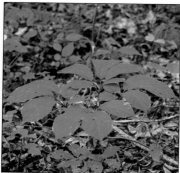

Ginseng (American)

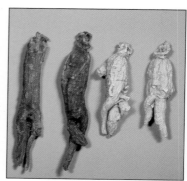

Ginseng (Asian)

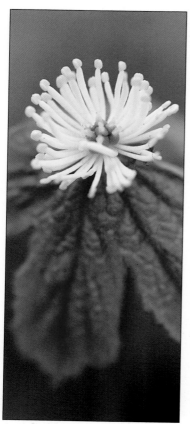

Goldenseal (flower)

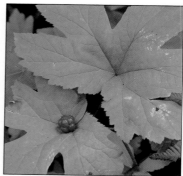

Goldenseal (leaf)

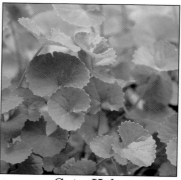

Gotu Kola

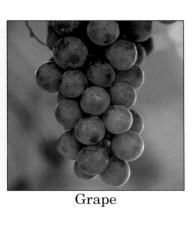

Grape

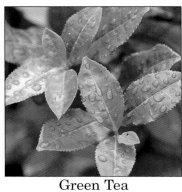

Green Tea

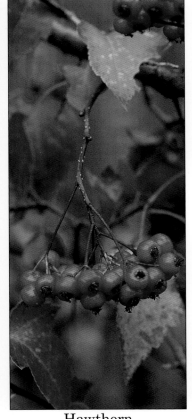

Hawthorn

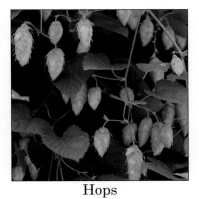

Hops

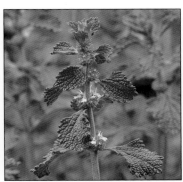

Horehound

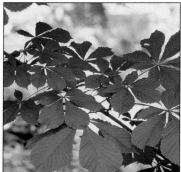

Horse Chestnut

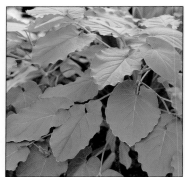

Kava Kava

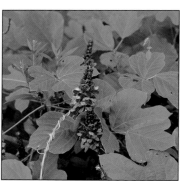

Kudzu

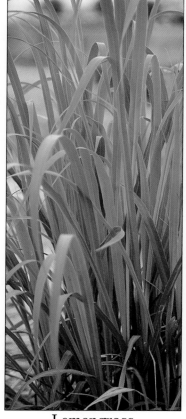

Lemongrass

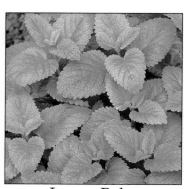

Lemon Balm

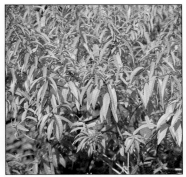

Lemon Verbena

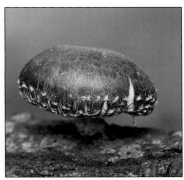

Lentinan

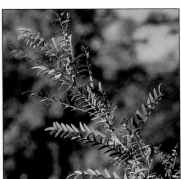

Licorice

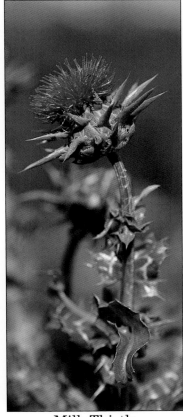

Milk Thistle

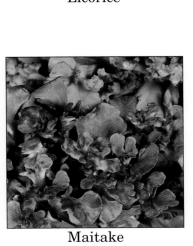

Maitake

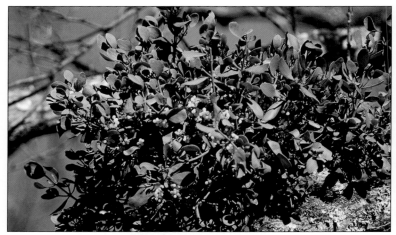

Mistletoe (American)

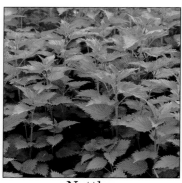

Nettles

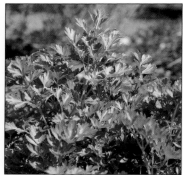

Parsley

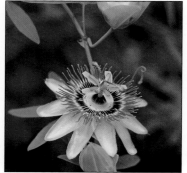

Passion Flower

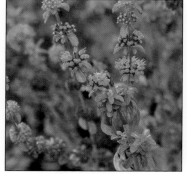

Pennyroyal

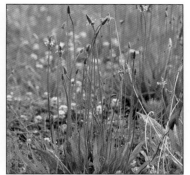

Plantain

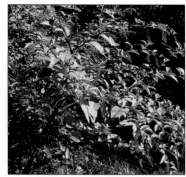

Pokeweed (flower)

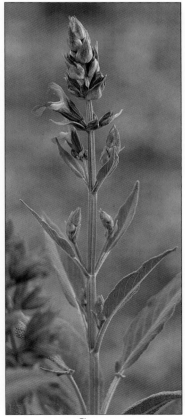

Sage

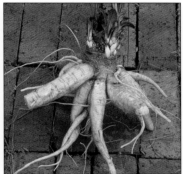

Pokeweed (root)

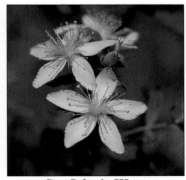

St. John's Wort

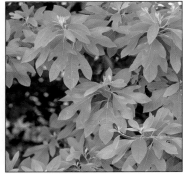

Sassafras

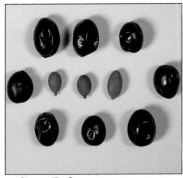

Saw Palmetto (berries)

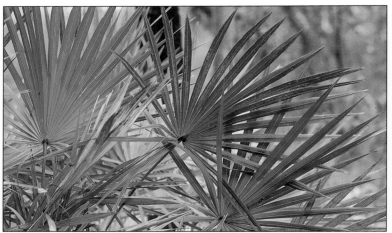

Saw Palmetto (leaves)

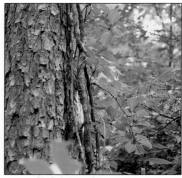

Schisandra (vine)

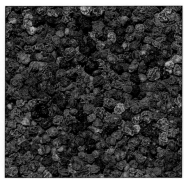

Schisandra (fruit)

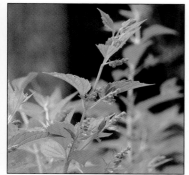

Scullcap

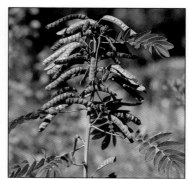

Senna

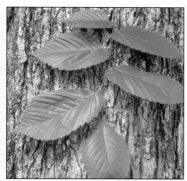

Slippery Elm

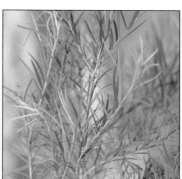

Tea Tree

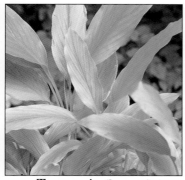

Turmeric (leaves)

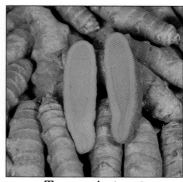

Turmeric (root)

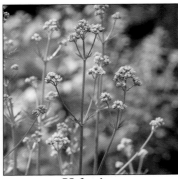

Valerian

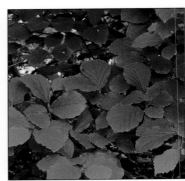

Witch Hazel

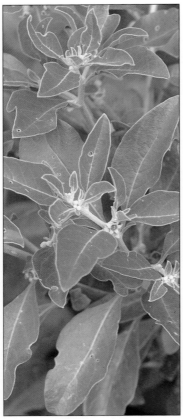

Withania

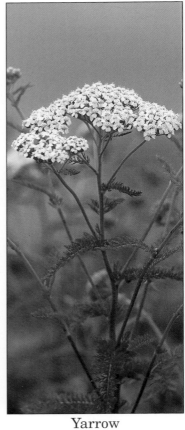

Yarrow

Therapeutic Index

The Therapeutic Uses Index cross references the multiple applications noted within *Guide to Popular Natural Products* monographs, which are presented alphabetically. The information contained in this index is intended to be a starting point when seeking information about natural products. It is imperative to read the entire monograph before taking any phytomedicinal or herb. Contact a qualified medical professional for serious or long-term problems.

The Therapeutic Uses Index entries are presented alphabetically. Boldface entries refer to the condition, followed by the monograph name in which the condition is discussed. The distinction between current and folkloric uses is designated by the following key:

  C – Clinical (Physiologic effects in humans and animals. Includes data from clinical studies. Information will be found within the pharmacology section of each monograph.)

  V – In vivo/In vitro (Preliminary studies show in vivo or in vitro action. Information will be found within the pharmacology section of each monograph.)

  H – Historic/Folkloric (Reviews the historical and folk uses of the topic. Information will be found within the history section of each monograph.)

  M – Multiple (Application of topic noted in more than one category within the monograph. Example: In the echinacea monograph, the immunostimulant properties of echinacea are cited as a folkloric application and for clinical use.)

Please remember the uses cited in this index are not FDA-approved uses. In addition, listing of potential uses are not endorsements or recommendations by Wolters Kluwer Health, Inc. Please use your own judgment and seek the advice of a health care professional before initiating therapy.

Antibacterial (cont.), see
Barberry, C
Calendula, V
Coltsfoot, V
Cranberry, C
Feverfew, V
Garlic, M
Hibiscus, C
Lemon Verbena, C
Mastic, C
Parsley, V
Passion Flower, V
Quassia, M
Schisandra, C
Scullcap, V
St. John's Wort, V
Stevia, C
Tea Tree Oil, C
Turmeric, C
Antibiotic, see
Goldenseal, C
Lemon Verbena, V
Yarrow, C
Antidepressant, see
Milk Thistle, H
St. John's Wort, M
Antidote, poisonous herbs, mushrooms, snakebites, see
Fennel, H
Antifungal, see
Angelica, C
Barberry, M
Garlic, V
Parsley, V
Purslane, M
Quassia, M
Sassafras, V
Scullcap, V
Terminalia, C
Antigonadotropic, see
Comfrey, C
Antihepatotoxic, see
Elderberry, C
Turmeric, C
Antihistamine, see
Eleutherococcus, C
Anti-infective, see
Aloe, M
Black Walnut, M
Echinacea, M
Lemon, M
Onion, H
Scullcap, C
Witch Hazel, C
Anti-inflammatory, see
Angelica, C
Artichoke, C

Anti-inflammatory (cont.), see
Barberry, M
Bupleurum, C
Butterbur, C
Calendula, M
Cat's Claw, H
Comfrey, C
Emblica, C
Evening Primrose Oil, C
Hibiscus, C
Horse Chestnut, C
Ma Huang, C
Milk Thistle, C
Nigella Sativa, M
Passion Flower, H
Plantain, H
Prickly Pear, M
Pycnogenol, M
Sarsaparilla, M
Saw Palmetto, C
Scullcap, C
Sour Cherry, M
St. John's Wort, M
Withania, H
Antimicrobial, see
Aloe, C
Bitter Melon, M
Black Cohosh, V
Bloodroot, V
Blue Cohosh, C
Emblica, C
Hops, C
Lemon, C
Lentinan, C
Methylsulfonylmethane, C
Nigella Sativa, M
Olive Oil, C
Onion, C
Parsley, H
Passion Flower, V
Pau D'Arco, H
Pawpaw, C
Purslane, M
Sage, C
Sassafras, V
Tea Tree Oil, C
Terminalia, C
Antineoplastic, see
Chaparral, H
Garlic, C
Ginger, H
Goldenseal, C
Mistletoe, V
Sassafras, C
Yarrow, C
Antioxidant, see
Artichoke, C

Antioxidant (cont.), see
Barberry, C
Chaparral, C
Garlic, C
Grape Seed, C
Hibiscus, C
Jiaogulan, C
Kudzu, C
Lemon, C
Lycopene, C
Milk Thistle, C
Nigella Sativa, C
Olive Leaf, C
Onion, C
Purslane, C
Rosemary, C
Sage, C
Sour Cherry, M
Turmeric, C
Antiprotozoal, see
Pau D'Arco, H
Antisecretory, see
Sage, C
Antiseptic, see
Garlic, C
Goldenseal, C
Lemongrass, H
Sage, H
Tea Tree Oil, M
Antispasmodic, see
Blue Cohosh, H
Butterbur, C
Chamomile, M
Dong Quai, M
Goldenseal, H
Hawthorn, H
Hops, C
Lemon Balm, M
Lemon Verbena, H
Lemongrass, H
Nettles, H
Red Clover, M
Rosemary, H
Sage, M
Valerian, C
Wild Yam, H
Antithrombotic, see
Chondroitin, C
Danshen, C
Garlic, C
Kava, C
Antitrypanosome, see
Pau D'Arco, H
Antitussive/Cough, see
Barberry, H
Bloodroot, H
Butterbur, H
Capsicum Peppers, C

Blood purifier, see
  Bloodroot, H
  Dong Quai, H
  Echinacea, H
  Eleutherococcus, C
  Fo-Ti, C
  Milk Thistle, M
Blood vessels, dilate, see
  Cat's Claw, C
  Hawthorn, C
Boils, see
  Pau D'Arco, H
  Slippery Elm, H
  Tea Tree Oil, H
Bone pain, see
  Cat's Claw, H
  Methylsulfonylmethane, C
Brain cancer, see
  Maitake, C
Breast cancer, see
  L-arginine, C
  Maitake, C
  Mistletoe, C
  Pawpaw, C
  Pycnogenol, C
  Red Clover, H
Breast pain, see
  Evening Primrose Oil, C
  Gamma Linolenic Acid, C
Breast size, increase, see
  Saw Palmetto, H
Bronchial asthma, see
  Gamma Linolenic Acid, M
Bronchitis, see
  Borage, H
  Chaparral, H
  Coltsfoot, H
  Ma Huang, M
  Milk Thistle, H
  Onion, H
Bronchodilator, see
  Cramp bark, M
Bruises, see
  Comfrey, H
  Danshen, C
  Parsley, H
  Prickly Pear, H
  Slippery Elm, H
  Witch Hazel, C
Burns, see
  Aloe, M
  L-arginine, C
  Chaparral, H
  Comfrey, H
  Olive Oil, M
  Passion Flower, H
  Tea Tree Oil, M

Burns (cont.), see
  Witch Hazel, H

Calcium channel
  blocker, see
  Coltsfoot, C
Cancer, see
  Barberry, H
  Bloodroot, C
  Bupleurum, C
  Calendula, H
  Cat's Claw, C
  Chaparral, M
  Cranberry, H
  Danshen, C
  Echinacea, C
  Elderberry, H
  Eleutherococcus, C
  Emblica, C
  Evening Primrose Oil, V
  Fo-Ti, C
  Gamma Linolenic Acid, C
  Garlic, C
  Ginseng, H
  Gotu Kola, C
  Green Tea, M
  Hibiscus, H
  Hops, H
  Jiaogulan, C
  Lemon, C
  Lentinan, C
  Lycopene, M
  Maitake, C
  Meadowsweet, H
  Melatonin, C
  Mistletoe, M
  Nettles, H
  Nigella Sativa, C
  Onion, C
  Parsley, H
  Pau D'Arco, H
  Pycnogenol, C
  Red Clover, C
  Reishi Mushroom, C
  Rosemary, C
  Scullcap, C
  St. John's Wort, H
  Turmeric, M
  Witch Hazel, H
Candida albicans, see
  Pau D'Arco, H
Canker sores, see
  Mace, H
Cardiac stimulant, see
  Ginger, C
Cardioprotective, see
  Brahmi, H
  Eleutherococcus, C

Cardioprotective (cont.),
  see
  Gamma Linolenic Acid, C
  Hawthorn, C
  Lemon, C
  Lycopene, C
  Olive Oil, C
  Onion, C
  Snakeroot, H
  Terminalia, M
  Ubiquinone, C
**Cardiovascular
  disease**, see
  L-arginine, C
  Black Cohosh, C
  Black Walnut, M
  Brahmi, H
  Eleutherococcus, C
  Evening Primrose Oil, C
  Hawthorn, M
  Hibiscus, H
  Jiaogulan, C
  Kudzu, C
  Lemon, C
  Lycopene, C
  Mistletoe, C
  Olive Oil, C
  Onion, C
  Pycnogenol, C
  Reishi Mushroom, C
  Snakeroot, H
  Sour Cherry, C
  Terminalia, M
  Ubiquinone, C
**Carminative/
  Flatulence**, see
  Angelica, H
  Capsicum Peppers, H
  Fennel, H
  Garlic, H
  Ginger, H
  Lemon Balm, H
  Lemon Verbena, H
  Licorice, H
  Parsley, H
  Rosemary, H
  Sage, C
  Turmeric, H
  Wild Yam, H
Cathartic/Purgative, see
  Aloe, M
  Black Walnut, M
  Dandelion, H
  Dong Quai, H
  Elderberry, H
  Flax, H
  Fo-Ti, C
  Hibiscus, M

Cathartic/Purgative (cont.),
see
Olive Oil, M
Parsley, H
Plantain, M
Pokeweed, H
Senega Root, H
Senna, M
Terminalia, C
Causalgia, see
Capsicum Peppers, C
Cellulitis, see
Ginkgo, C
Cerebral infarction, see
Pycnogenol, C
**Cervicitis,
trichomonal**, see
Tea Tree Oil, C
**Chemoprotective
agent**, see
Green Tea, V
Chickenpox, see
Chaparral, H
Chilblains, see
Ginkgo, H
Childbirth, see
Barberry, C
Blue Cohosh, H
Cramp bark, H
Dong Quai, C
Fennel, H
Parsley, H
Raspberry, H
Schisandra, H
Cholera, see
Barberry, H
Wild Yam, H
Choleretic, see
Turmeric, C
**Cholesterol levels, de-
crease**, see
Alfalfa, M
L-arginine, C
Artichoke, C
Black Cohosh, V
Cat's Claw, C
Emblica, C
Evening Primrose Oil, C
Flax, C
Fo-Ti, C
Garlic, C
Green Tea, V
Jiaogulan, C
Lemon, C
Lentinan, C
Maitake, C
Milk Thistle, C
Olive Oil, C

Cholesterol levels, decrease
(cont.), see
Plantain, C
Terminalia, C
**Circadian rhythm, modula-
tion**, see
Melatonin, C
Circulation, see
Danshen, M
Pycnogenol, M
Cirrhosis, see
Milk Thistle, C
**Climacteric
complaints**, see
Fennel, H
Passion Flower, H
CNS depressant, see
Nettles, C
CNS stimulant, see
Dong Quai, C
Ginseng, M
Ma Huang, C
Schisandra, C
Colds, see
Borage, M
Bupleurum, M
Chaparral, H
Flax, H
Horehound, M
Ma Huang, H
Meadowsweet, C
Witch Hazel, H
Colic, see
Parsley, H
Colitis, see
Cat's Claw, H
Dandelion, C
Ginseng, H
Witch Hazel, C
**Colon, adenomatous
polyps**, see
Green Tea, V
Colorectal cancer, see
Echinacea, C
Garlic, C
Pawpaw, C
**Congenital defects, pre-
vent**, see
Eleutherococcus, C
Congestion, see
Ma Huang, M
Horse Chestnut, H
Onion, H
Conjunctivitis, see
Calendula, C
Sassafras, C
Witch Hazel, H
Constipation, see
Aloe, M

Constipation (cont.), see
Black Walnut, M
Dandelion, H
Dong Quai, H
Elderberry, H
Flax, H
Fo-Ti, C
Hibiscus, H
Olive Oil, M
Parsley, H
Plantain, M
Pokeweed, H
Senega Root, H
Senna, M
Terminalia, C
Contraceptive, see
Bitter Melon, M
Cat's Claw, M
Gotu Kola, V
Melatonin, C
Quassia, C
Convulsions, see
Barberry, C
Kava, C
Snakeroot, H
Valerian, C
Corns, see
Tea Tree Oil, C
Cough/Antitussive, see
Barberry, H
Bloodroot, H
Butterbur, H
Capsicum Peppers, C
Coltsfoot, H
Flax, H
Horehound, M
Lemon Verbena, H
Lemongrass, H
Ma Huang, M
Onion, H
Reishi Mushroom, H
Schisandra, M
Senega Root, M
Tea Tree Oil, C
Crohn disease, see
Evening Primrose Oil, C
Cystitis, see
Hops, H
Olive Leaf, C
Tea Tree Oil, C
**Cytomegalovirus
inhibitor**, see
Nettles, V

Deafness, see
Garlic, H
Dementia, see
Ginseng, M

Demulcent, see
Flax, H
Olive Oil, M
Slippery Elm, C
Dental caries prevention, see
Grape Seed, C
Green Tea, V
Dental disorders, see
Bloodroot, M
Mastic, C
Nigella Sativa, H
Tea Tree Oil, H
Yarrow, H
Depression, see
Borage, H
Milk Thistle, H
SAMe, C
Schisandra, H
St. John's Wort, M
Dermatitis, atopic, see
Gamma Linolenic Acid, M
Diabetes, see
Alfalfa, H
Artichoke, C
Bitter Melon, M
Dandelion, H
Eleutherococcus, H
Evening Primrose Oil, C
Gamma Linolenic Acid, C
Ginseng, M
Maitake, C
Milk Thistle, C
Nettles, H
Olive Leaf, C
Pau D'Arco, H
Prickly Pear, C
Stevia, C
Diabetic neuropathy, see
Borage, C
Diarrhea, see
Barberry, C
Bovine Colostrum, C
Cat's Claw, H
Emblica, C
Goldenseal, H
Meadowsweet, C
Quassia, H
Raspberry, M
Sage, H
Schisandra, H
Witch Hazel, C
Dietary supplement, see
Alfalfa, M
L-arginine, M
Artichoke, C
Black Walnut, M
Evening Primrose Oil, C

Dietary supplement (cont.), see
Grape Seed, C
Lemon, M
Lentinan, H
Ma Huang, C
Methylsulfonylmethane, H
Olive Oil, M
Prickly Pear, M
Purslane, M
Digestive aid, see
Capsicum Peppers, H
Chamomile, H
Ginkgo, H
Goldenseal, H
Lemon Verbena, H
Meadowsweet, C
Olive Leaf, C
Onion, M
Purslane, M
Sage, H
Sarsaparilla, H
Snakeroot, C
Terminalia, M
Diuretic, see
Alfalfa, H
Artichoke, H
Borage, M
Brahmi, H
Cat's Claw, C
Cramp bark, H
Dandelion, M
Elderberry, H
False Unicorn, H
Ginger, H
Green Tea, M
Hibiscus, H
Hops, H
Horehound, H
Lemon, H
Licorice, H
Meadowsweet, H
Nettles, M
Olive Leaf, C
Parsley, H
Saw Palmetto, H
Senega Root, H
Snakeroot, C
St. John's Wort, H
Terminalia, H
Withania, H
Diverticulitis, see
Cat's Claw, H
Dizziness, see
Echinacea, H
Ginger, C
Gingko, C
Drunkenness, preventative, see
Evening Primrose Oil, C

Drunkenness, preventative (cont.), see
Ginkgo, H
Goldenseal, C
Kudzu, H
Dysentery, see
Cat's Claw, M
Emblica, C
Guarana, H
Kudzu, H
Parsley, H
Purslane, H
Schisandra, H
Witch Hazel, C
Dysmenorrhea, see
Black Cohosh, M
Blue Cohosh, H
Bupleurum, M
Calendula, H
Chaste Tree, C
Cramp bark, H
Danshen, M
Dong Quai, H
Evening Primrose Oil, C
False Unicorn, H
Fennel, H
Feverfew, H
Gingko, C
Goldenseal, H
Hops, H
Milk Thistle, H
Parsley, H
Pennyroyal, H
Pokeweed, H
Raspberry, H
Rosemary, H
Sage, H
Snakeroot, H
Wild Yam, H
Dyspepsia, see
Alfalfa, H
Artichoke, C
Black Cohosh, H
Emblica, C

Ear disorders, see
Garlic, H
Ginkgo, C
Olive Oil, M
Prickly Pear, H
Eczema, see
Nettles, H
Olive Oil, M
Terminalia, H
Witch Hazel, C
Eczema, atopic, see
Borage, H
Evening Primrose Oil, C

Gastrointestinal disorders (cont.), see
Ginger, H
Goldenseal, C
Lemon, C
Lemon Balm, M
Lemongrass, H
Licorice, H
Methylsulfonylmethane, C
Muira Puama, M
Nigella Sativa, M
Prickly Pear, M
Purslane, M
Schisandra, C

Gastrointestinal motility, see
Bovine Colostrum, C
Capsicum Peppers, H

Glycolysis, accelerate, see
Ginseng, C
Lemon, C

Gonorrhea, see
Cat's Claw, M

Gout, see
Barberry, H
Lemon, C
Sassafras, C
Senega Root, H
Slippery Elm, C

Graves disease, see
Lemon Balm, C

Growth stimulant, see
L-arginine, C
Kinetin, M

Gum inflammation, see
Bloodroot, C
Calendula, C
Witch Hazel, C

Gynecologic disorders, see
Bupleurum, M
Dong Quai, H
Gotu Kola, C

Hair preparations, see
Nettles, H

Hand cleanser, see
Grape Seed, C

Headache, see
Butterbur, C
Evening Primrose Oil, C
Feverfew, M
Green Tea, M
Nigella Sativa, M
Purslane, H
SAMe, C
Willow Bark, H

Healing agent, see
L-arginine, C

Healing agent (cont.), see
St. John's Wort, H
Yarrow, M

Heart disease, see
L-arginine, C
Black Cohosh, C
Black Walnut, M
Brahmi, H
Eleutherococcus, C
Evening Primrose Oil, C
Hawthorn, M
Jiaogulan, C
Kudzu, C
Lemon, C
Lycopene, C
Olive Oil, C
Onion, C
Reishi Mushroom, C
Snakeroot, H
Sour Cherry, C
Terminalia, M
Ubiquinone, C

Heart rate, lower, see
Cat's Claw, C

Hemorrhage, see
Chaste Tree, H
Ginseng, H
Milk Thistle, H
Turmeric, H
Witch Hazel, C

Hemorrhoids, see
Aloe, H
Cat's Claw, H
Comfrey, H
Horse Chestnut, H
Passion Flower, H
Peru Balsam, C
Plantain, C
St. John's Wort, H
Witch Hazel, M

Hepatic damage caused by psychotropic drugs, see
Milk Thistle, C

Hepatic disorders, see
Aloe, C
Artichoke, M
Bupleurum, M
Dandelion, H
Evening Primrose Oil, C
Gotu Kola, C
Milk Thistle, M
Parsley, H
Reishi Mushroom, M
SAMe, C
St. John's Wort, C
Terminalia, C
Turmeric, H

Hepatitis, see
Aloe, C

Hepatitis (cont.), see
Danshen, C
Milk Thistle, C
Reishi Mushroom, C
St. John's Wort, C
Turmeric, H

Herpes simplex, see
Lemon Balm, C
Slippery Elm, C
St. John's Wort, C
Tea Tree Oil, H

Herpes zoster, see
Capsicum Peppers, C

High blood pressure, see
L-arginine, C
Barberry, H
Bitter Melon, M
Black Cohosh, C
Borage, C
Cat's Claw, C
Dong Quai, H
Eleutherococcus, H
Evening Primrose Oil, C
Garlic, C
Gotu Kola, M
Hawthorn, H
Hibiscus, H
Jiaogulan, C
Kudzu, C
Lemongrass, H
Maitake, C
Mastic, C
Mistletoe, C
Olive Leaf, M
Olive Oil, C
Stevia, C
Ubiquinone, C

HIV/AIDS, see
Beta Glycans, C
Bitter Melon, C
Bovine Colostrum, C
Cat's Claw, C
Hibiscus, C
Lemon Balm, C
Nettles, V
St. John's Wort, C

Hormone replacement therapy, see
Red Clover, C

Human polymorpho-nuclear leukocyte (PMN), see
Milk Thistle, V

Hyperactivity, see
Evening Primrose Oil, C
Passion Flower, H

Hyperglycemia, see
Alfalfa, H

Guide to Popular Natural Products

Intestinal motility, see
Capsicum Peppers, H
Garlic, C
Hibiscus, M
Mistletoe, C
Intestinal parasites, see
Black Walnut, H
Cat's Claw, H
Chamomile, H
Curcurbita, H
False Unicorn, H
Horehound, H
Nigella Sativa, H
Purslane, H
Ischemia, see
Danshen, C
Pycnogenol, C
Itching, see
Aloe, H
Capsicum Peppers, C
Witch Hazel, H

Jaundice, see
Artichoke, H
Gotu Kola, H
Milk Thistle, H
Turmeric, H
Jet lag, see
Melatonin, C

Kidney disorders, see
Alfalfa, H
Cat's Claw, H
Evening Primrose Oil, C
Fo-Ti, C
Hibiscus, C
Milk Thistle, H
Nettles, C
Olive Leaf, C
Parsley, H

Labor, facilitate, see
Barberry, C
Blue Cohosh, H
Cramp bark, H
Dong Quai, C
Fennel, H
Parsley, H
Raspberry, H
Schisandra, H
Lacrimal gland atrophy, see
Evening Primrose Oil, C
Lactation, induce, see
Borage, H
Chaste Tree, C
Fennel, H

Lactation, induce (cont.), see
Milk Thistle, H
Laxative, see
Aloe, M
Black Walnut, M
Dandelion, H
Dong Quai, H
Elderberry, H
Flax, H
Fo-Ti, C
Hibiscus, M
Olive Oil, M
Parsley, H
Plantain, M
Pokeweed, H
Senega Root, H
Senna, M
Terminalia, C
Leprosy, see
Garlic, H
Gotu Kola, H
Sarsaparilla, M
Leukemia, see
Aloe, V
Eleutherococcus, V
Hibiscus, V
Milk Thistle, C
Pau D'Arco, H
Quassia, C
Terminalia, C
Lice, see
Parsley, H
Quassia, M
Lipid disorders, see
Artichoke, C
Bitter Melon, C
Eleutherococcus, C
Flax, C
Garlic, C
Jiaogulan, C
Prickly Pear, C
Terminalia, C
Liver cancer, see
Bupleurum, C
Evening Primrose Oil, V
Maitake, C
Liver cells, protective, see
Artichoke, M
Fo-Ti, C
Grape Seed, V
Milk Thistle, H
Schisandra, C
Withania, H
Liver disorders, see
Aloe, C
Artichoke, M
Bupleurum, M

Liver disorders (cont.), see
Dandelion, H
Evening Primrose Oil, C
Gotu Kola, C
Milk Thistle, M
Parsley, H
Reishi Mushroom, M
SAMe, C
St. John's Wort, C
Terminalia, C
Turmeric, H
Liver obstructions, see
Milk Thistle, H
Longevity, enhance, see
Gotu Kola, H
Melatonin, C
Reishi Mushroom, H
Low blood pressure, see
Cat's Claw, C
Hawthorn, M
Ma Huang, C
Mistletoe, C
Parsley, H
Turmeric, C
Valerian, C
Yarrow, C
Lung cancer, see
Maitake, C
Melatonin, C
Pawpaw, C
Lung disorders, see
Comfrey, H
Ginkgo, C
Ma Huang, M
Passion Flower, H
Schisandra, H
Senega Root, M
Lupus, see
Licorice, C

Malaria, see
Guarana, H
Olive Leaf, H
Pau D'Arco, H
Quassia, H
Snakeroot, H
MAO inhibitor, see
St. John's Wort, C
Mastalgia, see
Evening Primrose Oil, C
Measles, see
Kudzu, H
Quassia, H
Melanoma, see
Bloodroot, H
Melatonin, C
Pokeweed, H
Memory loss, see
Ginseng, C

Swelling (cont.), see
Ginkgo, H
Hibiscus, C
Horse Chestnut, C
Pokeweed, H
Sassafras, C
Withania, H
Sympathetic nervous system, see
Cat's Claw, C
Synovial fluid, alterations of, see
Pycnogenol, C
Syphilis, see
Pokeweed, H
Sarsaparilla, M
Slippery Elm, C

T **ardive dyskinesia**, see
Evening Primrose Oil, C
Teeth cleaning, see
Tea Tree Oil, H
Throat disorders, see
Black Cohosh, H
Bloodroot, H
Brahmi, H
Capsicum Peppers, C
Coltsfoot, M
Plantain, H
Pokeweed, H
Sage, H
Slippery Elm, C
Witch Hazel, C
Thrush, see
Pau D'Arco, H
Ticks, see
Lemon Verbena, C
Tonic, see
Dandelion, H
Lemon, H
Muira Puama, H
Rosemary, H
Sage, H
Schisandra, C
Scullcap, H
Yarrow, H
Tonsillitis, see
Capsicum Peppers, C
Pokeweed, H
Toothache, see
Bloodroot, M
Mastic, C
Nigella Sativa, H
Tea Tree Oil, H
Yarrow, H
Toxin poisoning, see
Fennel, H
Milk Thistle, C

Toxin protectant, see
Eleutherococcus, H
Tuberculosis, see
Fo-Ti, C
Hops, H
Witch Hazel, H
Withania, H
Tuberculosis of the lymph glands, see
Fo-Ti, C
Tumors, see
Beta Glycans, C
Bitter Melon, H
Cat's Claw, M
Echinacea, C
Eleutherococcus, H
Hibiscus, M
Lentinan, M
Meadowsweet, H
Melatonin, C
Parsley, H
Pawpaw, H
Pycnogenol, C
Quassia, C
Sour Cherry, C
St. John's Wort, C
Witch Hazel, H
Withania, H

U **lcerative colitis**, see
Evening Primrose Oil, C
Ulcers, see
Alfalfa, C
Bloodroot, H
Calendula, C
Cat's Claw, H
Danshen, C
Dong Quai, H
Gotu Kola, H
Licorice, C
Meadowsweet, C
Pau D'Arco, H
Urinary acidifier, see
Cranberry, M
Urinary deodorant, see
Cranberry, C
Urinary tract cancers, in women, see
Cat's Claw, M
Urinary tract disorders, see
Blue Cohosh, H
Cranberry, C
Flax, H
Onion, M
Purslane, H
Slippery Elm, H
Wild Yam, H

Uterine stimulant, see
Barberry, M
Blue Cohosh, H
Cramp bark, H
Dong Quai, C
Hibiscus, C
Mistletoe, C
Schisandra, H

V **aricella**, see
Chaparral, H
Varicose veins, see
Gotu Kola, C
Horse Chestnut, H
Milk Thistle, H
Witch Hazel, H
Vascular disorders, see
L-arginine, C
Ginkgo, C
Gotu Kola, C
Grape Seed, M
Horse Chestnut, C
Witch Hazel, C
Vasodilator, see
Dong Quai, C
Ginkgo, C
Horehound, C
Vertigo, see
Echinacea, H
Ginger, C
Gingko, C
Vision improvement, see
Fennel, H
Vitiligo, see
St. John's Wort, C
Vomiting, see
Gentian, H
Ginger, H
Lemongrass, H
Vomiting, induce, see
Bloodroot, H
False Unicorn, H
Pokeweed, H
Purslane, H
Senega Root, H
Withania, H

W **arts**, see
Bloodroot, H
Onion, M
Weakness, see
Ginseng, H
Pennyroyal, H
Weight loss, see
Chaparral, H
Fennel, H
Guarana, C

Primary
Index

Italicized page numbers indicate botanical photographs.